Neurocognitive Perspectives of Prosocial and Positive Emotional Behaviours

Theory to application

Neurocognitive Perspectives of Prosocial and Positive Emotional Behaviours

Theory to application

Edited by
Shashikanta Tarai and Arindam Bit
National Institute of Technology Raipur, India

IOP Publishing, Bristol, UK

ISBN 978-0-7503-3383-2 (ebook)
ISBN 978-0-7503-3381-8 (print)
ISBN 978-0-7503-3384-9 (myPrint)
ISBN 978-0-7503-3382-5 (mobi)

DOI 10.1088/978-0-7503-3383-2

Version: 20211201

IOP ebooks

British Library Cataloguing-in-Publication Data: A catalogue record for this book is available from the British Library.

Published by IOP Publishing, wholly owned by The Institute of Physics, London

IOP Publishing, Temple Circus, Temple Way, Bristol, BS1 6HG, UK

US Office: IOP Publishing, Inc., 190 North Independence Mall West, Suite 601, Philadelphia, PA 19106, USA

Shashikanta Tarai would like to dedicate this volume to his wife Pradipta *and daughter* Smrutirani *for their words of encouragement and continuous support throughout the writing and editing of this book.*

Arindam Bit wants to dedicate this book to his wife Soma *and daughter* Anishka *for their continuous support, incredible inspiration and unwavering understanding while writing every piece of this book. He also wants to acknowledge all his PhD and projects scholars for their support with the art and graphics of the chapters.*

Contents

Preface

Evolution of humanity is deeply rooted in persuasive skills of prosocial and positive emotional behaviours, actions and languages that guide our survival strategies. Prosocial behaviours (e.g., giving, helping, cooperating, sharing, establishing a friendship, donating, volunteering) of humans subsidise the social, political, economic harmony and development. Even our communicative verbal and non-verbal actions and emotions that are prosaically motivated facilitate and enhance the ingroup and outgroup socio-cultural relationship, collective identity and reconciliation. Our social interactions define the prosocial nature of who we are and what we do as humans. In this sense, we are prosocial-cooperative species. Our mind–brain that constitutes language has a socio-communicative ability to promote intra-group prosocial behaviour to minimise violence, horror, terror, aggression and unsocial behaviours.

The use of prosocial words such as caring, helping, sharing and denoting to others has a beneficial and utilitarian effect from our survival point of view. Therefore, the modern-day scientific and multidisciplinary research in psychology, biology, anthropology and sociology attempts to theorise prosocial behaviours, as opposed to unsocial behaviours, which benefit others. This book offers a comprehensive description, widespread application and a ready reference to the neurocognitive perspectives of prosocial and positive emotional behaviours and language. The research works and illustrations presented in this book describe the neuro-scientific and behavioural methods: electroencephalography (EEG), functional magnetic resonance imaging (fMRI), magnetic resonance imaging (MRI), electromyography (EMG) and functional near-infrared spectroscopy (fNIRS) to explain the neurocognitive mechanisms and neural biomarkers of prosocial and positive emotional behaviours in the human brain. Furthermore, it elaborates the spatial-temporal classifications in terms of the event-related potential (ERP) components such as P100, N170, N200, EPN, P300 and the brain regions, which are associated with prosocial and positive emotional stimuli.

This volume is organised into twelve chapters. All the chapters are devoted to the authors' research findings on neurocognitive, behavioural and biomedical outcomes of prosocial behaviours and language computation. It also dedicates comprehensive illustrations of how prosocial verbal and non-verbal activities have impacted the neural signatures in the brain, thereby modulating societal harmony and cooperation. The quantitative and computational approaches have been discussed and presented to categorise the neural biomarkers of prosocial behaviour and languages in the human brain. Chapter 1 introduces the neurocognitive signatures of prosocial and positive emotional behaviours and their social impacts on human evolution and language acquisition. The interpretation of current literature is discussed to understand better the neurocognitive computation of social cognition, empathy, moral decisions and actions, cooperative joint-action, persuasive skills and self-other prejudices that have impacted human development. Chapter 2 of this volume deals with the neurocognitive mechanisms of the brain's positive and negative action-emotion processing. We review the current literature to explain how our brain processes the emotion and action of linguistic (i.e., verbal: words, phrases and sentences) and non-linguistic (i.e., non-verbal: voice, tone, face, gestures, postures and eye movements) stimuli differently than non-emotional or neutral verbal and non-verbal stimuli. Chapter 3 illustrates the influence of the blood–brain barrier for induction of drugs and epigenetic factors (prosocial) for combating neurodegenerative disorders. Chapter 4 of this volume describes the neurocognitive mechanisms, clinical and neuropathological diagnosis of Alzheimer's disease (AD). The chapter offers insights into the biomarkers for neurodegenerative diseases (NDD) like AD, developing a possible interaction between neural and micro-vascular systems. Chapter 5 will provide an illustrative overview of correlation between prosocial elemental stimuli and peripheral neurons while evaluating human cognition at a higher level of neurological complexities. Chapter 6 illustrates the influence of Yogic exercises in conjunction with prosocial behavior for combating stress and depressive disorders associated with neurocognitive complexities. Chapter 7 illustrates the influence of blood-derived neurotrophic factors for therapeutic and pharmaceutic management of neurocognitive improvement. It also explains the mechanisms of synthesis of various neurotrophic factors while the brain is engaged in prosocial activities. Chapter 8 explains about the engineering aspects of the human brain, its biomechanical dynamics and characteristics of the developing brain under the influence of prosocial, antisocial, and clinical circumstances. Chapter 9 examines the processing of prosocial language and its impact on the human brain by applying EEG techniques. The band-frequencies of the delta, theta and beta, and the event-related potential (ERP) mechanisms of prosocial positive and antisocial negative communicative behaviors are illustrated during the processing of grammatically correct and incorrect English sentences. Chapter 10 illustrates the influence of pharmacological and epigenetic elemental factors in conjuction with prosocial elementary signatures on the therapeutic management of stress and mood disorder associated with higher level cognition. Chapter 11 presents the application of teachers' prosocial and positive emotional language, which modulates learners' neurocognitive and behavioural well-being in a classroom context. In this chapter, the underpinnings of the socio-cognitive theory of behaviour, cognitive neuroscience, social and emotional learning and positive psychology are interpreted in the light of current observations and findings. Chapter 12 provides the neurocognitive mechanisms of humans involved during the processing of prosocial–positive and antisocial–negative congruency and incongruency sentences. Most of the ERP incongruence results referring to P100 and P300 are discussed and interpreted in the light of current literature, focusing on the neurocognitive mechanisms of prosocial language that play a significant role in developing human cooperation, communication and joint attention for survival.

Moreover, this book highlights the theoretical and future-applied perspectives of the neurocognitive and behavioural mechanisms in communication, language teaching and learning, and stress management, reducing violence and conflict across the globe. It bridges the gap between the readerships of social and neural sciences by formulating social neuroscientific and computational methods. It contains an excellent scholarly overview on topics like neurocognitive mechanisms, the behavioural outlook of the brain, decision making, moral value judgement and the influence of emotional valence on neural plasticity. The scope of the book covers the subject area of neuroscience, behavioural and cognitive sciences, linguistics, computer science, information technology, biomedical engineering, medical sciences, psychology, biomimetic machine learning, brain sciences and socio-affective sciences. Indeed, this book intends to motivate the audience to emphasise the significance of prosocial investment of financial and knowledge resources, which can resolve territorial conflicts and thus can protect human civilisation from global threats. Therefore, this book will be of immense usage to researchers, academics, policymakers and experts to identify the beneficial approaches for establishing peace and prosperity across the globe. Furthermore, this book will be served as a reference book that will be useful to the laboratories of neuroscience, linguistics and cognitive sciences. Both experts and non-experts will find it beneficial to use the methods and findings illustrated in this volume.

Shashikanta Tarai, PhD
Arindam Bit, PhD

Editor biographies

Shashikanta Tarai

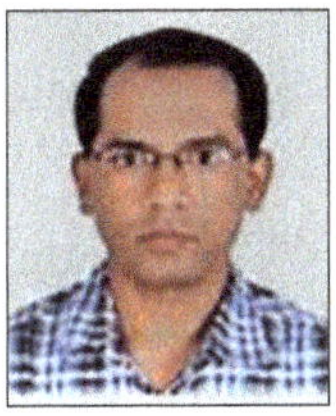

Shashikanta Tarai received his PhD from the Indian Institute of Technology Madras (IITM), Chennai, India. After his PhD, he completed his Postdoctoral Research at the Centre of Behavioural and Cognitive Sciences (CBCS), University of Allahabad, India. He was one of the awardees of the University Grant Fellowship (2006–2011) and Cognitive Science Initiative Fellowship (2012–2014) sponsored by the University Grant Commission and the Department of Science and Technology, Government of India. He is currently serving as Assistant Professor in the Department of Humanities and Social Sciences, National Institute of Technology Raipur, India. Dr Tarai published more than 20 research papers in peer-reviewed journals in the area of linguistics, neurolinguistics, psycholinguistics, and cognitive neuroscience of emotion and neurodegeneration. He served as an Associate Editor of the previewed Journal SN Social Sciences; he is currently serving as Editorial Board Member of the International Journal of Language and Linguistics. He presented his research accomplishments in Germany, Japan, Malaysia, Sri Lanka and the United Arab Emirates.

Arindam Bit

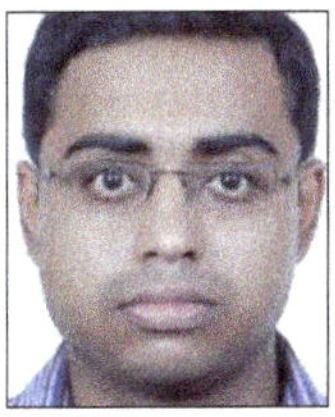

Arindam Bit received his PhD in Biofluidic Engineering at Jadavpur University, India. He is currently serving as Assistant Professor in the Department of Biomedical Engineering at the National Institute of Technology Raipur, India. He has more than 70 research publications in peer-reviewed journals. He served as guest editor to the Journal of Healthcare Engineering. He is a reviewer to many journals such as *Journal of Psycholinguistic Research*, *Journal of Cognitive Neurodynamics*, *Journal of Scientific Report-Nature*, *Journal of Medical & Biological Engineering & Computing*, *Progress in Computational Fluid Dynamics: An International Journal*, *Acta Biomechanics and Bioengineering*, and *Journal of Computer Methods in Medicine*. He is working in the field of healthcare technology, namely, tissue biomechanics, organoid modelling, and cognitive neuroscience. He is also a recipient of Marie Curie Individual Fellowship, and UK Royal Academy of Engineers awards.

List of contributors

Prastistha Bhagat
National Institute of Technology Raipur, G.E Road, Raipur, Pin 492010, India

Sayantani Biswas
National Institute of Technology Raipur, G.E Road, Raipur, Pin 492010, India

Arindam Bit
National Institute of Technology Raipur, G.E Road, Raipur, Pin 492010, India

Khemraj Deshmukh
National Institute of Technology Raipur, G.E Road, Raipur, Pin 492010, India

Tulika Ghosh
National Institute of Technology Raipur, G.E Road, Raipur, Pin 492010, India

Roopak Kumar
National Institute of Technology Raipur, G.E Road, Raipur, Pin 492010, India

Bharti Mishra
National Institute of Technology Raipur, G.E Road, Raipur, Pin 492010, India

Raghavendra Prasad
National Institute of Technology Raipur, G.E Road, Raipur, Pin 492010, India

Anbu Savekar
National Institute of Technology Raipur, G.E Road, Raipur, Pin 492010, India

Shashikanta Tarai
National Institute of Technology Raipur, G.E Road, Raipur, Pin 492010, India

Nishchay Verma
National Institute of Technology Raipur, G.E Road, Raipur, Pin 492010, India

Chapter 1

Neurocognitive signatures of prosocial and positive emotional behaviours: emerging research and social impact

Shashikanta Tarai, Roopak Kumar and Arindam Bit

The current chapter aims to analyze the recent literature on neural signatures of prosocial and positive emotional behaviours of humans that have a social impact on human evolution and language acquisition. From an evolutionary point of view, human group affiliations are described as ingroup love versus outgroup hate. However, the recent neurocognitive studies indicate that prosociality, cooperation and altruism in humans are not restricted to group-based explanations. Reanalyzing the current findings, we hypothesize that prosocial and positive emotional behaviours are not limited to the mere established concept of ingroup favouritism, but the tendencies of prosociality are changed according to interacting and communicative contexts of outgroup favouritism. Both these aspects of ingroup and outgroup prosocial and positive behaviours are computed in the medial-prefrontal (mPFC), the right dorsolateral prefrontal (rdlPFC) and the right inferior parietal (rIPL) regions. In this regard, the neural network path between mPFC and rdlPFC is enhanced during the processing of highly self-risk at the cost of prosocial-positive behaviours. However, the increasing rate of other needs heightens the neural connectivity between rIPL and rdlPFC regions. Overall, the rdlPF cortex plays a crucial role in processing self-interest along with other needs. These regions of interest (ROI) have broadened our conceptualization of the neuro-cognitive computation of social cognition, empathy, moral decisions and actions, cooperative joint-action, persuasive skills and self-other prejudices that have impacted human progress and development.

1.1 Introduction

Humans are uniquely cooperative, ultra-social and cultural beings (Henrich and Muthukrishna 2021). We domesticate language and culture to establish inter- and intra-group cooperation that positively impacts our biological, neurological, psychological, social and economic developments (Somel *et al* 2013). Our cognition or mind emerged due to the early development of cooperative-communicative skills (Eisenberg *et al* 1983). Animals or other species have a minimal repertoire of sexual, genetic and communicative collaborative interactions to only the closest kith and kin. An experimental study conducted on extremely cooperative species—wolves—established that, in cooperative interactions, the relational factors play a far more significant role than other cooperation driving factors like motivation and cognitive abilities (Dale *et al* 2020). That humans are innately social and hardwired to be divisive or unifying is an attribute of evolutionary development validated by historical evidence (Tooby 2018). Therefore, this innate paradigm highlights the implications of prosociality in humans from the neurocognitive and behavioural points of view (Buss and Von Hippel 2018). Prosocial behaviours are a set of actions designed to help or benefit others at a self-cost. They are considered a selflessly motivated action instead of a selfish action (Jensen 2016).

Previous literature exemplifies that prosocial behaviour can be studied using multilevel approaches such as meso, micro and macro levels. The meso level study deals with the helper–consumer dyads in an exact context, whereas the micro-level approach focuses on the origins of prosociality along with the sources of differences in these predispositions. The macro-level study investigates those prosocial functional actions related to groups and organizations (Penner *et al* 2005). Generally, the prosocial behaviours in humans appear in various forms like informing, sharing, comforting or helping. The intentions and actions that account for prosocial behaviours provide necessary information for establishing a need for others, hugging to comfort someone in distress, and sharing resources with someone deprived of those resources (Jensen 2016). Cooperative features in humans are unique because cooperation can be traced even in a large group of unrelated individuals. This type of cooperation is rare in other species (Kappeler and Van Schaik 2006). Social norms and third-party judgments play a crucial role in maintaining large-scale collaboration and collaboration among family, kin, and friends (Mathew *et al* 2013). However, humans manifest more excellent prosocial behaviour towards the ingroup when the decision is in the public interest, which is inclusively beneficial to all ingroup members, even by neglecting factors like interactions of group members, the concealment of the verdict, the economic cost of the ingroup. Such ingroup preference-based prosociality evolves as a spontaneous and instinctive social profile to favour ingroup members by disregarding personal reputation and financial incentives (Everett *et al* 2015). In this regard, a study conducted among 287 children of 5–10 years old found that prosocial behaviour is associated with lower competitive motivation and higher empathy in an intergroup competition. With increasing age, the strengthening of co-relations occurs positively between prosocial cooperation and competitiveness. Thus, prosocial cooperation and empathy can influence prosocial attitudes even towards outgroup members (Abrams *et al* 2015). The well-organized forms of group-biased behaviour like religious or racial prosociality are studied as a complex co-evolutionary phenomenon that includes genetic and cultural processes (Galen 2012). The psychological repertoire in humans that have been evolved in the process of natural selection resulted in hypervigilance ability not only to detect the intention of agents and their states of mind but also to manage prosocial reputations (Simpson and Beckes 2010). Moralizing Gods in religious groups created a greater degree of prosocial tendencies, leading to more extensive and stable cooperative groups (Norenzayan and Gervais 2012).

1.1.1 Acquisition of prosocial and unsocial behaviour

From the acquisition point of view, children around the globe first acquire prosocial behaviours and actions. The development of prefrontal cortical circuitry is responsible for the development of sharing and helping behaviours. Thus, individuals become sufficiently able to produce prosocial behaviour encoding self versus others (Steinbeis 2018). Diesendruck and Benozio (2012) examined children's behaviour during their interactions within a group versus outgroup members regarding self-identification, reciprocity expectations, and reputation management. It is found that children act pro-socially towards the ingroup while unsocially towards outgroup members. The study concluded that children did not develop a selfish nature, but they seemed to develop a groupish character. Thus, we build our cultural group loyalty from a young age and define the regulatory mechanisms for pro- and antisocial behaviours.

Additionally, language development and accusation is primarily affected by prosocial features of interaction with others (Lieven 2013). Children learn to copy homophilic preferences from the behavioural repertoire of the group they grow within. Consequently, homophilic preferential tendencies positively impact social mechanisms for establishing prosocial cooperation (Haun and Over 2015). A study conducted to assess the change in prosocial perception among 5–6-year-old children towards immigrants (McLoughlin and Over 2019) has found that children do not share their emotions and feelings with immigrant victims, but their perceptual mechanisms are affected by the victims' negative emotions. Another experiment, conducted on 136 children, revealed that children's donating behaviours regarding kindness, generosity and affection, and non-kindness, non-affection and non-generosity are influenced by previous information about the recipients. This result reveals that children share more resources with generous, affectionate and kind recipients than non-generous, non-affectionate or non-kind recipients (Blakey *et al* 2019). The prosocial over antisocial or unsocial preferences among preschool children indicates a common neurocognitive substrate that promotes sharing behaviours and expectations. Such prosocial tendencies are due to attentional mechanisms or processes and the evaluation of prosocial behaviours performed by others (Paulus 2015).

1.1.2 Mate selection strategy and altruism

Socio-evolutionary psychology considers the mating choices for identifying the potential sexual partners based on their prosocial behaviours towards a potential mate. The altruistic preferences towards attractive individuals are always motivated by prosocial behaviours (Bhogal *et al* 2019). Research consisting three studies among 681 participants revealed that mating strategies influence the helping attitudes in males. Males tend to manifest greater helping attitudes toward beautiful and physically attractive women than their male counterparts. Therefore, prosocial behaviours can be observed in the context of costly mate signal theory and mate–mating strategies (Schwarz and Baßfeld 2019) for both men and women, who show greater desirability towards altruistic partners for long-term partner relationships.

Conversely, there are inconsistent results for predicting the partner selection behaviours based on the physical attractiveness of partners (Farrelly and King 2019). However, the costly signal theory proposes that choosing to cooperate with an altruist is beneficial, which can be predicted the partner's behaviours. People always prefer and consider altruists over neutralists because heroic altruists establish a long term romantic relationship with female partners. This consideration may be due to the honest altruism signals and kindness, coupled with parenting abilities. These qualities are desirable in mates for their reproductive success (Norman and Fleming 2019). The research based on 199 participants shows that both genders (men and women), who have non-financial altruistic behaviours towards potential mates, prefer to share their resources more with the physically attractive opposite sex. Thus, prosocial behaviours may influence mate choice irrespective of lovely or non-attractive potential mates (Bhogal *et al* 2019).

1.1.3 Social phenomena and contextual cues of prosocial events, actions and behaviours

Gilbert and Basran (2019) suggest that antisocial and prosocial strategies are two major dimensions of social competition. Antisocial or unsocial strategies are self-centred, threat sensitive and aggressive, tactically used for threatening, intimidating or bullying and injuring or killing competitors. On the other hand, *prosocial* sharing and cooperating emit low or no threat to social signals, resulting in stimulation of physiological systems. Furthermore, prosocial stimulation is linked with the release of oxytocin and the activation of the vagus nerve of the parasympathetic system. This finding regulates the processing of threat stimuli and facilitates general well-being by enhancing the immune system due to the enlargement of the limbic system.

A cross-cultural experiment involving 586 Italian and Kosovo participants revealed that prejudices play an essential role in prosociality. These culturally divergent participants demonstrated a reluctance to receive help from outgroup members and were even sceptical of the prosocial motives of outgroups (Borinca *et al* 2021). However, the extent of bias towards ingroup members for altruistic behaviour is still unclear (Everett *et al* 2015). A study reveals that the withheld assistance strengthens negative intergroup expectations that generate distrust and fuel intergroup conflicts. Contrariwise, the prosocial actions elicit reciprocity resulting in more harmonious relations, even with outgroup members. Thus, the processes of recategorization, which is commonly found in the ingroup identity model, can affect intergroup attitudes and prosocial behaviours (Dovidio *et al* 2009). However, stronger emotions are observed while making such decisions that deviate from maximum monetary rewards. When weighing financial interests, individuals encounter instinctive and contemplative motivations as they face emotional arousal and social dilemmas (Jaber-López *et al* 2014).

The monetary gain or reward referring to prosociality demands emotional predisposition of gratitude and guilt. The appreciation maintains ongoing prosocial interactions while any responsibility obstructs and repairs the prosocial interactions (Vaish and Hepach 2020). In the western context, any positive feeling promotes prosocial behaviour, and persons with higher dispositional awe manifest greater prosocial tendency. Individuals with feelings of cheerful awe volunteer more often for strangers than participants with feelings of adverse awe (Guan *et al* 2019). Further, some studies have found an association between prosociality and gender. This association also emerges as an essential factor that affected the results of research on prosociality. For example, the study found that social framing reinforces prosocial behaviours, especifically in women; conversely, such encouraging reflections decrease any prosociality (Espinosa and Kovářík 2015).

Along with gender, some studies have found that socioeconomic class also affects prosocial behaviours. Although the lower socioeconomic groups or classes face scarcity in the distribution of resources, the greater exposure to threat manifests in the reduction of self-control. They simultaneously show the most vital commitment towards egalitarian values and greater feelings of compassion. The experiment revealed that individuals belonging to the lower socioeconomic class show more generous, charitable, trusting and helpful behaviours than those belonging to the upper class (Piff *et al* 2010). Data obtained from 136 countries suggest that prosocial relating to monetary spending fosters greater and larger happiness irrespective of cultures and the economy's status and indicates a deeply ingrained human nature of experiencing reward by helping others (Aknin *et al* 2013). Similarly, a study has been conducted on 305 Polish bone marrow donor youths, analyzing their personality traits, observed past-prosocial behaviours, family functionality and self-esteem, which have positively impacted their donating behaviours. However, the past literature suggests that prosocial behaviours have also been enforced for enhancing reward in the context of donation (Tuszyńska-Bogucka 2019).

1.1.4 Discourse of social and self-centred behaviours

In political and social discourse, the spoken textual analysis of 124 million words used in US congress between 1996 and 2014 suggests that the decline of prosocial language receives strong public disapproval (Frimer *et al* 2015). This means that prosocial language poses a direct and independent effect on public social approval. A recent study reveals that individuals with higher callous-unemotional (CU) personalities respond quickly to antisocial behaviours, while lower CU traits are associated with delayed response to antisocial behaviour (Dotterer *et al* 2021). A study conducted on 312 participants found that prosocial behaviours may sometimes direct self-serving goals. Expressing gratitude is prosocial in nature, but at the same time, it may indicate the practice of increased social intelligence for impression management (Gulliford *et al* 2019). A simulation study finds that the preventions of antisocial rewarding and the maintenance of cooperation largely depend on prosocial behaviours' contextual functions. However, using the lens of a game theory of social communicative-interactions, Dos Santos and Peña (2017) suggest that increased reward funds support the preservation of prosocial rewarding; nevertheless, the spatial structures may sometimes select contrary to prosocial rewarding. Therefore, additional prosocial reward mechanisms are required even in a spatially structured population to prevent antisocial or unsocial rewarding to combat the deterioration in cooperation. Prosocial individuals are marginally acted against anger and exhibit retaliation, while unsocial selfish individuals are encouraged by negative emotions like anger to react across constant interactions, which break down the cooperative situation or context (Skatova *et al* 2017). Physical appearance is another factor that influences prosocial preferences. The brain region, the amygdala, manifests a definite neural response to abnormal or anomalous faces, resulting in explicit biases against individuals with anomalous physique. Thus, people, especially those who belong to a high socioeconomic class, show less empathic concern and minimal prosocial attitudes towards individuals with facial abnormalities (Workman *et al* 2021).

1.1.5 Neurocognitive studies on prosocial-positive and unsocial negative behaviours

The bio-energetic-cognition loop is a mechanism that develops cooperative abilities in humans and protects children from energy shortage during the neural maturation period. Children require a high energy intake compared to adults for neurocognitive maturation as a four-year-old child uses 50% of total energy expenditure (TEE) while an adult utilizes $\approx$12%. Moreover, making up of the brain of a four-year-old child $\approx$6% is much higher than 2% in an adult, which increases the costs of synaptic neuron maturation. Therefore, the cooperative abilities in humans protect toddlers during the potentially vulnerable period of neuron maturation by fulfilling the need for high energy food intake (Skoyles 2012). Further, the multi-attribute drift-diffusion model reveals that ventral striatum, temporoparietal junction (TPJ), and ventromedial prefrontal cortex (vmPFC) play a crucial role in altruistic choices, which may predict why and when any individual practises generous behaviour and with what reaction time (Hutcherson *et al* 2015).

Human empathy mediates the development of prosocial behaviours when the sympathetic nature towards others' distress is coupled with a drive for their welfare. Disruption, atypical development, and functional defects in the neural circuits are responsible for processing and integrating the distress cues with decision value (Decety *et al* 2016). Prosociality is also influenced by socially relative reward and evaluation based on competition and comparisons between ourselves and others. The shared neural networks in the medial prefrontal cortex and the dopamine-related subcortical areas have been involved in the process of reward valuation in humans and primates (Isoda 2021). The right amygdala has negatively been associated with the severity of antisocial behaviours and callous-unemotional traits.

Furthermore, the probabilities of functional deficits in the brain arise during the acute threat response, cognitive control and social cognitions (Dugré *et al* 2020). The proper functioning of neural circuits and coordinated brain activity disturbances may lead to impairments in prosocial interactions, resulting in other pathological conditions like autism spectrum disorder, addiction or depression (Walsh *et al* 2021). Deactivation of the ventral striatum (VS) and activation of the dorsal posterior medial frontal cortex (dorsal pMFC) along with anterior insula (AI) have been observed when an individual's response deviates from group opinions. Therefore, deviant response in dorsal pMFC may predict people's behavioural adjustments regarding social conformity and public approval (Wu *et al* 2016).

The current analysis aims to summarise and reanalyze the existing literature; more specifically, the contemporary researches published between 2010 and 2021 on neurocognitive and behavioural signatures related to prosocial and positive emotions in humans. Relying on an extensive literature survey, we predict that:

Meta-hypothesis 1: Though prosociality in conventional studies has been greatly attributed to the evolutionary aspects of ingroup love and outgroup hate, recent research has added new dimensions based on individual differences within group functionalities that pose several challenges to conceptualize empathy and altruism.

Meta-hypothesis 2: Neurocognitive studies reveal the activation patterns of the brain's different regions and neural networks when responding to other prosocial and antisocial stimuli depending on the experimental conditions.

1.2 Methodological design

A meta-analysis is a methodological tool that analyses several primary studies conducted on similar research problems (Timulak 2014, Borenstein 2021). It provides a systematic opportunity to re-assess and compares already completed studies on similar topics (Allen 2009, Field and Gillett 2010). The meta-analyses techniques are incrementally used in neurocognitive studies (Hopwood and Schutte 2016, Wu *et al* 2016, Bjornestad *et al* 2018). The current analysis has been performed in the following steps to ensure maximum transparent and comprehensive reporting of the results and conclusion regarding previous studies conducted on prosociality related themes; (i) the database searches and extraction according to the guidelines of the preferred reporting items for systematic reviews and meta-analysis (PRISMA) (Hutton *et al* 2015, Moher *et al* 2015), (ii) the quality appraisal of the included studies, (iii) the adoption of an established analytic framework (Sera *et al* 2019, Borenstein 2021).

A database was searched online by using search engines like Google Scholar and ISI Web of Science by entering different keywords, including prosociality, prosocial, antisocial behaviour, altruism, empathy, and cooperation. The search resulted in 861 articles published from 2010 to June 2021, out of which we downloaded 280 papers based on the title review. We included those studies only if they adopted experimental methodology in controlled and experimental conditions to measure the behavioural or neural outcomes in response to experimental designs. Psychological and neurological outcomes included changes in attitudinal and behavioural patterns and the activation of specific brain region/s or neural networks in response to lab-controlled stimuli. The following inclusion criteria, as depicted in figure 1.1, were further applied to the downloaded articles; (a) assessment of the abstract to fit in the selected theme of the current paper, (b) publications based on one scientific experiment method including behavioural and neurological aspects, (c) prosocial studies conducted only on humans, excluding other primates and animals, (d) participants free from psychiatric or neurological abnormalities (except one paper where the study discusses behavioural changes observed in brain-damaged patients).

The current analysis systematically reviews the methods, number of participants, outcomes, and conclusions of thirty four published papers (N = 34). All the remaining articles not fulfilling the criteria were excluded from the study. Out of 34, 33 papers were cross-sectional and included participants from different age groups, genders, and locations as listed in table 1.1.

1.2.1 Meta-themes and analysis

The studies selected for the analysis of positive (trust, empathy, cooperation, etc) and negative (enmity, anxiety, anger, aggression, threat, etc) emotions and actions indicate various psychological outcomes and neural activation patterns. Finally,

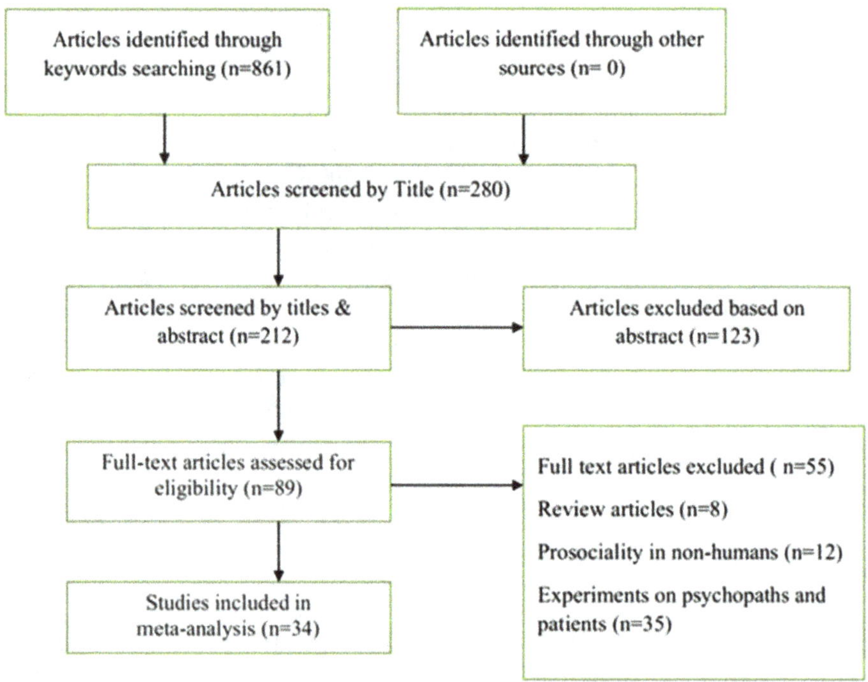

Figure 1.1. The flow chart depicts the selection criteria of published literature based on PRISMA (Preferred Reporting Items of Systematic Reviews and Meta-Analysis).

Table 1.1. The number of studies and the relevant methods are listed as per the recent studies.

Serial	Authors	Methods/frameworks (behavioural experiments)	Subjects (female)	Mean age
1	Li *et al* (2019)	Dictator game, manipulation check, behavioural experiments questionnaire	447 (269)	18.9
2	Vermue *et al* (2019)	Trust game	361 (198)	29.04
3	House *et al* (2020)	Dictator game (DG)	1248 (415)	9.76
4	Song *et al* (2020)	Sharing task; instrumental and empathic helping	283	2.8
5	Margana *et al* (2019)	2 prosocial trait (low and high) × 2 attractiveness (low and high) × 2 relationship type (long-term and short-term) within subjects factors, online survey, questionnaire, Likert scale	198	19.56
6	Moore *et al* (2013)	Rating opposite-sex for short- and long-term relationships, priming	67 (32)	21.8
7	Skatova *et al* (2017)	Shared use game, social value orientation questionnaire	118 (70)	21.43
8	Stiff *et al* (2019)	Pro-sociality scale questionnaires, group discussion	539 (384)	21.29
9	Tuszyńska-Bogucka (2019)	Bandura's social cognitive framework, personality inventory (TIPI), family Apgar, prosocial behaviours questionnaire (PBQ), self-reported altruism (SRA)	234 (193)	22.36
10	Anlı (2019)	Prosocial behavioral intentions scale (PBIS), altruism scale (AS), Toronto empathy questionnaire (TEQ), adult prosocialness scale (APS) and social appearance anxiety scale (SAAS)	993 (609)	19.94
11	Gulliford *et al* (2019)	Multi-component gratitude measure (MCGM), Tromsø social intelligence scale (TSIS), positive affect negative affect scale (PANAS), gratitude resentment and appreciate scale (GRAT-S)	347 (184)	32
12	Jaber-López *et al* (2014)	Physioeconomics, electrodermal activity	93	NA
13	Mayer *et al* (2019)	Experimental vignette study, the survey on Likert	540 (337.2)	42.69

(*Continued*)

Table 1.1. (*Continued*)

Serial	Authors	Methods/frameworks (behavioural experiments)	Subjects (female)	Mean age
14	Piff *et al* (2010)	An online questionnaire, dictator game, subjective SES, manipulation of relative social class exp., trust game, memory task, manipulation check, distress exp.	442	NA
15	Frimer *et al* (2014)	Goal task, aspiration index, prosocial role-play, selfish role-play experiment, idealism versus realism experiment	636 (296.3)	33.4
16	Hein *et al* (2010)	Natural group manipulation, fMRI, empathic concern scale	16	29.8
17	Ferschmann *et al* (2019)	Five items are self-reported by following the prosocial subscale questionnaire based on strengths and weakness, MRI, cortical thickness (CT) analyzes	169 (92)	17.7
18	Workman *et al* (2021)	Online survey, dictator, game, ultimatum game, fMRI study	430 (181)	30.6
19	Wittmann *et al* (2016)	Minigame exp., questionnaire, MRI scan	24 (9)	25
20	FeldmanHall *et al* (2015)	Pain versus gain task, interpersonal reactivity index (IRI), fMRI	17 (11)	23.3
21	Hu *et al* (2017)	The interactive dice game, fMRI experiment, loss aversion gamble task	160 (101)	20.94
22	Reimers *et al* (2017)	Ultimatum game (UG), fMRI experiment, saliva analysis to measure secretion patterns of testosterone	43 (43)	26.4
23	Telzer *et al* (2011)	fMRI, family assistance task questionnaires about family obligation preferences	25 (13)	20.2
24	Muscatell *et al* (2012)	fMRI scan, social status measure, neuroimaging task	38 (22)	16.41
25	Cao *et al* (2015)	fMRI scan during viewing painful visuals, affective priming task (own versus others' race), level of contact with other-race: questionnaire, explicit group identification task	30 (18)	23.17
26	Lamm *et al* (2015)	fMRI experiment, visuo-tactile stimulation	50 (50)	26.5

27	Eskenazi *et al* (2015)	Shared intentions (SI), parallel intentions (PI), individual intention (II) stimuli experiments, echo-planar imaging blood-oxygenation-level-dependent (EPI-BOLD) fMRI	21 (9)	22
28	Ashar *et al* (2017)	fMRI during the processing of the donation task relating to suffering of others, empathic care and distress rating questionnaire, emotions' rating experiment (online)	66 (40)	30.1
29	Sui *et al* (2015)	Stimuli based personal and reward associations tasks to two brain damaged patients, left (vmPFC) cortex and insula, and TP cortex	2	NA
30	Cacioppo *et al* (2015)	Social and emotional stroop tasks, EEG	70 (30)	23.59
31	Hu *et al* (2015)	fMRI exp., behavioural experiment (dictator game), psycho-physiological interaction (PPI) analysis	120 (78)	23.15
32	Lukinova and Myagkov (2016)	The welfare game (WG) is based on the prisoner's dilemma (PD) payoffs, the ultimatum game (UG), fMRI	25 (13)	NA
33	Hackel *et al* (2017)	Decision-making task, face memory task, free choice and forced-choice monetary allocation experiment, neuroimaging	50 (33)	20.9
34	Balconi *et al* (2019)	The joint social task, cooperative task experiment, perception questionnaire, Likert scale, fNIRS measurements	32 (32)	22.59

the selected articles were divided into three categories based on the adopted methodological tools and designs and results: (i) measuring of psychosocial and behavioural effects on participants in the controlled experimental environments (economic games, questionnaires, etc); (ii) tracing activation of specific or the combination of different regions of the brain during prosocial decisions and acts (fMRI, EEG, etc); and (iii) researches that include both, aspects of behavioural psychology as well as neural analysis of the brain during prosocial, nonsocial or antisocial stimuli processing.

An extensive literature survey provided an insight into the various thematic trends prevalent in academic discourse on prosociality, as represented in table 1.2. Relying on previous studies, we categorized the selected articles into three themes:

Table 1.2. The thematic contents are described as per the behavioural results and outcomes of the studies.

Authors' serial	Thematic focus	Findings/outcomes
1	Geo-social mobility and group favouritism	Migration/mobility reduces ingroup favouritism.
2	Trust-violation and group behaviour	Trust-violation reduces ingroup biases, increases chances for trust development on novel or outgroup members.
3	Prosocial behaviour and social norms	Responsiveness to norms shapes prosocial behaviour.
4	Toddlers, treats and happiness	Sharing and instrumental help both are emotionally rewarding.
5	Heroism, altruism and relationship desirability	Heroism and altruism increase desirability, mate selection preference for reproductive success.
6	Prosocial behaviours in potential partners	Helping behaviours make a person more attractive and desirable as a potential long-term partner.
7	Guilt and prosocial behaviours	Prosocial demonstrate more guilt for faulty decisions or actions.
8	Institutions, individuals and prosociality	Pro-sociality is affected by both institutional context and individuals' dispositions or personalities.
9	Prosociality and potential organ donors	A strong positive relationship exists between prosocial decision (here organ donation) and personality traits.
10	Prosocial behavioural intentions scale (PBIS), empathy, altruism	A positive correlation between PBIS, kindness and generosity.
11	Gratitude, pride and social intelligence	Gratitude fosters greater self-monitoring and social intelligence.
12	Unethical behaviours and emotional arousal	Anxiety increases when someone performs unethical behaviour and waits for inspection and punishment.
13	Moral language and prosocial motivation	Moral language draws more significant resources related to social issues.
14	Altruism and lower class	Individuals of lower socioeconomic classes are more egalitarian and altruistic in behaviours.
15	Actors, agents and prosociality	The actor acts to maintain its group affiliation, whereas the agent looks for the basic survival needs.

(1) ingroup, outgroup, individual self-interest and prosociality; (2) impact of prosocial behaviours; and (3) neurocognitive processing of prosocial and altruistic stimuli. The data analysis was performed at quantitative and qualitative levels based

on the categorization of the articles under themes. Since we have selected a broader theme of prosociality, the studies were first tabulated according to the methodological frameworks, participants' group size, results, themes and conclusion.

1.3 Results

1.3.1 Ingroup, outgroup and individual prosociality

1.3.1.1 Actors and agents involved in prosociality

As a watched self, the actor inclines to be morally ethical, while the self agent as an executor intends to be self-centred. The selfish individual, as an actor or agent, is dedicated to serving adaptive functions. The actor acts to maintain their group affiliation, whereas the agent looks for their basic survival needs. Idealistic priming makes agents more moral, whereas, after realistic priming, actors turn more selfish. In this regard, the study also found that females demonstrate less selfish tendencies than males as agents (Frimer *et al* 2014). A trust game experiment showed that individuals initially manifest ingroup favouritism, but trust-violation reduces the ingroup biases and increases the chances of trust development on the novel or outgroup members. The trust-recovery phase resumes ingroup investment without discriminating against the novel group members. When it comes to trust in an unknown group member, people strongly rely on their past experiences with group members. People respond intensely to the negative interactions of trustworthy ingroup partners and more positive interactions with the distrustful outgroup partners (Vermue *et al* 2019). Giving favourable treatment enhances happiness among toddlers. They feel happier after instrumental help. However, toddlers' happiness remains unaffected even after positive feedback or being thanked (Song *et al* 2020), as shown in table 1.2.

1.3.1.2 Heroism, altruism and lower-class people

Contrary to high-class people, people belonging to the lower socioeconomic class have a strong tendency of prosociality and generosity towards strangers and persons in distress. Despite limited resources and subordinate rank, they are more willing to help others in need, even at the cost of self-loss. The lack of economic resources and subjective perceptions of being subordinate in rank influence their prosocial behavioural patterns and positively inspire them to adopt more egalitarian social values and actions (Piff *et al* 2010). The prosocial traits such as heroic acts and altruistic motives cause an upsurge in relationship attraction that ultimately follows a mating strategy among humans. Demonstration of generosity increases desirability for highly attractive than less attractive males. However, the manifestation of heroism increases desirability for highly attractive males but preferably for short-term relationships (Margana *et al* 2019). The theory of sexual selection seems to be another mechanism that may likely explain the maintenance and choices of prosocial behaviours in our species. Demonstrating helping behaviours makes an individual more desirable and favourable as a potential long-term partner (Moore *et al* 2013).

1.3.2 Impact of prosocial behaviours on group genesis and development

1.3.2.1 Prosocial behaviours preserve social norms

Adult prosocial behaviour is synchronized with what society judges as correct social norms. Development of responsiveness to novel social norms among children follows a similar pattern across cultures. Variability in prosocial behaviours develops in middle childhood according to the responsiveness to the standards. Responsiveness to socially normative information shapes prosocial behaviour, which is valid across societies (House *et al* 2020). People often change their behaviour in reaction to how other members behave by following group norms. Unfair conduct of group members amplifies anger among others. Moderate and prosocial individuals react less than selfish people when they get angry at others' dishonest behaviour. Moreover, people with prosocial behaviours demonstrate more guilt while moderators display more instrumental guilt for wrong decisions or actions. Guilt plays a critical emotional role in encouraging human cooperation (Skatova *et al* 2017).

Pro-sociality is a complex phenomenon that is affected by both institutional context and individuals' dispositions or personalities. Individual factors include empathic concern and perspective stance, while institutional factors involve affective organizational commitment along with role clarity (Stiff *et al* 2019). Charitable behaviours and active prosocial actions have been observed among potential organ donors. Agreeableness and conscientiousness also play a crucial role in making prosocial decisions and in triggering prosocial behaviours. However, women are more inclined to donate organs, but emotions in the family, especially love, kindness and concern, exert the most noteworthy influence on organ donating behaviour. There is a strong optimistic correlation between prosocial decisions and personality traits. These include self-esteem, consciousness, agreeableness, prosocial intention, and a functional relationship among family members (Tuszyńska-Bogucka 2019). In a Turkish study, the interactive association between prosocial behavioural intentions scales (PBIS) and adult prosocialness scale (APS) was found to be highly significant, but PBIS and social appearance anxiety scale (SAAS) did not yield a significant correlation.

On the other hand, PBIS showed a positive correlation between empathy and altruism (Anlı 2019). The experience and endorsement of gratitude foster greater social intelligence and self-monitoring. Social intelligence, which is measured in terms of information processing, social skills and awareness scales, was enhanced after the intervention of gratitude factors. In contrast, the intervention of pride resulted in reduced levels of social information processing and social awareness (Gulliford *et al* 2019). Negative emotional arousal has been linked only with unethical behaviours because it is a reliable marker of anxiety detection when an individual performs unethical behaviour and waits for inspection and punishment by other group members (Jaber-López *et al* 2014). When people use moral language to promote organizational vision and mission, they draw greater attention towards resources like money and time related to social issues. Moral language is more effective than economic language because it is composed of the moral values of the organization or company. This situation can be analyzed in the context of prosocial motivation and anticipated guilt (Mayer *et al* 2019).

1.3.3 Neurocognitive processing of prosocial and altruistic stimuli

To help ingroup members, people even opt to harm themselves. Individuals display greater empathy for ingroup members. The left anterior insula (AI) of the brain are accountable for empathy-related ingroup biases. The magnitude of responses in the AI predicts costly helping behaviours when witnessing someone in pain. So, shared activation in the AI (left) has been found while empathizing with the pain of others and during the processing of nociceptive stimuli in self. Strong activation of the brain signal in the right nucleus accumbency (NAcc) has been found when we see the pain of an outgroup member.

Moreover, the impression of the outgroup members modulates the empathy-related AI responses and NAcc activation when witnessing the outer members in pain. The activation of the empathy co-related insula may provoke costly altruism, whereas aggressive signals in the nucleus accumbens can reduce the helping propensity (Hein *et al* 2010). Prosocial behaviours have been found to increase with age. The interaction between positive-prosocial behaviours and age-linked brain development showed some robust clusters in different regions of the brain; the right temporal cortex, the dlPFC, the frontal gyrus (IFG), the mPFC, the temporal junction (TPJ) and the dACC, as is illustrated in figure 1.2. Across all age groups, the low prosocial marks were co-related with the thinner cortex, while the high prosocial marks were linked with the thicker cortex. Thus, prosociality is associated with a higher rate of cortical thinning at the time of early developmental adolescence. This process shows attenuation in the transition phase of young adulthood in the brain regions, which are responsible for social cognition and behavioural control (Ferschmann *et al* 2019).

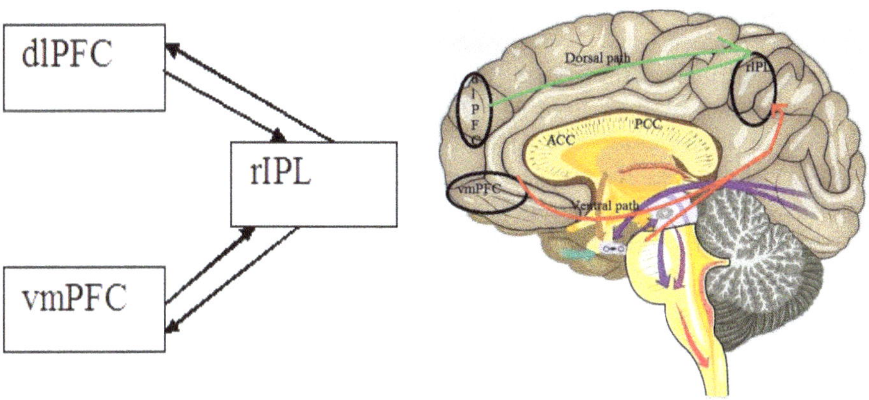

Figure 1.2. Depicts the ventral and dorsal neural-path ways that connect from the ventromedial prefrontal cortex (vmPFC) to the right inferior parietal lobe (rIPL) and from dorsolateral prefrontal cortex to the rIPL during the processing of self and other related stimuli.

1.3.4 Judging individuals with facial anomalies

Individuals with facial anomalies (some form of irregularities and scars) were rated as less trustworthy, less gratifying, less attractive, and more nervous than individuals with attractive or average-looking faces. People with the highest socioeconomic status (SES) are least inclined to prosocial behaviour towards individuals with facial anomalies. When looking at an anomalous face, brain activations have been increased in the bilateral amygdala, bilateral fusiform, the right orbitofrontal cortex (OFC), the right hippocampus, the left inferior frontal gyrus (IFG), the left inferior parietal lobe (IPL) and the right superior occipital cortex. The right fusiform gyrus was found highly activated when encountering highly arousing faces, i.e., the novel beautiful and anomalous faces. The change of signals was positively related in the area of the left amygdala during justice beliefs towards others (Workman *et al* 2021).

During the evaluation of cooperative teamwork, the estimation of self-ability can be increased or decreased according to the performances of other members. So, the self-other emergence phenomenon is evident during cooperative acts. Self and other related signals have been observed in ACC in social contexts (Wittmann *et al* 2016). The bilateral right temporoparietal junction (TPJ), which is linked with emotional perspective-taking and theory of mind, is activated when we observe someone's pain. Similarly, the empathic concern activates the anterior temporal lobe (aTL) and the right DLPFC. Decreasing guilt is linked with an enhanced BOLD signal in the ACC region, associated with costly altruism and increasing empathic concern. Why are humans prone to help others (even strangers) in need, even at their own cost? The readiness to help strangers is driven by an individual's other-oriented empathic concern (FeldmanHall *et al* 2015).

The rate of helping is higher in two conditions if the helper senses no self-risk circumstances and observes the other's needs. Other-need and self-risk contain separate as well as overlapping brain regions. More excellent connectivity between rIPL and rDLPFC has been found associated with an increased rate of helping in the condition of high others' needs, the neural paths are depicted in figure 1.2. rDLPFC causally influences both self-risk and other-need, while rIPL affects only other-need during altruistic decisions. Overall, the network of MPFC, rIPL, and rDLPFC influences the altruistic behaviour of humans (Hu *et al* 2017). A study based on the converged method of behavioural economics, endocrinology and neuroimaging reveals that in self-oriented people testosterone promotes AI responsivity, which may enhance the signals during the processing of norms-abiding behaviours. In the case of altruists, testosterone levels have been positively related to the activation in sgACC/vmPFC, when our brain responds to unfair offers proposed by outgroup members (Reimers *et al* 2017).

1.3.5 Family obligations and prosociality

During any prosocial decision, individuals with low and subordinate family obligations demonstrate activation of the brain around or even below zero, indicating that they do not recruit brain regions responsible for self-control. Individuals who are more inclined to help their family show more excellent connections between ventral striatum and brain areas engaged in mentalizing and self-control, which ultimately cause a sense of reward when helping the family. The costly prosocial decisions or behaviours are not automatic as these involve neural activation in the regions responsible for self-control (Telzer *et al* 2011). In the presence of social information, individuals belonging to low status spontaneously pay greater attention to their mental or psychological states. Low-status individuals show greater neural activity in DMPFC, MPFC and precuneus/PCC brain regions when they receive information about others (Muscatell *et al* 2012), as shown in figure 1.2. People identify their group members more positively with faster reaction times than other group members. The ingroup racial bias in empathic behaviours is prone to changes with increased exposure and daily life contacts with other-race people due to greater empathic activation in ACC, as depicted in figure 1.2. However, people continue to perceive the pain of own-race suffering more highly than individuals from other races (Cao *et al* 2015). People can distinguish between pleasant touch and an unpleasant touch of empathy. Friendly touch activates the mOFC, occipital areas, and parietal visual cortex, whereas unpleasant touch stimuli recruit a larger network, including the right amygdala, anterior, middle cingulate cortex, and anterior frontoinsular cortex (Lamm *et al* 2015), as presented in table 1.3. The perception of social interactions of shared goals and intentions recruits different brain regions than the perception of social interactions with verity independent or self-regulating intentions. Social interactions signal upcoming shared intentions, which activate corresponding social scripts, causing activation in the posterior cingulate cortex (PCC) and bilateral temporal poles (Eskenazi *et al* 2015), as represented in table 1.3.

1.3.6 Impact of empathic care during distress and suffering

Distinctions between distress and empathic care have been labelled as ‘feeling for’ versus ‘feeling with’ or more simply expressed as compassion versus empathy. Empathic caring behaviour has been found related to the activation in the ventromedial frontal cortex and orbitofrontal cortex. These regions are also associated with positive prosocial, empathetic and emotional behaviours. Activities in the posterior cingulate are a key node of mentalizing that gets activated when observing emotional suffering and have also been noted during empathic care. Empathic distress may be associated with mirroring processes in the somatosensory and premotor systems. Thereby empathic distress provokes negative arousal when observing others in suffering (Ashar *et al* 2017). A temporoparietal cortex damaged patient showed hyper self-bias effects while another patient with damaged left vmPFC and insula demonstrated hypo self-bias tendencies. This study indicates that brain lesions can alter self-bias tendencies according to the site of damage (Sui *et al* 2015). When lonely individuals are predisposed to negative social stimuli, their brain microstates are evoked approximately 200 ms earlier than the reaction time of less lonely individuals. Socially positive and unsocially negative stimuli or words recruit similar brain regions responsible for processing pleasant stimuli. The negative social lexicons in the Stroop task activate brain regions responsible for orienting and

Table 1.3. The neurological findings are summarised according to the thematic focuses of studies.

Authors' serial	Thematic focus	Activation observed in region/s
16	Ingroup pain	Left AI.
17	Prosocial behaviour and age-related cortical development	The left dlPFC, the rdACC, the rdmPFC, the rIFG, the rpSTC, the TPJ.
18	Judging individuals with facial anomalies	Bilateral fusiform, amygdala, right latOFC, right hippocampus, right VS, left IFG, the rSCC, left IPL and bilateral IPS. Right fusiform gyrus.
19	Self-other emergence during teamwork	pgACC and area 9.
20	Others' pain, empathic concern	Anterior temporal lobe (aTL), bilateral right temporoparietal junction (TPJ).
21	Altruistic decisions in no self-risk and high other-need conditions	rdlPFC, MPFC and rIPL.
22	Norms-abiding behaviour	AI, sgACC/vmPFC.
23	Family obligations and prosociality	Ventral striatum and areas engaged in mentalizing and self-control.
24	Low-status individuals' response to social information	Mentalizing regions of DMPFC, MPFC and precuneus/PCC.
25	Racial bias in empathic behaviours	Greater empathic activation in ACC.
26	Empathic and unpleasant touch	Pleasant touch activates mOFC, occipital areas and parietal visual cortex.
27	Social interactions of shared intentions	Bilateral temporal poles, precuneus/posterior cingulate (PCC).
28	Empathic care and distress	(Empathic care) medial OFC, vmPFC, VS, septal region, precuneus/posterior cingulated. (Empathic distress) premotor and somatosensory systems.
29	Hyper, hypo self-bias in brain lesions patients	Temporo-parietal cortex damaged patient was hyper self-biased, left vmPFC and insula impaired patient was hypo self-biased.
30	Loneliness levels affecting response to positive and nonsocial words	Negative social lexicons activated brain regions related to executive control, mechanisms of visual perception, xtrastriate, fusiform, AF and DPC extending towards dorsal anterior cingulated and frontal eye field.
31	Punishing and helping conditions	Neural association and connectivity increase between right lPFC and bilateral striatum during cooperation and help, whereas the vmPFC and the lPFC during penalty and punishment.

32	Sociality and cooperation	(Sociality) superior and inferior frontal gyri, parahippocampal gyrus and anterior cingulate. (Cooperation) Brodmann (BA) 8 and 9.
33	Group-level self-investment versus group-level self-affiliation	Ventral striatum, medial orbito-frontal cortex region.
34	Experiential sharing	DLPFC and DPMC areas.

controlling the executive function of visual attention, including extrastriate, fusiform, dorsolateral prefrontal and anterior prefrontal cortex. In contrast, in the Stroop task, social words activated those brain regions involved in the theory of mind, social cognition and executive control of attention (Cacioppo *et al* 2015).

1.3.7 Helping and punishing conditions

The striatum region, which is considered a part of humans' reward system, gets more significant activation during the recognition and evaluation of the rewarding conditions. Therefore, helping any stranger and thwarting a criminal are inherently rewarding for humans. The bilateral striatum has been found activated during the processing of stimuli related to permitting and punishing. The neuronal connectivity was increased between the right lPFC and the bilateral striatum during the processing stimuli associated with help. However, the left lateral prefrontal cortex and vmPFC are activated when processing stimuli related to punishment. Empathically, highly concerned people show greater activation in the fronto-parietal regions. Such individuals opt to help others and decide faster to assist others (Hu *et al* 2015). Sociality also provokes activation in the superior and inferior frontal gyri, parahippocampal gyrus and anterior cingulate cortex, shown in table 1.3. The act of cooperation causes increases in the signals in DLPFC, Brodmann (BA) 8 and 9, though the BA 9 areas function concerning attention and working memory (Lukinova and Myagkov 2016). Greater activation in the medial orbitofrontal cortex region has been observed when an individual makes prosocial choices.

Observing another ingroup member win money rather than one's self may cause displeasure even among group members. Thus, social identity or group affiliation may not always cause a mandatory positive response towards the ingroup. Members' motivational orientation may influence their reactions to their group, resulting in mitigation or strengthening of the sense of shared group membership. Group-level self-investment instead of group-level self-affiliation was linked with increased responses in the ventral striatum when witnessing gains to one's own group (Hackel *et al* 2017). The exchange of an experiential gift causes a significant activity that is increased in DLPFC and DPMC. The cortical actions in DLPFC increase after receiving the experiential gift, indicating a possibility of experience sharing. A greater sense of bonding between the donor and receiver is also activated in DLPFC, which is responsible for establishing interpersonal and social relationships (Balconi *et al* 2019), as table 1.3 shows.

1.4 Discussion

This chapter provides prosocial and positive emotional behaviours trends, analyzing the behavioural, psychosocial and neurocognitive academic discourses. Conventionally, the prosocial behaviours were analyzed under evolutionary psychology and cognitive sciences theories based on group affiliation. Neuroscience literature defines the brain network such as the dPCC, the vmPFC, the dPCC, the dlPFC and the MCC involved in the processing of prosocial and positive emotional behaviours. Behavioural literature on prosociality, cooperation and altruism indicates that humans' prosocial and positive behaviours are not restricted to group-based explanations only. Thus, we derived our first hypothesis: though prosociality in conventional studies has been greatly attributed to the evolutionary aspects of ingroup love and outgroup hate, recent research has added new dimensions based on individual differences within group functionalities that pose challenges to the established concepts of empathy and altruism. Our results based on the analysis of 34 behavioural and neurological studies support our hypothesis-1 and indicate that prosociality in humans is a complex phenomenon that cannot be analyzed only under the delimitation of the dichotomy of ingroup versus outgroup conflicts.

1.4.1 Group-based prosocial behaviours

Positive social decisions resolve the psychological conflict between the self versus ingroup members and the self versus other outer-group members. For example, cross-cultural research conducted by House *et al* (2020) on eight diverse societies suggests that the mind influences the development of prosocial behaviour to respond to the normative information of the concerned society. The prosocial behaviours of adults are conditionally anticipated by what fellow members of the society judge to be correct for the social norm. Social variables of prosocial behaviour evolve in middle childhood with children's responsiveness to the cultural norms. Hackel *et al* (2017) suggest that social identities and subjective values may influence the neural representations in this context. Individuals' investment in ingroup, a motivational component related to social identification, triggers a tendency towards ingroup biased prosociality. Li *et al* (2019) revealed that residential mobility is another crucial factor that shapes the prosocial behaviour towards ingroup or outgroup members. It is observed that stable individuals demonstrate stronger intentions in favour of ingroups than their outgroup counterparts. Frequent migration increases individual identity distinctiveness from the affiliated ingroup and consequently reduces ingroup favouritism and prosocial behaviours. The findings of the previous study suggest that the trust behaviour of the participants were not only guided by the initial group attitudes but also the behavioural towards unknown or novel individuals, which were adjusted based on the earlier group experiences. However, participants showed a change in behaviour after experiencing incongruent interactions with novel partners (Vermue *et al* 2019). Some studies find self-survival strategies without losing group affiliation and benefits. The tension between selfish motivation and moral appearance rises to two motivated selves: the selfish agent who is an executor of selfishness and the moral actor who has often watched the self that tends to be moral. This selfish agent and moral actor duality may analyze the implicit and explicit conflicting behaviours, answering why humans behave better when feeling that they are watched by others (Frimer *et al* 2014). However, after seeing an ingroup member in pain, the self reports empathic concern and activates the anterior insula that provokes help for others. Conversely, the outgroup members in pain can be predicted by activation of nucleus accumbens. Thus, the activation of empathy-based insula motivates the self for helping others. The tendency to help others decreases the antagonistic signals in nucleus accumbens (Hein *et al* 2010). When we see individuals in pain belonging to our race, our anterior cingulate cortex (ACC) is more activated than any other brain area. However, the level of contact with non-own- race individuals may also influence such activation in the ACC. The ACC area can also manifest higher activation when we see non-race people in pain (Cao *et al* 2015).

1.4.2 Happiness of self-reward, feeling others' pain and mating preferences

In the case of Dutch and Chinese young children, studies have shown that participants exhibit more happiness after instrumental helping and giving treatments to others than receiving treatments from others. Positive social feedback, including thought processes, is also affected by the happiness of toddlers. These observations indicate that sharing and instrumental helping are emotionally rewarding. These findings support the evolutionary explanation of prosocial behaviour across cultures (Song *et al* 2020). A study conducted to investigate intra- and inter-brain activities while performing a prosocial behavioural-gift exchange revealed an increase in oxygenated haemoglobin in both donor and receiver brains, especially in the dorsolateral prefrontal cortex region (DLPFC). An experiment has shown that, as a result of gift exchange, the brain activity of both donor and receiver was more synchronized in the areas of dorsal premotor cortex DPMC (Balconi *et al* 2019), as depicted in table 1.2. The empathic concern trait motivates costly altruism guided by the activities in the ventral tegmental area (VTA), caudate, and subgenual anterior cingulate cortex. These key regions promote caregiving to others and social attachment (FeldmanHall *et al* 2015). The right dorsolateral prefrontal cortex (rDLPFC) is the central node that integrates and modulates the motives for self-interest and others' requirements. In contrast, the network of the inferior parietal lobe (IPL), the medial prefrontal cortex (MPFC) and DLPFC plays a crucial role during the altruistic decision-making process (Hu *et al* 2017). Strong emotions have been observed while making such decisions that deviate from the maximization of monetary reward. Emotional arousal faces a social dilemma and goes through a conflict between instinctive and contemplative motivations while weighing pure monetary interests (Jaber-López *et al* 2014). The highest activities in the right inferior frontal gyrus and the medial prefrontal cortex (mPFC) have been observed while making economic decisions in a high social compared to a low social condition (Lukinova and Myagkov 2016).

Prosocial behaviours are driven by both social cognition as well as deliberate efforts. A more significant functional coupling was found between the regions responsible for self-control and reward processing in the ventral striatum in individuals with stronger family preferences (Telzer *et al* 2011). Apart from family obligations, socioeconomic status is also an essential variable in prosocial studies. People belonging to lower socioeconomic status are more likely to involve neural circuitry (DMPFC, MPFC, precuneus/PCC) engaged in thinking or mentalizing about others' feelings and thoughts (Muscatell *et al* 2012). However, altruistic and positive prosocial behaviours can also be studied from the perspective of the social evolution of mate selection strategy. Altruistic behaviour signals good genes and is likely to attract potential mates of the opposite sex (Moore *et al* 2013). Women are attracted to men having heroic and altruistic behaviours. Additionally, such preference becomes more potent if the male is comparatively more attractive than unattractive. As a result, the prosocial traits received higher choices (Margana *et al* 2019).

1.4.3 Cooperation, prosocial conditions and brain activation

Studies suggest that the performance of others contextually influences the estimation of one's own abilities. The pregenual ACC tracks one's own self-performance while the dorsomedial frontal area tracks others' performances (Wittmann *et al* 2016). Even the joint actions activate temporal poles and precuneus, and parallel intentional interactions activate the ventral striatum. The temporal poles and precuneus support the mental state reasoning, and the former is more associated with retrieving social memories (Eskenazi *et al* 2015). However, loneliness triggers short-term self-preservation that enhances the implicit vigilance for social threats. In this context, lonely brains perform quicker to differentiate negative social stimuli from unsocial stimuli (Cacioppo *et al* 2015).

Furthermore, maintaining social norms requires a simultaneous act of punishing violators and helping victims by society. In both these acts, the bilateral striatum gets more activation in the region strongly associated with reward processing. The lPFC and bilateral striatum are more activated during positive stimuli like help and cooperation than the left PFC and vmPFC, which are activated during the processing of punishment stimuli. The greater activation in the frontoparietal regions is marked in individuals who show high empathic concern and preferences to help victims and punish violators (Hu *et al* 2015). Others' suffering may trigger both empathic care and distress. Empathic care is allied with the mOFC and nucleus accumbens activities, while empathic distress is linked with activities in the somatosensory and premotor cortex (Ashar *et al* 2017). The human brain can even distinguish between empathic driven pleasant versus unpleasant touch of others. The medial orbitofrontal cortex (OFC) is associated with the experience of friendly communication and the proper fronto-insular cortex responses while experiencing unpleasant touch (Lamm *et al* 2015). It is also observed that the rate of cortical thickening and thinning may be associated with prosocial behaviours across different age groups. The high prosocial behaviour was linked with more significant cortical thinning in the early to middle adolescence age, and then attenuation was observed during the transition into young adulthood (Ferschmann *et al* 2019). Thus, these arguments are presented in different behavioural and neurological experiments, which support our hypothesis-2 that neurocognitive studies reveal the activation patterns of the brain's different regions and neural networks paths when responding to different prosocial or antisocial stimuli on the experimental conditions.

1.5 Conclusion

In this chapter, we presented recent trends in the field of prosocial and positive emotional studies, which broadly define the evolutionary aspects of group identity and affiliations contributing to ingroup love versus outgroup hate. Prosocial behaviours demand more significant social, cognitive, emotional intelligence, and emphatic skills, which broaden our neural networks at the global level. The neural network connecting the dorsolateral prefrontal cingulate cortex (dlPFC) and ventromedial prefrontal cortex (mvPFC) is devoted to and activated during the computation of prosocial and positive behaviours. Our behavioural observations reveal that prosocial cooperation and altruism in humans are not restricted to group-based analysis only. The summary of the studies has expanded our understanding of social cognition, empathy, moral decisions-actions, cooperative acts, and persuasive skills that positively impact our brain–mind. We conclude that prosocial and positive behavioural investment can reduce unsocial habits, behaviours and activities. So we should not give up the prosocial intrinsic nature of humans; we need to promote prosocial and positive emotional linguistic behaviours across the globe.

References

Abrams D, V de Vyver J, Pelletier J and Cameron L 2015 Children's prosocial behavioural intentions towards outgroup members *Br. J. Dev. Psychol.* **33** 277–94

Aknin L B, Barrington-Leigh C P, Dunn E W, Helliwell J F, Burns J, Biswas-Diener R, Kemeza I, Nyende P, Ashton-James C E and Norton M I 2013 Prosocial spending and well-being: cross-cultural evidence for a psychological universal *J. Pers. Soc. Psychol* **104** 635

Allen M 2009 Meta-analysis *Commun. Monogr.* **76** 398–407

Anlı G 2019 Adaptation of the prosocial behavioural intentions scale for use with Turkish participants: assessments of validity and reliability *Curr. Psychol.* **38** 950–8

Ashar Y K, Andrews-Hanna J R, Dimidjian S and Wager T D 2017 Empathic care and distress: predictive brain markers and dissociable brain systems *Neuron* **94** 1263–73

Balconi M, Fronda G and Vanutelli M E 2019 Donate or receive? Social hyper scanning application with fNIRS *Curr. Psychol.* **38** 991–1002

Bhogal M S, Farrelly D and Galbraith N 2019 The role of prosocial behaviours in mate choice: a critical review of the literature *Curr. Psychol.* **38** 1062–75

Bhogal M S, Bartlett J E and Farrelly D 2019 The influence of mate choice motivation on non-financial altruism *Curr. Psychol.* **38** 959–64

Bjornestad J, Lavik K O, Davidson L, Hjeltnes A, Moltu C and Veseth M 2020 Antipsychotic treatment–a systematic literature review and meta-analysis of qualitative studies *J. Mental Health* **29** 513–23

Blakey K H, Mason E, Cristea M, McGuigan N and Messer E J 2019 Does kindness always pay? The influence of recipient affection and generosity on young children's allocation decisions in a resource distribution task *Curr. Psychol.* **38** 939–49

Borenstein M, Hedges L V, Higgins J P and Rothstein H R 2021 *Introduction to Meta-Analysis* (New York: Wiley)

Borinca I, Falomir-Pichastor J M, Andrighetto L and Durante F 2021 Outgroup prejudice and perceptions of prosocial intergroup behaviours *Eur. J. Soc. Psychol.* **51** 40–53

Buss D M and Von Hippel W 2018 Psychological barriers to evolutionary psychology: ideological bias and coalitional adaptations *Arch. Sci. Psychol.* **6** 148

Cacioppo S, Balogh S and Cacioppo J T 2015 Implicit attention to negative social, in contrast to nonsocial, words in the Stroop task differs between individuals high and low in loneliness: evidence from event-related brain microstates *Cortex* **70** 213–33

Cao Y, Contreras-Huerta L S, McFadyen J and Cunnington R 2015 Racial bias in neural response to others' pain is reduced with other-race contact *Cortex* **70** 68–78

Dale R, Marshall-Pescini S and Range F 2020 What matters for cooperation? The importance of social relationship over cognition *Sci. Rep.* **10** 1–14

Decety J, Bartal I B A, Uzefovsky F and Knafo-Noam A 2016 Empathy as a driver of prosocial behaviour: highly conserved neurobehavioural mechanisms across species *Phil. Trans. R. Soc.* B **371** 20150077

Diesendruck G and Benozio A 2012 Prosocial behaviour towards ingroup and outgroup members *Encyclopedia on Early Childhood Development* 2nd edn (Montreal: CEECD)

Dos Santos M and Peña J 2017 Antisocial rewarding in structured populations *Sci. Rep.* **7** 1–14

Dotterer H L, Tomlinson R C, Burt S A, Weigard A S, Klump K L and Hyde L W 2021 Neurocognitive abilities associated with antisocial behaviour with and without callous-unemotional traits in a community sample *Neuropsychology* **35** 374

Dovidio J F, Gaertner S L, Shnabel N, Saguy T and Johnson J D 2009 Recategorization and prosocial behaviour: common ingroup identification and a dual identification *Psychology of Helping: New Directions in Intergroup Prosocial Behaviour* (Malden, MA: Wiley-Blackwell)

Dugré J R, Radua J, Carignan-Allard M, Dumais A, Rubia K and Potvin S 2020 Neurofunctional abnormalities in antisocial spectrum: a meta-analysis of fMRI studies on Five distinct neurocognitive research domains *Neurosci. Biobehav. Rev.* **119** 168–83

Eisenberg N, Lennon R and Roth K 1983 Prosocial development: a longitudinal study *Develop. Psychol.* **19** 846

Eskenazi T, Rueschemeyer S A, de Lange F P, Knoblich G and Sebanz N 2015 Neural correlates of observing joint actions with shared intentions *Cortex* **70** 90–100

Espinosa M P and Kovářík J 2015 Prosocial behaviour and gender *Front. Behav. Neurosci.* **9** 88

Everett J A, Faber N S and Crockett M J 2015 The influence of social preferences and reputational concerns on intergroup prosocial behaviour in gains and losses contexts *R. Soc. Open Sci.* **2** 150546

Everett J A, Faber N S and Crockett M 2015 Preferences and beliefs in ingroup favouritism *Front. Behav. Neurosci.* **9** 15

Farrelly D and King L 2019 Mutual mate choice drives the desirability of altruism in relationships *Curr. Psychol.* **38** 977–81

FeldmanHall O, Dalgleish T, Evans D and Mobbs D 2015 Empathic concern drives costly altruism *Neuroimage* **105** 347–56

Ferschmann L, Vijayakumar N, Grydeland H, Overbye K, Sederevicius D, Due-Tønnessen P, Fjell A M, Walhovd K B, Pfeifer J H and Tamnes C K 2019 Prosocial behaviour relates to the rate and timing of cortical thinning from adolescence to young adulthood *Dev. Cogn. Neurosci.* **40** 100734

Field A P and Gillett R 2010 How to do a meta-analysis *Br. J. Math. Stat. Psychol.* **63** 665–94

Frimer J A, Aquino K, Gebauer J E, Zhu L L and Oakes H 2015 A decline in prosocial language helps explain public disapproval of the US Congress *Proc. Natl Acad. Sci.* **112** 6591–4

Frimer J A, Schaefer N K and Oakes H 2014 Moral actor, selfish agent *J. Pers. Soc. Psychol.* **106** 790

Galen L W 2012 Does religious belief promote prosociality? A critical examination *Psychol. Bull.* **138** 876

Gilbert P and Basran J 2019 The evolution of prosocial and antisocial competitive behaviour and the emergence of prosocial and antisocial leadership styles *Front. Psychol.* **10** 610

Guan F, Chen J, Chen O, Liu L and Zha Y 2019 Awe and prosocial tendency *Curr. Psychol.* **38** 1033–41

Gulliford L, Morgan B, Hemming E and Abbott J 2019 Gratitude, self-monitoring and social intelligence: a prosocial relationship? *Curr. Psychol.* **38** 1021–32

Hackel L M, Zaki J and Van Bavel J J 2017 Social identity shapes social valuation: evidence from prosocial behaviour and vicarious reward *Soc. Cogn. Affect. Neurosci.* **12** 1219–28

Hopwood T L and Schutte N S 2017 Psychological outcomes in reaction to media exposure to disasters and large-scale violence: a meta-analysis *Psychol. Violence* **7** 316

House B R *et al* 2020 universal norm psychology leads to societal diversity in prosocial behaviour and development *Nat. Human Behav.* **4** 36–44

Haun D and Over H 2015 Like me: a homophily-based account of human culture *Epistemological Dimensions of Evolutionary Psychology* (New York: Springer) pp 117–30

Hein G, Silani G, Preuschoff K, Batson C D and Singer T 2010 Neural responses to ingroup and outgroup members' suffering predict individual differences in costly helping *Neuron* **68** 149–60

Henrich J and Muthukrishna M 2021 The origins and psychology of human cooperation *Ann. Rev. Psychol.* **72** 207–40

Hu J, Li Y, Yin Y, Blue P R, Yu H and Zhou X 2017 How do self-interest and other-need interact in the brain to determine altruistic behaviour? *Neuroimage* **157** 598–611

Hu Y, Strang S and Weber B 2015 Helping or punishing strangers: neural correlates of altruistic decisions as third-party and of its relation to empathic concern *Front. Behav. Neurosci.* **9** 24

Hutcherson C A, Bushong B and Rangel A 2015 A neurocomputational model of altruistic choice and its implications *Neuron* **87** 451–62

Hutton B *et al* 2015 The PRISMA extension statement for reporting of systematic reviews incorporating network meta-analyzes of health care interventions: checklist and explanations *Ann. Intern. Med.* **162** 777–84

Isoda M 2021 Socially relative reward valuation in the primate brain *Curr. Opin. Neurobiol.* **68** 15–22

Jaber-López T, García-Gallego A, Perakakis P and Georgantzis N 2014 Physiological and behavioural patterns of corruption *Front. Behav. Neurosci.* **8** 434

Jensen K 2016 Prosociality *Curr. Biol.* **26** R748–52

Kappeler P M and Van Schaik C P 2006 *Cooperation in Primates and Humans* (Berlin: Springer)

Lamm C, Silani G and Singer T 2015 Distinct neural networks underlying empathy for pleasant and unpleasant touch *Cortex* **70** 79–89

Li W Q, Li L M W and Li M 2019 Residential mobility reduces ingroup favouritism in prosocial behaviour *Asian J. Soc. Psychol.* **22** 3–17

Lieven E V 2013 Language acquisition as a cultural process *Cultural Evolution: Society, Technology, Language, and Religion* (Cambridge, MA: MIT Press) pp 269–83

Lukinova E and Myagkov M 2016 Impact of short social training on prosocial behaviours: an fMRI study *Front. Syst. Neurosci.* **10** 60

Margana L, Bhogal M S, Bartlett J E and Farrelly D 2019 The roles of altruism, heroism, and physical attractiveness in female mate choice *Pers. Individ. Differ.* **137** 126–30

Mathew S, Boyd R and Van Veelen M 2013 Human cooperation among kin and close associates may require enforcement of norms by third parties *Cultural Evolution: Society, Technology, Language, and Religion* (Cambridge, MA: MIT Press) pp 45–60

Mayer D M, Ong M, Sonenshein S and Ashford S J 2019 The money or the morals? When moral language is more effective for selling social issues *J. Appl. Psychol.* **104** 1058

McLoughlin N and Over H 2019 Encouraging children to mentalize about a perceived outgroup increases prosocial behaviour towards outgroup members *Dev. Sci.* **22** e12774

Meleady R and Seger C R 2017 Imagined contact encourages prosocial behaviour towards outgroup members *Group Process Intergroup. Relat.* **20** 447–64

Moher D, Shamseer L, Clarke M, Ghersi D, Liberati A, Petticrew M, Shekelle P and Stewart L A 2015 Preferred reporting items for systematic review and meta-analysis protocols (PRISMA-P) 2015 statement *Syst. Rev.* **4** 1–9

Moore D, Wigby S, English S, Wong S, Székely T and Harrison F 2013 Selflessness is sexy: reported helping behaviour increases desirability of men and women as long-term sexual partners *BMC Evol. Biol.* **13** 1–8

Muscatell K A, Morelli S A, Falk E B, Way B M, Pfeifer J H, Galinsky A D, Lieberman M D, Dapretto M and Eisenberger N I 2012 Social status modulates neural activity in the mentalizing network *Neuroimage* **60** 1771–7

Norenzayan A and Gervais W M 2012 The cultural evolution of religion *Creating Consilience: Integrating Science and the Humanities* (New York: Oxford University Press) pp 243–65

Norman I and Fleming P 2019 Perceived attractiveness of two types of altruist *Curr. Psychol.* **38** 982–90

Paulus M 2015 Cognitive development: the neurocognitive basis of early prosociality *Curr. Biol.* **25** R47–8

Penner L A, Dovidio J F, Piliavin J A and Schroeder D A 2005 Prosocial behaviour: multilevel perspectives *Annu. Rev. Psychol.* **56** 365–92

Piff P K, Kraus M W, Côté S, Cheng B H and Keltner D 2010 Having less, giving more: the influence of social class on prosocial behaviour *J. Pers. Soc. Psychol* **99** 771

Reimers L, Büchel C and Diekhof E K 2017 Neural substrates of male parochial altruism are modulated by testosterone and behavioural strategy *NeuroImage* **156** 265–76

Schwarz S and Baßfeld L 2019 Do men help only beautiful women in social networks? *Curr. Psychol.* **38** 965–76

Sera F, Armstrong B, Blangiardo M and Gasparrini A 2019 An extended mixed-effects framework for meta-analysis *Stat. Med.* **38** 5429–44

Simpson J A and Beckes L 2010 Evolutionary perspectives on prosocial behaviour *Prosocial Motives, Emotions, and Behavior: The Better Angels of our Nature* (Washington DC: American Psychological Association) pp 35–53

Skatova A, Spence A, Leygue C and Ferguson E 2017 Guilty repair sustains cooperation, angry retaliation destroys it *Sci. Rep.* **7** 1–11

Skoyles J 2012 Human neuromaturation, juvenile extreme energy liability, and adult cognition/cooperation *Nat. Preced.* 1–1

Somel M, Liu X and Khaitovich P 2013 Human brain evolution: transcripts, metabolites and their regulators *Nat. Rev. Neurosci.* **14** 112–27

Song Y, Broekhuizen M L and Dubas J S 2020 Happy little benefactor: prosocial behaviours promote happiness in young children from two cultures *Front. Psychol.* **11** 1398

Steinbeis N 2018 Neurocognitive mechanisms of prosociality in childhood *Curr. Opin. Psychol.* **20** 30–4

Stiff C, Rosenthal-Stott H E, Wake S and Woodward A 2019 Student prosociality: measuring institutional and individual factors that predict prosocial behaviour at university *Curr. Psychol.* **38** 920–30

Sui J, Enock F, Ralph J and Humphreys G W 2015 Dissociating hyper and hypoself biases to a core self-representation *Cortex* **70** 202–12

Telzer E H, Masten C L, Berkman E T, Lieberman M D and Fuligni A J 2011 Neural regions associated with self control and mentalizing are recruited during prosocial behaviours towards the family *Neuroimage* **58** 242–9

Timulak L 2014 Qualitative meta-analysis *The SAGE Handbook of Qualitative Data Analysis* (London: SAGE Publications)

Tooby J 2018 The emergence of evolutionary psychology *Emerging Syntheses in Science* (Boca Raton, FL: CRC Press) pp 67–76

Tuszyńska-Bogucka W 2019 'Be the match'. Predictors of decisions concerning registration in potential bone marrow donor registry in a group of Polish young adults as an example of prosocial behaviour *Curr. Psychol.* **38** 1042–61

Vaish A and Hepach R 2020 The development of prosocial emotions *Emot. Rev.* **12** 259–73

Vermue M, Meleady R and Seger C R 2019 Member-to-member generalization in trust behaviour: how do prior experiences inform prosocial behaviour towards novel ingroup and outgroup members? *Curr. Psychol.* **38** 1003–20

Walsh J J, Christoffel D J, Wu X, Pomrenze M B and Malenka R C 2021 Dissecting neural mechanisms of prosocial behaviours *Curr. Opin. Neurobiol.* **68** 9–14

Wittmann M K, Kolling N, Faber N S, Scholl J, Nelissen N and Rushworth M F 2016 Self-other mergence in the frontal cortex during cooperation and competition *Neuron* **91** 482–93

Workman C I, Humphries S A, Hartung F, Aguirre G K, Kable J W and Chatterjee A 2021 Morality is in the eye of the beholder: the neurocognitive basis of the 'anomalous-is-bad' stereotype *Ann. NY Acad. Sci.* **1494** 3–17

Wu H, Luo Y and Feng C 2016 Neural signatures of social conformity: a coordinate-based activation likelihood estimation meta-analysis of functional brain imaging studies *Neurosci. Biobehav. Rev.* **71** 101–11

Chapter 2

Processing of emotion and action verbal and non-verbal stimuli: neural signatures in the human brain

Shashikanta Tarai, Tulika Ghosh and Arindam Bit

Our brain processes the emotion and action of linguistic (i.e., verbal: words, phrases and sentences) and non-linguistic (i.e., non-verbal: voice, tone, face, gestures, postures and eye movements) stimuli differently than non-emotional or neutral verbal and non-verbal stimulus. However, the question arises of how our brain perceives and anticipates the meaning of emotions, whether they are verbal or non-verbal means of stimuli, based on prior actions or events. The neural signatures related to events and emotions are synthesised, summarised and interpreted across electroencephalographic and neuroimaging studies. The results confirm that our brain anticipates happy, sad and angry emotions based on prior positive and negative actions and events. Across studies, participants performed various emotion and action recognitions, match–mismatch and value judgement tasks to capture the behavioural response time and accuracy, time and regions of neural activations. Also, they performed word judgement tasks in which emotion words matched or mismatched with the prior action or event words. Positive emotional pictures or words, especially happy emotions, were processed faster with higher accuracy than sad or angry words or images when the emotional stimulus was incongruent with prior negative actions or events. The analysis of event-related potentials (ERPs) and neuroimaging data (ND) across studies revealed the modulation of the early P100 and the early posterior negativity (EPN), the P300 and the late positive complex (LPC), the late posterior positivity (LPP), and N400 components in the frontal, temporal, central, centro-parietal, parietal and occipital lobes. These regions are involved and activated during the processing of both verbal and non-verbal stimuli

doi:10.1088/978-0-7503-3383-2ch2

of emotions and actions. It is observed that the human brain automatically anticipates feelings based on action-oriented goals.

2.1 Introduction

Human events and actions are strongly associated with feelings and emotions (Chen *et al* 2016). Emotions are closely interrelated with action because they are the causal control of movements or activities (Reis and Gray 2009, Frijda 2010). For example, anyone can feel happy while celebrating and rejoicing a marriage or birthday party. However, someone can fight when they usually face cruelty or anger. The human brain processes emotions based on contextual cues of actions or events. In this regard, activities are some of the reactions to emotions. To analyse the processing of any emotion, whether it is positive (happy and joy) or negative (sad, anger, disgust, fear), it is indispensable to study the contextual cues of events or actions that lead to emotion. For example, positive and rewarding events trigger happy emotions, including organising a party or winning a race, whereas adverse events trigger sad emotions such as losing a game or attending a funeral party. In this sense, emotions are usually a valenced reaction to relevant action stimuli directed to target events (Ekman 1993, Frijda 1994). The distinct patterns of appraisals and evaluation tendency of positive and negative events are associated with emotional valences of emotions (Levenson *et al* 1990, Lazarus 1991). Our survival strategies are also grounded and motivated by positive events or actions that trigger positive emotions. Emotion and action or events are entangled and intertwined with each other (Ferri *et al* 2013). Every event or activity is related to emotion, and every emotion is also a reaction to an event (Frijda 1986, 2006, Damasio 2003). Motor behaviours that are bodily activities of actions are strongly associated with emotions (Hajcak *et al* 2007).

2.1.1 Action and emotion in socio-communicative contexts

In a socio-communicative context, linguistic behaviours also exhibit event or action verbs that lead to the exception and anticipation of different valences of emotions. Our embedded parallel and interconnected model predicts the thought (T) of action/event (X, Y) through the emotional reaction (ER) to action or event (X2, Y2). The prediction is based on the perceptual performance (P), consequence (C) and perpetual appraisal (PA), as depicted in figure 2.1. In language, an emotional word matches with the event or action verbs in a sentence. This chapter examines the existing psycholinguistic, neurolinguistics, and cognitive psychology and neuroscience perspectives of action and emotion processing across studies. The main objective is to generalise the way our brain processes the expectancy violation between event or action and emotion, leading to incongruence in the verbal and non-verbal domains of communication.

2.1.2 Expectancy violation between action and emotion

The expectancy violation between action and emotion may alter and modulate the neural time-course of processing in the brain. Numerous behavioural and neurophysiological studies support the integration of emotion and action processing in the

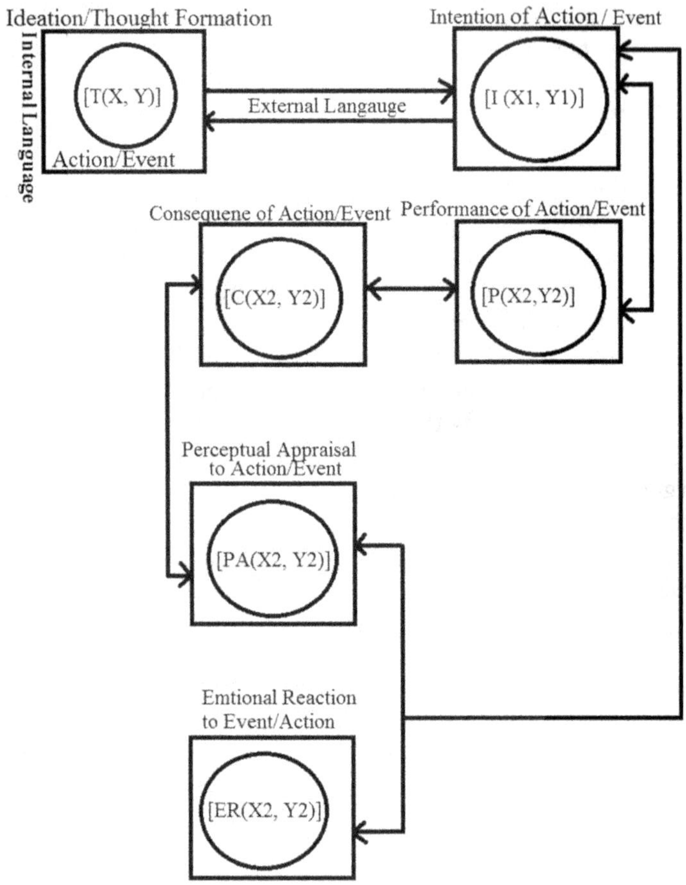

Figure 2.1. The embedded parallel model predicts the emotional reaction, i.e., [ER(X2, Y2)] to the bodily performance of action or events [P(X2, Y2)] through intention [I(X1, Y1)] of action/event thought [T(X, Y)].

human brain. For instance, neurophysiological research shows that the positive action of holding a suitcase and the adverse negative action of throwing a bag are strongly associated with positive 'happy' and negative 'angry' emotions, respectively (Ferri *et al* 2013). These behavioural bodily actions linked with happy and angry faces are processed in the motor frontal, temporal and occipital regions, suggesting higher activations for actions embedded with emotions (Ferri *et al* 2013). Further, a study using the Transcranial Magnetic Stimulation technique (TMS) also validated that the pleasant and unpleasant facial expressions evoked significantly greater neural activation than neutral images (Hajcak *et al* 2007). At the non-verbal level, though most studies have examined the integrational processing of emotion and action by using pictorial forms, a few studies have only focused on the association of action and emotion by employing verbs and adjectives at the verbal level. Synthesising literature on the processing of both these verbal and non-verbal stimuli of emotion and actions, the neural signatures that diverge due to different tasks, stimulation, paradigms, methods and results are interpreted to state the implications and future directions of the previous studies.

2.1.3 Neuroimaging studies on action and emotion

Studies have shown that the somatic motor and premotor cortex that include the frontal and central areas of the human brain plan for effortful and voluntary actions, movements, behavioural strategies and evaluation of activities (Martin and Chao 2001, Pulvermüller 2005). These areas also process the action words and pictures referring to arms, legs and faces (e.g., hold, kick or eat) (Pulvermüller *et al* 2001, Grezes *et al* 2003, Hauk *et al* 2004, Tettamanti *et al* 2005, Peelen *et al* 2012). Using the non-invasive method of data acquisition techniques like functional magnetic resonance imaging (fMRI) and electroencephalogram (EEG), studies have mainly found the rapid processing of action words within 200–300 ms in the frontocentral regions of the brain when the participants are asked to judge the action and neutral words (Pulvermüller *et al* 2001, Boulenger *et al* 2006, Hauk *et al* 2008). Moreover, the action words in a sentence like she grasps, he jumps, and she walks activate the left temporal cortex (LTC), posterior middle temporal Gyrus (pMTG) and superior temporal sulcus and (STS) (Davis *et al* 2004, Deen and McCarthy 2010, Rueschemeyer *et al* 2010, Crepaldi *et al* 2011, Willms *et al* 2011, Bedny *et al* 2012). Most of these studies emphasise the attentional processing of semantic information of isolated words and pictures of action and emotions in the central, centro-parietal and parietal regions by employing various neural-imaging (e.g., fMRI, MEG and EEG) techniques. However, the activation of areas of the brain (e.g., somatotopic motor, premotor and frontocentral regions) and the time of course of processing have not been integrated and summarised across studies that are varied based on stimulus, tasks and paradigms. Therefore, a thorough understanding of findings on emotion and action is intended to provide a unique platform for establishing cutting-edge inquiry that may reflect the growing importance of action and emotion studies in the domain of cognitive neuroscience.

2.1.4 EEG studies on action and emotion words

Using EEG technique, studies have found that, in comparison with neutral words, inspirational and emtional words evoked higher amplitudes because the meaning of emotive words takes immense attention with higher cognitive resources from the point of view of evolutionary significance, survival strategies and involuntarily attention (Lang *et al* 1997, Kissler *et al* 2006, Paulmann and Kotz 2008, Citron 2012). Similarly, the experiments on lexical and semantic decision tasks established the sequential time courses of the emotional arousal, valence and detail processing of emotional word meaning. Our brain recognises the content of emotional arousal much faster and earlier than the valences of emotion (Schirmer and Kotz 2006). The detailed conceptualisation of the meaning of emotional words and their contextual uses in terms of knowledge extraction occurs in the later stage of processing (Phillips *et al* 2003). After the onset of the word, the neural time course of valences of both written and spoken emotional words occurs either at 200 ms or between 300 and

800 ms (Herbert *et al* 2008, Kissler *et al* 2009, Kissler and Herbert 2012). Further, the analysis of neural time course shows that pleasant words evoke higher amplitude as compared to unpleasant words in the early posterior-negative (EPN: 200–300 ms) and the late positive components (LPC: 300–600 ms) (Junghöfer *et al* 2001). The amplitude of these two components (EPN: 200–300 ms and the LPC: 450–800 ms) was higher in frontal, medial-temporal, central, parietal, occipitotemporal and centro-parietal regions of the brain (Cuthbert *et al* 2000, Zald 2003, Schupp *et al* 2004, Sergerie *et al* 2008). Specifically, the late component is associated with the detailed processing of emotional words with a more extensive semantic network than neutral or non-emotional words (Dillon *et al* 2006, Fischler and Bradley 2006). If there is a mismatch between emotion and action, it will be interesting to observe how our brain processes emotion based on action, which may process much faster and earlier than isolated independent emotional words in the EPN and LPC components.

Neurolinguistic literature has emphasised the event-related potential (ERP) components related to online semantic and syntactic violations of sentence comprehension (Schacht and Sommer 2009a). However, the processing of emotional words based on semantic violation of preceding actions or events has not been compared and interpreted with the processing of non-emotional words both at the verbal and non-verbal levels, employing a semantic judgement task (Bayer *et al* 2010). So far, at the verbal level, it is observed that the semantic violation related to the perception of phrase structure, sub-categorisation, the number and case agreement produces the 'syntactic positivity shift' or P600 component (Hagoort *et al* (1999), for a review). However, the semantic violation associated with integrating multiple words (e.g., nouns and adjectives; verbs and adverbs) produces the higher negative deflection of N400 (Kutas and Federmeier 2000, Hagoort 2003, Zhang *et al* 2006). In this domain, the lexico-syntactic violation referring to either gender or number agreement provokes early posterior negativity (EPN) between 300 to 500 ms or the left anterior negativity (LAN) (Friederici *et al* 1996).

Despite lexical studies on emotion and non-emotion, the neural mechanisms of emotion and action are not well understood. This chapter interprets the behavioural time-course of syntactic, semantic and lexico-syntactic processing of emotion and action by following the linguistic tasks and paradigms. It also links the time course of processing with the regions of the brain. The comparative assessments of different components of emotions and actions would provide a substantive clue to cognitive mechanisms, which either may process much faster than the neurolinguistics components such as EPN (200–300 ms), LAN (200 ms), N400 (300–400 ms) and P600 (400–600 ms). The faster response to emotions may be due to the context of events or action verbs in a sentence. The event or action verb in a sentence represents a contextual cue to the emotion by which our brain can recognise and retrieve the semantic category of emotional words from a vast array of verbal or non-verbal networks. The congruency task certainly provides evidence of the relational and interdependency of cognitive mechanisms of emotion and action. The task of emotional face incongruence is well established in the domain of neurocognitive science (Righart and De Gelder 2008). After the onset of the stimulus, the congruency effect of emotional face and body integration begins at 115 ms in the occipital regions (Meeren *et al* 2005). However, after the onset of the object, the effect of action and object incongruency occurs at around 300 ms (Sitnikova *et al* 2003). This component prompted us to search the relevant studies and integrate the early and late processing of verbal and non-verbal stimuli to determine whether integration of action and emotion congruency occurs within 100 ms.

2.1.5 Aim of the current chapter

This chapter discusses the findings of behavioural, neuroimaging or neuropsychological studies on emotion and action processing in the human brain. In this direction, we integrate the methodological insights and findings of previous EEG and fMRI studies. First, we introduce the relevance of empirical and theoretical backgrounds of emotion and action studies in the introduction. Second, the methodological insights of EEG and fMRI studies on emotion and action specify the problems and issues related to experimental tasks and paradigms. Third, significant findings, including the different types of ERP components, brain regions, and hemispheric laterality, are summarised to find out the current state of research. Fourth, the findings of the previous studies are integrated and interpreted in the light of competing for the verbal and non-verbal stimulus of action and emotion that facilitate spatio-temporal top-down modulation of neural mechanisms and bottom-up sensory inputs. Fourth, the current hypothesis on action and emotion processing interprets and explains the research gaps for the future direction of study. Finally, the concluding inferences emphasising temporal aspects of processing are drawn with relevance to the implication of cognitive mechanisms of action and emotion studies.

2.2 Methodology

2.2.1 Participants: exclusion and inclusion criteria

Most of the studies on action or event verbal and non-verbal stimulus processing have selected healthy right-handed participants by following the purposive sampling technique (Urgesi *et al* 2010, Alemanno *et al* 2012, Bedny *et al* 2012, Hirschfeld *et al* 2012, Peelen *et al* 2012, Pulvermüller 2018, Casiraghi *et al* 2019, Kuhnke *et al* 2020, Pisu *et al* 2020). Similarly, a large number of cognitive studies on emotional, verbal and non-verbal stimuli have also considered healthy right-handed infant and adult participants by certifying the purposive judgement sampling technique (Borod *et al* 2000, Leppänen *et al* 2007, Bayer *et al* 2010, Ferri *et al* 2010, Abbassi *et al* 2011, Weinberg *et al* 2012, Smith *et al* 2013, Saarimäki *et al* 2016, Chen *et al* 2019, Ren *et al* 2019, Wu *et al* 2019, 2020, 2021, Yang *et al* 2020, Schindler *et al* 2021). A few studies have either focused on action and emotion or emotion and action integrated processing in the brain of healthy adult and infant participants (Moseley *et al* 2012, Ferri *et al* 2013, Hepach and Westermann 2013, Yu and Kitayama 2019, Eben *et al* 2020, Guex *et al* 2020, Mennella *et al* 2020, Ruba *et al* 2020). Most of these studies have primarily selected male participants with less representation of females. Therefore, we should consider equal proportional representative samples of males and females, which may provide a stable result and unbiased gender interpretation on the processing of action and emotional stimuli. It is also correct to observe the average age of participants across studies that may influence the processing effects of action and emotion stimulus. From the point of view of the population, it is essential to classify and categorise the processing effects of action and emotion by considering the age of infant, adult and old participants. Except for the abnormal and patient studies, other studies exclude participants who suffer from a neurological or psychiatric disorder and drug abuse. If the participants showed any excessive rate of artefacts and electrical noise in the acquisition of EEG and fMRI data, those participants also needed to be excluded from the study at the time of pre-processing of data. All participants signed a written consent form, and they were also paid for their participation in the experiment. In some cases, they voluntarily participated to complete the task of the investigation without any payment. All the experimental studies are conducted with prior approval of the Institute/University/Organisational Ethics Committee.

2.2.2 Materials: verbal stimulus

In many studies, the actions or events are classified based on verbal and non-verbal stimuli. Verbal stimuli include linguistic units such as words, phrases and sentences, whereas non-verbal stimuli comprise the non-linguistic such as picture, body postures, facial expression, gestures, voice and tone. In the domain of language, action or events broadly refer to the verb. For example, the study of Klepp *et al* (2017) has selected German verbs (48 disyllabic verbs) referring to the action of hand ('greifen' to grasp) and foot ('laufen' to walk). They also include 48 abstract verbs ('erraten' to guess). The frequency of the occurrence of the verb is determined by using the Leipzig Corpora, which is available at http://wortschatz.uni-leipzig.de (Biemann *et al* 2007). In the study, participants are asked to regulate and adjust the experimental slide bars with a scale of a numerical value to express their feeling of actions related to the leg, foot, and arm and hand that the action verb offered.

Similarly, in a recognition and decision task, participants are asked to recognise whether a word is a noun or verb ('is it a verb? Or noun?'), while attending 140 verbs and 120 sets of nouns (Muraki *et al* 2020). In this case, verbs are classified based on their embodiment ratings (Sidhu *et al* 2014), emotional ratings (Warriner *et al* 2013), and cognitive ratings. In valence ratings, participants recognise the degree of happiness or unhappiness, whereas, in the embodiment ratings, they are asked to rate whether a verb refers to an action or state related to the human body. The low rating is indicated as unhappy in these ratings, and the high rating is specified as happy. In embodiment rating, the more subordinate verbs do not involve the human body, whereas the higher rating verb quickly involves the human body. Cognitive ratings of verbs affect the rating of mental actions or processes related to thought and experience, in which the numerical scale from 1 to 7 represents minus cognitive to fully-plus cognitive. Like verbs, nouns are also classified as the high body-object interaction (BOI) and low BOI (Tillotson *et al* 2008, Bennett *et al* 2011). The study of Fan *et al* (2017) includes the total 24-word stimuli of L2 English comprising six positively and six negatively emotional words. The remaining 12 words are emotionally identical to L1 Chinese symbolic characters. The frequency of L2 English emotional words is drawn from the British English Corpus (http://www.natcorp.ox.ac.uk), whereas the frequency of L1 Chinese words is selected from the Chinese dictionary (Liu *et al* 2012). Using the frequency conversion formula (e.g., 100 000 000/25 000 000 = the current frequency rate of L1 words or the actual frequency rate of L1 words) and applying the t-test, the study does not indicate any significant differences between L2 words and L1 words. Another study presents the human characters and their actions from 24 stories (mean story length = 70 words) (Deen and McCarthy 2010). Each reported story is presented in 172 seconds with a 10 s period of interval between stories. Participants were instructed to read and comprehend each tale. The reading time for each story is synchronised with the scanning time of functional magnetic resonance (fMRI). The story contains some action words like 'John walked' or 'Jane grasped'. Alemanno *et al* (2012) have also used the Italian sentences consisting of two factorial designs: concreteness (2 level stages: hand-related action; sentences with abstract verbs) and separate polarities (2 level stories: assertive; negative) to find out the processing of action (write, brush, walk, applaud, iron) and abstract (think, imagine, envy, innovate) verbs. The sentence stimulus (160 sentences) are constructed by using the first person singular pronoun (I) and verb with affirmative (80 affirmatives: 40 hand-related, 40 abstracts) and negative polarity (80 negatives: 40 hand-related, 40 abstracts).

For an auditory recognition task, a study has selected the high-movement action verbs, the intermediate-movement or motion verbs referring to the dynamic state and bodily-physical functions, and the low-motion mental verbs (Bedny *et al* 2012). It also has selected the high motion or movement nouns (animals), the intermediate motion-related nouns (tools), and the low-movement or motion nouns (inanimate natural) for both control and experimental groups. Each category has 50-word pairs. Shebani and Pulvermüller (2013) have also selected 72 words that include 36 arm-hand action related verbs (e.g., grab, braid and clap) and 36 leg-foot action related verbs (e.g., hop, kick and step). The study of Fields and Kuperberg (2012) has also chosen 222 groups of two-sentence states: 2 self-bearing situations (self and other) and three motional situations (neutral, pleasant and unpleasant). For example, there are some categories of sentences like enjoyable (e.g., 'A man who knocks on the room door, he has a gift in his hand'), unpleasant (e.g., 'A man who knocks on the room door, he has a gun in his hand'), and neutral (e.g., 'A man who knocks the room door, he has a tray in his hand'). In a lexical perception of task, 200 words and 100 sentences are selected based on the six-point scale of emotionality from 0 (not at all) to 5 (extremely) (Borod *et al* 2000). Bayer *et al* (2010) have selected 328 syntactically and semantically German correct sentences by following the structure like (e.g., [determiner or article—actor of the action—auxiliary verb—determiner/article—object]—[verb]; e.g., [Die (the)—Frau (woman)—will (will)—den (the)—Mann (man)] [anrufen (call)]). In these types of stimuli, the sentence-final verbs vary based on their emotional connotations (neutral, negative). The valence and arousal emotional words are rated on a five-point scale, using a self-assessment manikin (SAM; Bradley and Lang 1994). Using the pseudo-words, meaningful words and emotional pictures match and mismatch, the study of Kuchinke and Mueller (2019) has tested the congruency and incongruence of emotional words and pictures. Emotional images are chosen from the International Affective Picture System (IAPS; Lang *et al* 2008). Chen *et al* (2019) have also used 60 positive and 60 negative emotional words in English and Chinese. In addition, 180 alphabetically correct but meaningless nonsense words (i.e., pseudo-words) are also selected from each language. The study of Wu *et al* (2020, 2021) has taken 40 negative emotional laden words, 40 negative emotional label-words, 40 positive emotional label-words and 40 positive emotional laden-words, which are were either matched or mismatched with their written strokes, arousal and frequency. The target experimental words were randomised and allocated to the four mask-priming words (positive emotional-laden words, negative emotion-laden words, negative emotion-label words, and positive emotion-label words). A neuroimaging (fMRI) study has included meaning variables of words covering action relatedness, concreteness, sensorimotor imageability, and coupled with emotional arousal and valences (Osgood *et al* 1975, Bradley and Lang 1994, Moseley *et al* 2012). Participants are asked to respond to a question like 'Is this word typically conveying the meaning of an emotion?', comprehending the emotional words (rile, dread, spite), words related to facial expressions (chew, grunt and gnaw) and arm-foot related words (grasp, peel and carve). These are the categories of verbs that reflect sensory-motor emotion and feelings like scream, wail, dread and spite. Yang and Shu (2012) have also taken 48 single character Chinese action related verbs such as ge (cut) nie (pinch), wa (dig), sao (sweep) and reng (throw) as the experimental stimulus. Participants are asked to read and comprehend the words without giving any behavioural judgment or response during the fMRI recording. In another study, 36 Finnish emotional words representing surprise, sadness, anger, happiness, disgust and fear are employed to elicit emotions (Saarimäki *et al* 2016). The emotional words are also sub-classified within six categories: disgust (sickening, yucky, disgusted, bilious, repelled, nauseous), surprise (confused, bemused, wondering, surprised, astonished, amazed), sadness (gloomy, depressed, heavyhearted, sorrowful, unhappy, sad), happiness (pleased, delighted, cheerful, merry, happy, joyful), fear (afraid, frantic, frightened, anxious, nervous, restless) and anger (annoyed, cranky, angry, fierce, displeased, furious) (Toivonen *et al* 2012).

2.2.3 Materials: non-verbal stimulus

Like verbal-linguistic stimulus, many studies have employed non-verbal stimuli such as picture, voice, and body language of action and emotion. A magnetic resonance imaging (MRI) study has used action related expressions (Lingnau and Petris 2013) that display the shoulders, head, hands, knees, elbows, feet and hips. For example, the human actions of throwing, kicking a ball, punching, and kicking someone are considered target stimuli for collecting behavioural responses and neural signatures. Many psychophysics studies have extracted anger from the dance and gestures (Pollick *et al* 2002, 2001) and consider them as the stimulus. However, the study of Grosbras and Paus (2006) has compared the neutral and angry movement of the body, following the video clips as the stimuli, to design a two-way factorial ANOVA body parts (two hands and face) and emotional states (neutral and angry). Similar dynamic video databases are also used to evoke basic emotions such as disgust, fear, happiness, sadness, and neutral stimuli in an fMRI experiment (Tettamanti *et al* 2012, Saarimäki *et al* 2016). Participants were asked to watch the movie as they would view the TV. During fMRI scanning, they have no active task to perform. The video clips are presented in random order. Studies have also used various facial stimuli depicting disgust, anger, fear, sadness and happiness (Ekman and Friesen 1976, Borod *et al* 1994, Borod *et al* 2000). Pictorial forms of emotions that are available in the database of International affective picture system (IAPS) are selected based on 25 high-pleasant arousings (PH), 25 low-pleasant arousings (PL), 25 high-unpleasant arousings (UH), 25 low-unpleasant arousings (UL), and 25 neutral (NL) stimulus (Leite *et al* 2012). Even studies have selected the emotional face from the database of Chinese affective faces (Gong *et al* 2011, Fan *et al* 2017) to understand the neural processing of emotions. Most of the studies have either given identification, recognition and description tasks of facial expressions, prosodic, lexical and sentential tasks. In the prosodic recognition task, the auditory spoken stimuli of emotional tones recorded from professional actors are selected for the study (Borod *et al* 1994). Kensinger *et al* (2007) and Barrett and Kensinger (2010) have used 42 neutral and 42 individual fear disgust and neutral facial expressions.

Another study used 450 positive, negative and neutral images ($150 \times 3 = 450$) from Affective Picture System (IAPS; Takehara *et al* 2020) and the International and the Open Affective Standardised Image Set (OASIS; Benedek *et al* 2017). Before the experiment, participants ($N = 20$) rated the emotional images considering their arousal and valances scores. After the scoring test, 90 pictures are selected (30 from each category) and used in the study (Takehara *et al* 2020). Positive images include smiling children and puppies, which elicit happy emotions, whereas the negative emotions that represent disgust and fear have the scene of an unsanitary toilet, a robbery and an accident scene. Neutral pictures include the objects and landscapes representing crosswalks, memo pads and electric outlets (Takehara *et al* 2020). Previous studies have also used the database of the California Facial Expressions (Dailey *et al* 2001), representing fearful, happy and disgusted faces (Smith and Kirby 2011). A set of 180 emotional coloured images comprising 60 neutral, 60 fear and 60 sad are acquired from the emotion picture system (Marchewka *et al* 2014, Pugh *et al* 2021), standardized emotional images (Kurdi *et al* 2017) and International Affective Picture System (Lang *et al* 1999).

Similarly, the facial expressions of stimuli comprising grey recolour emotional photographs of individuals ($N = 8$; females $= 4$) portraying neutral, happy and fearful expressions are adapted from the study of Ekman and Friesen (1976) (Sato *et al* 2017). The beginning point of emotional expressions is considered neutral expressions that start from a neutral (0%) scale to emotional (100%) expressions. Portugal *et al* (2020) have employed eight-four emotional pictures that are obtained from IAPS and the Getty Images® (http://www.gettyimages.com) (Lang *et al* 2005). These 84 pictures contained two sets, such as threat and neutral stimuli (42 images from each). Out of 42 pictures, 21 pictures represent a threat in which the gun is either away from or towards the participants. The study of Hepach and Westermann (2013) has used movie clips showing a female and male actor waving or saying Hello baby; I'm [actor's name] with either neutral, happy, or angry emotional expressions. The time duration of each video clip is kept short at 4 seconds. Ferri *et al* (2013) have also used video clips referring to coloured movies of emotion-action (EA) of face, arm and torso of either male or female actor expressing anger and happiness coupled with grasping one of four objects such as a bottle, pencil case, receiver or CD cases placed on a table. These clips comprise angry action (AA), happy action (HA), and neutral action (NA) with angry face (AF), happy face (HF) and neutral face (NF). The verbal and non-verbal stimuli have been used to conduct many cognitive neuroscience studies on action and emotion. However, emotions and actions have been integrated only by using non-verbal pictures or video stimuli.

2.2.4 Stimuli presentation procedures and behavioural tasks

Most behavioural, EEG, MRI and fMRI experiments have been conducted in a dark sound-attenuated room. Participants are seated facing a white or black monitor screen from a distance of between 90 and 100 cm. With the help of psychological software 'E-Prime' and Lab Chart, both the verbal-linguistic (e.g., words, phrases, sentences and discourses) and non-verbal (e.g., picture, image, scene, voice, tone and body language) stimuli are presented to the participants for performing their desired target-task. For example, Klepp *et al* (2017), in their behavioural study relating to the specific body-part interact with an action verb and motor behaviour, have used the trail with a fixation cross followed by either a foot verb, an abstract verb or a hand verb which lasted for 300 ms. Participants fixate on the centre of the monitor screen during the experiment. Stimuli are displayed either simultaneously or one after another at a fixed duration (e.g., 500 ms/200 ms) with an interval of 1000 ms between stimuli, as shown in figure 2.2(a, b). Stimuli were randomised either block-wise or within a block of trails to evade any form of regular response patterns from the participants. At the end of each trial, a white or black blank screen appeared as an indication to participants to accomplish their behavioural target tasks.

In most studies, participants were asked to visualise, read or comprehend the verbal and nonverbal stimulus (figure 2.2). Then, they were asked to respond either by pressing left or right keys according to their desired match and mismatch, congruency and incongruence or negative and positive emotion and action tasks. Studies have kept the response time either finite or infinite. To get participants familiarised with the task and response, practice trials were given to each participant. It ensured that the response accuracy and time should not be varied because of the unfamiliarity of non-verbal and verbal emotion and action trails.

2.2.5 EEG, fMRI recording and pre-processing of signals

Most of the experiments were conducted using HydroCel™ Geodesic Sensor Net of EGI, EMG, TMS and TRIO scanner instruments. In addition, brain images were collected using EEG, MRI and fMRI scanners. Different EEG channels' montages, including 128, 30, and 16 electrodes, are used for recording the EEG signals, as

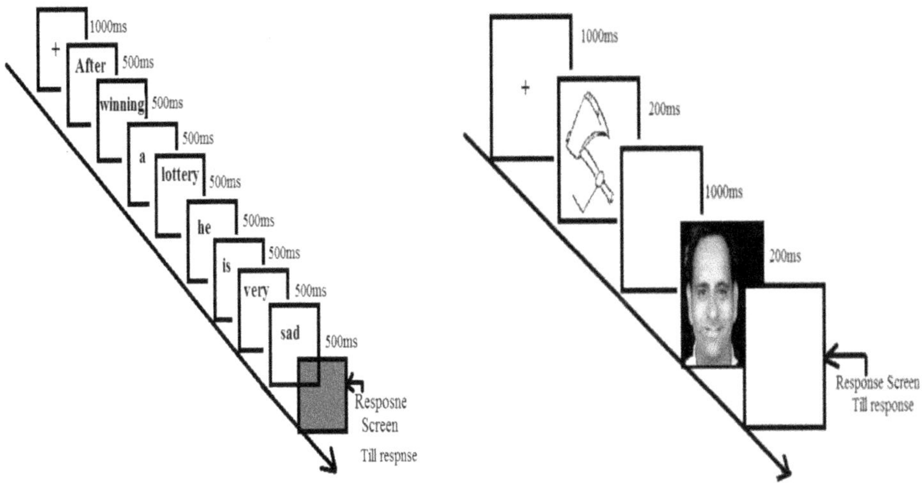

Figure 2.2. Schematic diagram of (a) verbal incongruent and (b) non-verbal incongruent between action and emotional stimuli sequences trial presentation.

shown in figure 2.3. The recording of motor-evoked potentials (MEPs) was conducted by involving the performance of both flick and grasp actions. For this, the recording of EMG was executed by using Ag/AgCl cup electrodes (Urgesi *et al* 2010).

Evoked signals were flittered with band-pass frequency (20 Hz to 2 kHz) and digitised using EMG equipment. MRI signal was obtained using a 32-channel Siemens Trio scanner (Cracco *et al* 2019). The EMG sampling rate of the signal was kept at 20 kHz. Before recording the TMS pulse, a pre-stimulus test was done to check the presence of EMG activity. The image acquisition was primarily performed on a 3.0-T Scanner (Yang and Shu 2012). In the case of EEG, the impedance connectivity of electrodes is always kept below 5 KΩ. The recording was usually conducted with an online band-pass of 0.1 Hz to 100 Hz with a 250 Hz sampling rate. The central 'Cz' electrode was selected as a referential channel to all EEG channels. All the EEG signals were locked with a specified time to the target critical emotional words during the pre-processing of signals and segmented as experimental conditions. The ocular and muscular artefacts were removed using a band-pass frequency range from 0.3 to 20 Hz. Averaged EEG signal that was free from electrical noise was used to measure the visualisation of ERP across subjects. ERP signals are measured and calculated by segmenting the mean amplitudes (−100 or −200 ms before the onset of stimulus), covering the time windows of interest (+800 or 900 ms after the onset of stimulus). The average baseline EEG signals were visualised to inspect how the change of the ERP waves significantly varied across the brain regions based on the experimental conditions.

The average ERP amplitudes (μv) concerning positive or negative deflections were obtained across experimental conditions such as positive and negative emotions and actions and their integration at the verbal and non-verbal levels. For example, the

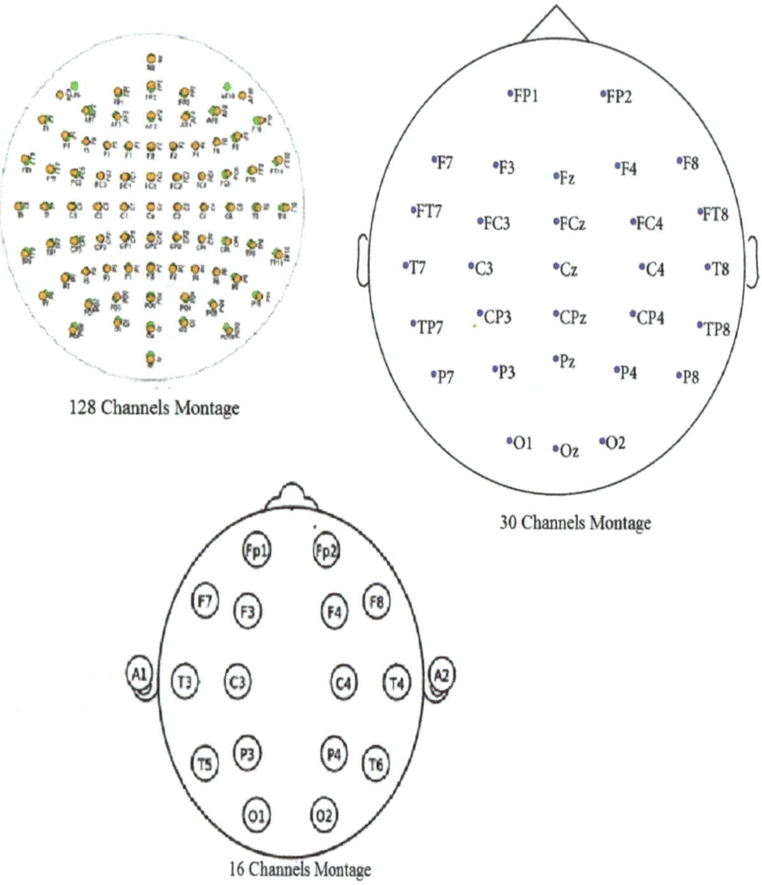

Figure 2.3. Different montages referring to the number of channels such as 128, 30 and 16 are represented from the point of view of their electrode points related to the scalp of the brain.

whole-brain regression analysis was formed using the EEG lab for the EEG recording, whereas the voxel-wise regression analyses were used in fMRI recording. The study of both cases used the regression models of congruent and incongruent. Four stimulus-based regressions were conducted, following the experimental conditions: bio-congruent, bio-incongruent, non-bio-congruent, non-bio-incongruent (Deen and McCarthy 2010). Moreover, the association between the positive event and happy emotion (PEV-HE congruent) and the negative event with sad emotion (NEV-SE congruent) are segmented to observe their interaction with their incongruent counterparts, such as negative events with happy emotion (NEV-HE Incongruent) and positive events with sad emotion (PEV-SE Incongruent). A series of descriptive and linear regression statistics such as two-ways ANOVAs and four-ways ANOVAs were computed to understand the brain's statistical effect of processing emotion, action, and combinations. These statistical effects are distributed mainly over the average amplitudes (μv) in the right and left sides of pre-frontal, frontal, temporal (T), central (C), parietal (P), centro-parietal (CP), occipital (O) regions and parieto-occipital (PO). The laterality factors of hemispheres such as left and right hemispheric sides are involved in executing a three-way ANOVA on the average amplitudes of ERP components. Tukey posthoc measurement is also performed for different factorial evaluations, observing the interaction effect of the experimental conditions. Event-related potentials that show the modulation of amplitudes ($\mu\nu$) are primarily measured and presented within the timeline of P100 (47–143 ms), P300 (255–483 ms) and N400 (300–400 ms). Early cognitive component P1 was estimated within time windows from 50 ms to 150 ms, by following the time window of P100 in the context of emotional word processing: Herbert *et al* (2008) P1 (80–130), Scott (2009a) P1 (80–120), Kessler *et al* (2009) P1 (80–130), and Sass *et al* (2010) P1 (88–128). P300 was measured between 255 ms and 483 ms, like the component reported in Herbert *et al* (2006) P3 (250–400) and Scott (2009a) P3 (300–450).

2.3 Analysis of behavioural results

2.3.1 Behavioural results

The retrieval of perceptual emotion and action related motor features, both pictorial and auditory stimuli, is always task-dependent. Participants accurately attend to the stimuli by following the target tasks (92.28%) (Kuhnke *et al* 2020). A three-factorial repeated measure ANOVA with different task factors (sound judgment, lexical decision and action judgement), action (low and high) and sound (low and high) show the significant main effect of task, sound and action, revealing higher judgment accuracy for soft sounding words and high action words than high sound and low action words (Kuhnke *et al* 2020). Post-hoc analysis of response accuracy does not show any effect of task factors. However, the response time (ms) also reveal the interaction effect with tasks, sounds and actions, suggesting a faster response to low rating action words with high rating sound than high rating action words with a soft or low rating sound. Furthermore, the main effect of actions reveals shorter responses for high rating action than low rating action words, whereas the main result of sound indicated faster responses for high rating sound than low rating sound words.

Further, in the emotional recognition task, the main effect of emotion is significant, having a high recognition accuracy for anger than fear faces. Similarly, the accuracy is higher for high intensity than for low emotion (Vilarem *et al* 2020, Grèzes *et al* 2021). During a passive reading task, action words (AW) related to arms and face are rated higher than emotional words (EW) about arms and face (Moseley *et al* 2012). The neutral pictures are processed faster than threat pictures (Portugal *et al* 2020). The response ratings of meaningfully incorrect and correct sentences have differed based on the presence and absence of harmful and high-arousal and neutral and low-arousal verbs. In the context of the actor-object phrase, the ratings are higher for target neutral than negative verbs (Bayer *et al* 2010). Semantically incorrect sentences take more time to process than semantically correct sentences. The response time for the picture joy is faster than sad emotional pictures (Chen *et al* 2016). Emotional pictures primed with labelled emotional words are more accurately judged and recognised (0.95) than those primed with emotional-laden words (0.92). Positive emotional photos (694.32 ms) are processed faster with

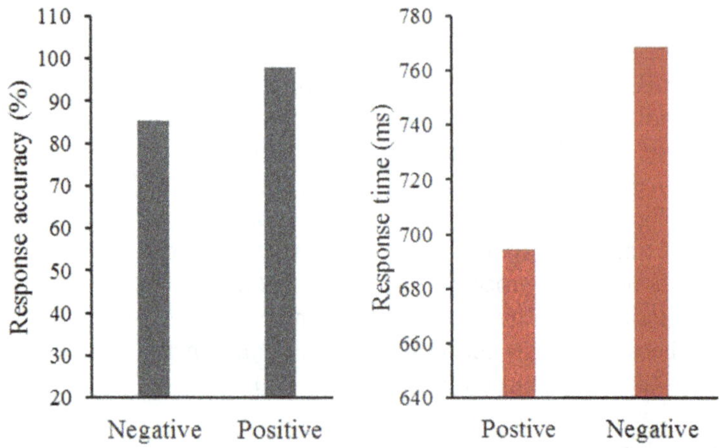

Figure 2.4. The representative figures show that positive emotional words and pictures are processed faster with high accuracy than negative emotional words and pictures.

higher accuracy than negative (768.84 ms) emotional images (Wu *et al* 2019, 2020), as represented in figure 2.4. It is observed that an emotional picture and positive emotional words are processed faster with high accuracy than negative emotional words (Wu *et al* 2021). Positive emotional words such as happy, joy and pleasant are computed much quicker than neutral words such as work, sit, and day and negative or unpleasant words such as sad, angry and disgust (Kanske and Kotz 2007), as shown in figure 2.4.

The response time for neutral words is slower than the emotional words (Fischler and Bradley 2006). In the emotional face and word congruency task, the emotional face and word incongruence in Chinese L1 (first language) is processed slower with lower accuracy than the response time and accuracy of the emotional face and words incongruence in English L2 (Second language) (Fan *et al* 2017). The higher reaction time and lower accuracy rate in the case of Chinese L1 indicate the interference of emotional words on the emotional face in the Stroop conflict task. The Stroop conflict of emotional face-word is fairly found in both L1 and L2 tasks in the Chinese context. The contexts and environment are routinely encoded during emotion perception. The accuracy or recognition rate is higher when the context is matched or congruent with emotions (Barrett and Kensinger 2010). Overall, happy faces are better recognised than other non-emotional neutral, emotional fear and disguised faces (Smith and Kirby 2011). Most of these behavioural results reveal higher behavioural response accuracy and faster response time for positive emotions and events or actions than negative ones. In the context of congruency and incongruence or match and mismatch of action and emotions tasks, the high accuracy and faster response time for congruent than incongruent trials are found across studies. Happy words and pictures, including positive actions, have a more considerable behavioural processing advantage than sad words and pictures couple with negative actions. Based on prior actions or emotions, the human can predict the preceding feelings or actions in their day-to-day life. In a communicative context, humans often anticipate emotional words based on prior actions or events verbs. Thus, the verbal and non-verbal stimulus of action helps us perceive and navigate the forthcoming emotional words in a discourse influenced by the primary event verb. Positive event verbs more rapidly process than negative event verbs in a sentence.

2.4 Analysis of ERP results

2.4.1 Regions of brain involved in action and emotion processing

Most of the neurophysiological studies have found the action observations, perceptions and executions in the premotor areas of the brain. Action or events words are processed in the frontal and frontocentral motor cortex when the participants read the action or event words in a sentence (Gallese *et al* 1996, Gallese and Lakoff 2005), as shown in figure 2.5. Action-related words activate the premotor and motor areas of the brain (Pulvermüller and Fadiga 2010), as shown in figure 2.5. Many neuroimaging studies have found activations in the left hemispheric sides of the frontal regions when participants silently read or listen to the activities related to verbs (Hauk *et al* 2004, Tettamanti *et al* 2005). Sentences with action verbs are processed in the left frontal and pre-central (premotor areas) and frontoparietal regions of the brain (Tettamanti *et al* 2008), as shown in figure 2.5. Specifically, the differences between hand-related action-verbs and abstract verbs are observed over midline fronto-central (FCz), the left frontocentral (FC3) and central (C3) electrodes, suggesting higher amplitudes for action verbs than abstract verbs (Alemanno *et al* 2012). The right and left hemispheric prefrontal cortex (PFC) and the left-dorsal premotor cortex are involved in several competing actions or events related to outcomes or goals (Lingnau and Petris 2013).

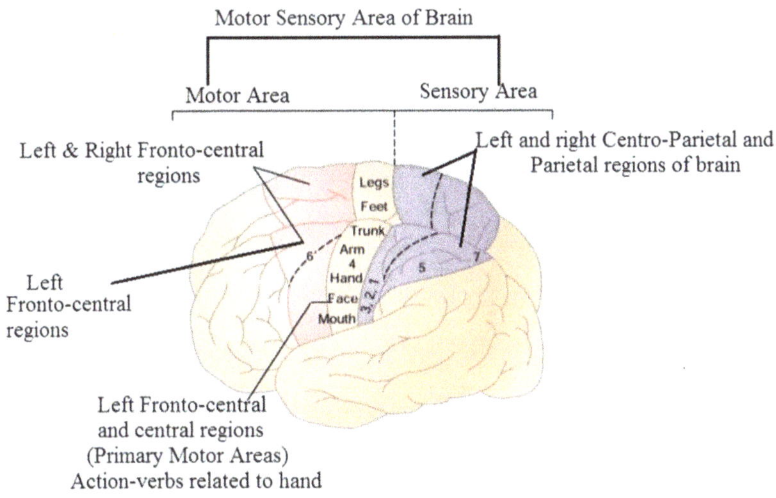

Figure 2.5. The brain's motor-sensory areas comprising frontocentral, central, centro-parietal and parietal regions brain process the action and emotion verbal and non-verbal stimuli.

Early sensorimotor activations between 155 and 174 ms have been associated with action verbs (Vanhoutte *et al* 2015). However, the abstract verbs are processed outside the sensorimotor regions, especially in the pre-frontal cortex in the early and late components (Dalla Volta *et al* 2014). For example, the early component of P100 (50–150 ms) demonstrates that when event or action verbal words are either matched or mismatched with emotional words, an interaction effect between positive and negative events or action verbs with happy and sad words is significant in the left and right hemispheric side of central and frontoparietal, centro-parietal regions of the brain, as shown in figure 2.6.

The left frontocentral and bilateral fronto-central motor systems are strongly activated and stimulated when processing action-related words and phrases (Pulvermüller and Fadiga 2010, Kemmerer *et al* 2012) shown in figures 2.5 and 2.6. Furthermore, the actions related to objects, either in words or pictures, are processed in the inferior left-parietal lobe (Binkofski and Buxbaum 2013, Osiurak 2014, Chen *et al* 2018). In the domain of language, Glenberg and Kaschak (2002) and Rueschemeyer *et al* (2010) have found the action oriented-sentences compatibility effect (ACE), which shows that participants are quick to accomplish an event or action that is matched rather than mismatched to the movement of the body.

2.4.2 Analysis of P100 (50–150 ms)

The processing of action verbs usually interferes with the concurrent movement within 200 ms (Boulenger *et al* 2006). Pulvermüller *et al* (2005) have shown the early activation of action words in P100, which peak appears at about 130–150 ms in the fronto-central, central and centro-parietal electrodes and is represented in figure 2.6. The positive ERP waves from 128 to 150 ms show higher amplitudes for the processing of fearful faces with actions than the processing of neutral faces in the

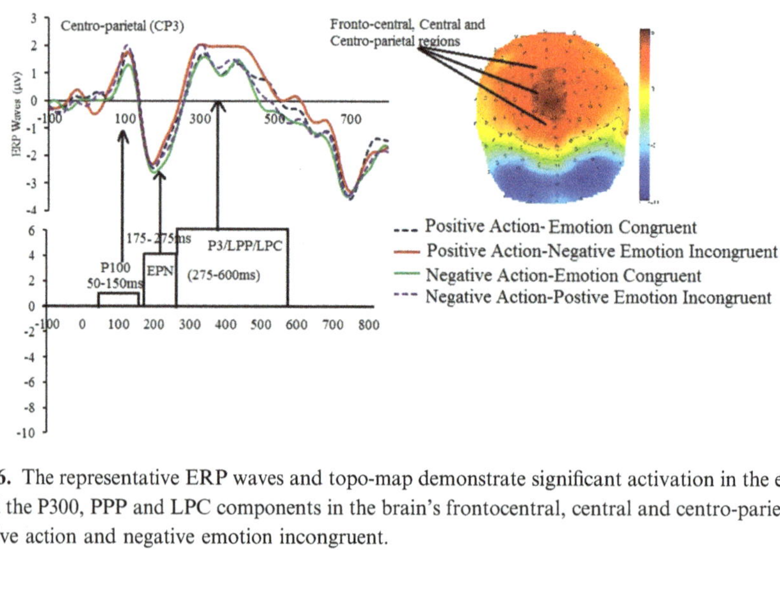

Figure 2.6. The representative ERP waves and topo-map demonstrate significant activation in the early P100, EPN and the P300, PPP and LPC components in the brain's frontocentral, central and centro-parietal regions for positive action and negative emotion incongruent.

temporal or amygdala regions of the brain (Guex *et al* 2020). The facial emotional expressions such as happy, sad and angry are processed in the early component of P100 (Haxby *et al* 2000, Herrmann *et al* 2005). It is observed that the amplitudes of early component that is reported in P1 (80–120 ms) are higher for emotional valence words than neutral words (Scott *et al* 2009b). In the parietal, parieto-occipital and occipital regions, the amplitudes of the early positive component are higher within time windows of 100–150 ms (Batty and Taylor 2003, Foti *et al* 2010, Luo *et al* 2010), which are more significant for emotional than neutral expressions. The early amygdala activity spreads from occipital to parietal regions when our brain processes the affective contents, emotional faces, and words relevant to actions or events (Krolak-Salmon *et al* 2004, Goldstein *et al* 2007, Jenison *et al* 2011). This suggests that the incongruence effect between event or action words and emotional words is significant in the early P100 component. Reading negative hand-action or event sentences enhances the more extensive neuronal activation than positive hand-related actions (Alemanno *et al* 2012). Event or action is embodied with emotions, and their integrations enhance the early neuronal activity associated with language. The early activations of the brain's motor, premotor and supplementary motor regions are related to hand-related action (Candidi *et al* 2010, Fernandino and Iacoboni 2010, Müller *et al* 2011). Parietal and premotor areas are predominantly activated when participants perform actions or actions are performed by others (Lingnau and Petris 2013). Though the articulation of speech or perception words is related to language-motor priming, the neurons of motor or premotor areas play a crucial role in processing action-related verbs (Klepp *et al* 2017). The early recognition of action or event words occurs around 250 ms, following bottom-up modulations of the sensory-motor areas (Ubaldi *et al* 2015), whereas the top-down modulations of detail processing of action or event slow down the processing that occurs in 300 ms in the pre-frontal regions of the brain, as figure 2.6 shows. The principles of motor control enrich the action perception and execution mechanisms in the parietal-premotor brain networks (Rizzolatti and Sinigaglia 2016, Hilt *et al* 2020). Further, the ventral route of the Middle Temporal Gyrus (MTG) and the anterior Inferior Frontal Gyrus (aIFG) accomplish the processing of action-perception, anticipation and comprehensions (Flanagan and Johansson 2003, Kilner *et al* 2004, Beauchamp and Martin 2007). The action-emotion is also processed in the dorsal route by following the Inferior Parietal Lobe (IPL) and the posterior Inferior Frontal Gyrus (pIFG) (Schütz-Bosbach and Prinz 2007). Further, similar to the processing of action or event words (like murder, scream, explosion and faeces) in motor, premotor, frontocentral motor areas, the semantic processing of emotional words (like fear, dread and spite) also activate the central and centro-parietal regions (Kemmerer and Gonzalez-Castillo 2010, Moseley *et al* 2012). Early binding of emotion and action interaction occurs around 200 ms after the stimuli. This early binding activates in the premotor and motor areas of the human brain (Conty *et al* 2012). Taken together, a growing body of literature supports the idea that emotional perception is contextually action sensitive and dependent; their interaction is activated in the motor-related central areas of the brain (Portugal *et al* 2020).

Many studies have identified the modulation of emotion in the P100 component when perceiving fearful and angry faces (Foti *et al* 2010, Blechert *et al* 2012, Herbert *et al* 2013, Smith *et al* 2013, Bublatzky *et al* 2014). Effects of angry, fearful and happy expressions that exhibit in P100 also depend on the characteristics of participants, suggesting higher amplitudes of P1 for only low-shy participants (Jetha *et al* 2012). Furthermore, the P1 amplitudes have been observed during the processing of fearful faces (Batty and Taylor 2003, Foti *et al* 2010, Luo *et al* 2010, Frühholz *et al* 2011, Itier and Neath-Tavares 2017). This result suggests that the processing of the fearful face is automatic because it enhances visual processing and captures early and rapid attention in comparison to other emotional expressions (West *et al* 2011, Pessoa and Adolphs 2010, Denefrio *et al* 2017, Li *et al* 2018). In addition to the processing of fearful faces, the P1 amplitudes are enlarged for happy, angry and disgusted faces (Conty *et al* 2012, Sel *et al* 2014, Zhang *et al* 2014, Hagemann *et al* 2016).

2.4.3 Analysis of early posterior negativity (EPN: 175–275 ms)

The early posterior negativity (EPN) is a negative-going deflection that falls between 175 and 275 ms occurring in the temporal-occipital regions of the brain (Schupp *et al* 2006, Foti *et al* 2010), as is represented in figure 2.6. The amplitudes of EPN are primarily enhanced during the processing of emotional faces compared to neutral faces in the temporal and occipital cortex (Leppänen *et al* 2007, Mühlberger *et al* 2009). From 200 to 300 ms, it is more sensitive to fear and anger faces representing threat than neutral and pleasant faces at lateral parietal and occipital sites (Holmes *et al* 2008, Hajcak *et al* 2012, Müller-Bardorff *et al* 2018, Wu *et al* 2019). Not only faces but fear and anger words are also processed in this early component starting around 200 to 400 ms after the stimulus (Herbert *et al* 2008, Kissler *et al* 2009, Ferré and Sánchez-Casas 2014). EPN reflects the voluntary allocation of attention caused by verbal and non-verbal emotional stimulus (Schupp *et al* 2007). Moreover, the amplitudes of EPN are higher for happy, angry, sad and fearful faces than neutral faces (Blechert *et al* 2012, Faja *et al* 2016, Itier and Neath-Tavares 2017, Peltola *et al* 2018, Bublatzky *et al* 2014). During the salient reading task of emotional words, the EPN component, whose peak falls within a time window of 200–300 ms, has an occipital and temporal distribution of scalp, and its amplitude is more significant for emotionally valence words (negative and positive) than neutral or non-emotional words (Kissler *et al* 2009). This peak also remains during the emotional judgment or recognition task (Scott *et al* 2009b, Hinojosa *et al* 2010, Citron *et al* 2011), the written word recognition task (Hinojosa *et al* 2010) and the emotional related Stroop conflict task (Franken *et al* 2009, Herbert *et al* 2010). This result suggests that the EPN (200–300 ms) indexes automatic and implicit processing of emotional, verbal materials (Hinojosa *et al* 2010, Kissler *et al* 2006, Martín-Loeches 2007) in the right sides of the frontotemporal and occipital regions of the brain (Junghöfer *et al* 2001, Schupp *et al* 2006). This result is aligned with the computation of emotional stimuli in the right-hemispheric sides of the brain. However, several studies have found the EPN effect in the left hemispheric sides of the brain because of the involvement of language-related regions (Kissler *et al* 2007). This reveals that early components can distinguish left and right hemispheric differences between neutral and emotional stimuli (Junghöfer *et al* 2001, Schupp *et al* 2003). EPN differences are consistently detected for angry and fearful words and faces, whereas they are less found in the case of happy or joyful faces (Karl *et al* 2016, Mavratzakis *et al* 2016, Wu *et al* 2019).

2.4.4 Negative event and emotion processing in P300, LPC and LPP (275–600 ms)

The late ERP effect of emotion, which falls within the time range of P300 (275–600 ms), is classified as the late positive complex (LPC) and the late posterior potential (LPP), as shown in figure 2.6. The LPC and LPP, which are positive-going slow waves, are higher for negative and positive emotional pictures than the neutral pictures (Schupp *et al* 2004a, 2004b, Fischler and Bradley 2006, Herbert *et al* 2006, Schacht and Sommer 2009b). The higher motivational significance of emotional arousal enhances the LPC/LPP amplitudes that sustain elaborate processing (Cuthbert *et al* 2000). Negative emotional words such as sadness, worry, and anxiety evoked higher amplitudes of LPC than positive emotional words in central regions of the brain (Wu *et al* 2021). This means that negative or unpleasant words enhanced larger LPC amplitudes than positive or pleasant words (Bernat *et al* 2001, Zhang *et al* 2017). It is higher over central and parietal or centro-parietal regions within 300 ms (Weinberg and Hajcak 2011). Similarly, some other studies have shown the differential enhancements of LPP amplitudes as an exhibition of fearful, disgust and angry faces, which elicit larger LPP than sad, happy and neutral faces (Foti *et al* 2010, Luo *et al* 2010) from 300 to 1000 ms in the central and parietal electrodes (Santos *et al* 2008, Frühholz *et al* 2011, MacNamara *et al* 2012, Wu *et al* 2019). LPP modulations have been associated with the motivational relevance of images (Weinberg and Hajcak 2010) and with continual elaborative and computational processing (Hajcak *et al* 2010, Weinberg and Hajcak 2011). This evidence indicates that angry and fearful faces are exclusively more relevant than other positive emotional faces (Schupp *et al* 2004). Furthermore, the arousal ratings for sad and happy images are lower than angry and fearful images, and the LPP is more prominent for more arousing pictures (Cuthbert *et al* 1996). Therefore, the LPP is particularly profound and complex to restraints to different types of emotional, verbal and non-verbal stimuli (Weinberg and Hajcak 2010). We may observe that happy faces appear more frequently than sad or angry faces in our daily life, and due to the higher degree of the LPP are impactful to the low occurrence of negative emotional frequency (Hajcak *et al* 2012, Weinberg *et al* 2012), thereby the happy emotion fails to enhance the amplitudes of LPP.

Further, the late positive complex (LPC) and the late posterior positivity (LPP) peak between 400 and 600 ms and have centro-parietal scalp distributions, as shown in figure 2.6. This component is primarily aligned with the verbal, emotional stimuli and, more explicitly, to the valences of emotion. The amplitudes of LPC and LPP are frequently higher for emotional stimuli than neutral ones (Carretié *et al* 2008, Hinojosa *et al* 2010), revealing sustained processing. Moreover, amplitude differences are also observed between negative and positive stimuli (Herbert *et al* 2008, Kissler *et al* 2009). This impact also has more advantages over negative words than neutral or positive emotional words (Hofmann *et al* 2009, Gootjes *et al* 2011). This is due to emotional stimuli that are more prominently, effortlessly and rapidly processed. Even emotional stimuli require less sustained devotion, attention and judgment or evaluation than neutral stimuli. In most cases, the neutral stimuli demand less motivation; therefore, they are less significant and may need a more effortful evaluative process than emotional stimuli. The critical point here is that the amplitudes of LPC seem to discriminate positive and negative emotional valences over the EPN. Thus, LPC and LPP, which belong to a more prominent positive component of P300, are more generally related to attentional mechanism relevant to emotional stimulus. Therefore, the enlarged amplitudes of LPC are detected when participants attend the happy, angry, and fearful faces (Foti *et al* 2010, Andreatta *et al* 2012, Blechert *et al* 2012, Herbert *et al* 2013, Smith *et al* 2013, Bublatzky *et al* 2014, Yoon *et al* 2016).

Several other studies have found LPP and P300 components modulations, which showed higher amplitudes for happy and angry expressions (Tortosa *et al* 2013, Liu *et al* 2012, Zhang *et al* 2014, Karl *et al* 2016, Wu *et al* 2019). For example, in the face detection task, the event-related potential amplitudes from 300 to 374 are significant for threat and anger than neutral faces (Guex *et al* 2020). Similarly, the main effect of action pictures related to threat and fear is substantial in the ERP windows from 378 to 404 ms. Moreover, the late P300 (250–480 ms) is significant for the action or event, which shows higher amplitudes for the adverse event than the positive event, and is observed in the left and right hemispheric sides of parietal, occipital and parieto-occipital regions of the brain. However, the main effect of emotional words, which shows higher amplitudes of P300 for sad words than happy words, is significant in the right hemispheric sides of the centro-parietal regions of the brain. In the right and left sides of the parietal, parieto-occipital and occipital areas, the P300 amplitudes are modulated by processing positive event verbs and negative event verbs when they are matched or mismatched with happy and sad words. This result indicates that there are higher amplitudes of P300 for the positive event and happy emotion congruency. However, there is no significant effect of P300 amplitudes that can differentiate between the negative event and happy words incongruent and negative event and sad words congruent. In left-hemispheric sides of centro-parietal regions, the P300 amplitudes are higher for negative events than positive events. Tragic words show higher amplitudes like adverse events than positive emotional words in the left-hemispheric sides of centro-parietal regions. The action frequency increases when the positive action is consistently paired with a positive outcome or reward, but it decreases when the action is linked with a negative effect (Prével *et al* 2021). The study of Conty *et al* (2007) has established a relationship between P300 and its related subcomponents such as P3a and P3b in the centro-parietal regions of the brain. It is observed that the early portion of the LPP is closely resembled by P300 or P3a and P3b (Nieuwenhuis *et al* 2005). Compared to the P300 component, the LPP or LPC is a broad and sustained positivity, which always goes beyond the time frame of the P300 (Weinberg and Hajcak 2011).

2.4.5 Analysis of N400 (350–700 ms)

One of the late ERP waves associated with the semantic violation is called the negative deflection of N400, which occurs between 350 and 700 ms at the pre-frontal, frontal, central, fronto-central and centro-parietal regions, as depicted in figure 2.7. This negative deflection has been classified as semantic processing of linguistic verbal stimulus (Kutas and Hillyard 1983, 1984, Kutas and Federmeier 2000). The semantic congruency effect between the target emotional word and the priming word is exhibited in the N400 component (Williamson *et al* 1991, Kiehl *et al* 1999). The human mood and feeling can modulate the amplitudes of the N400 component when the positive mindset is semantically integrated with negative attitude in either congruent or incongruent contexts during the processing of sentences (Federmeier *et al* 2001). For example, during the processing of unpleasant and joyful-pleasant adjectives, the amplitudes of N400 are more reduced for lovely and joyful adjectival words than unpleasant words (Kiefer *et al* 2007). The pleasant adjectives are connected with condensed N400 amplitudes compared to unpleasant adjectives (Herbert *et al* 2008). In semantic processing, incongruent sentences elicit higher amplitudes of N400 than congruent sentences in the frontocentral regions (Kanske and Kotz 2007, Kiefer *et al* 2007), as shown in figure 2.7. Thus, the N400 represents the lexical access and evaluation (Lau *et al* 2008), including the lexico-semantic unification and combinatorial processes (Kutas and Federmeier 2000), which facilitate the lexical-semantic processing of emotional stimuli (Kanske and Kotz 2007). Even the effect of N400 is significant in the frontal, temporal and central regions of the brain when the participants process the angry prosodic meaning, which is incongruent with happy word meaning (Tarai and Srinivasan 2019).

Here the interference of prosody with word meaning increases the amplitudes of N400, which underlies the word-prosody Stroop conflict. This word-prosody Stroop

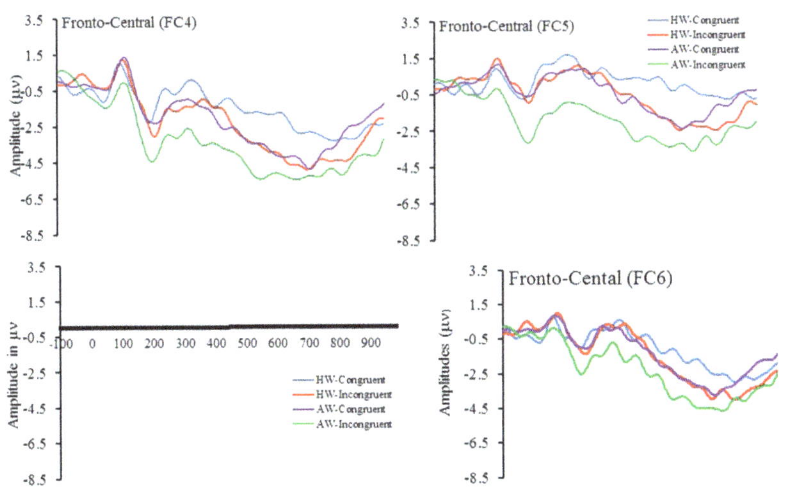

Figure 2.7. The main effect congruency shows higher N400 (350–700 ms) amplitudes incongruent than congruent in frontocentral regions of the brain.

effect, like colour-word Stroop, is exhibited in the previous study of Schirmer and Kotz (2006) and Ishii *et al* (2010). This N400 effect is retained in the cross-modal study between emotional face and prosody incongruency (Paulmann and Pell 2010). Moreover, the N400 component is described as a conflict-control negative deflection and cognitive component, which is linked with the elaborate lexico-semantic violation and prosody-semantic congruency in the domain of audio-visual paradigms (Kutas and Federmeier 2000, Kutas and Federmeier 2011, Brunellie're *et al* 2019, Petit *et al* 2019).

2.5 Discussion

In this chapter, we describe the behavioural and neurophysiological studies that have emphasised action and emotion processing. From the point of view of response accuracy (%) and time (ms), most of the behavioural results have shown the high action words are processed faster with higher accuracy than low action words. Action words related to arms and face were rated higher than emotional words about arms and face. This result suggests that the verbal and non-verbal stimulus of action words or faces enhance, anticipate and determine the perceptual ability of forthcoming emotional words in discourse. Positive events or action verbs are more rapidly processed than negative events or action verbs in a sentence. From the point of view of neurophysiological findings, it is observed that the premotor and motor areas of the brain are convoluted during the processing of events or action words and pictures. More specifically, the action and event words are processed in the fontal and frontocentral motor cortex. The activation in the left-hemispheric sides of the frontal, pre-central (premotor areas) and frontoparietal regions of the brain is higher than right-hemispheric sides when processing action- or event-related verbs in a sentence. EEG studies have found the modulation of P100 amplitudes within time windows from 50 to 150 ms during the perception of negative emotions and action verbs in the frontocentral and central electrodes. The amplitudes of P100 are higher for fearful faces with actions than neutral faces in the amygdala regions of the brain. Even the posterior parts of the brain, i.e., the parietal and premotor areas, are primarily activated during the performance of actions. This early component supports the idea that recognition of emotions is contextually motion-sensitive and dependent, which is exhibited in the motor-related central areas of the brain. In addition to the early P100 component, studies have found that the negative deflection of early posterior negativity (EPN), which falls within the time windows of 175 and 275 ms, primarily occurs in the temporal-occipital regions of the brain during the processing of emotional faces. The amplitudes of EPN are more sensitive to fear and anger faces representing threat than neutral and pleasant faces at lateral parietal and occipital sites. EPN amplitudes are allocated for the voluntary distribution of attention caused by verbal and non-verbal emotional and action stimuli. EPN, the late posterior positivity (LPP) and the late positive complex (LPC), which belong to the P300 family of components, are associated with emotion and action processing. The amplitude of late positive complex is higher for negative than positive emotions in the centro-parietal regions.

In the left-hemispheric sides of centro-parietal regions, the P300 amplitudes are higher for negative events than positive events. Compared to the P300 component, the LPP or LPC is a broad and sustained positivity that goes beyond the time windows of P300, as shown in figure 2.6. Like these late positive components, the semantic violations of emotional valences are associated with the negative N400 component in the brain's frontocentral, central and centro-parietal regions. This negative deflection of N400 is classified as a conflict-control negative deflection associated with elaborate lexico-semantic violation and prosody-semantic congruency. Taken together, these psychophysiological shreds of evidence demonstrate the anticipation of emotion processing based on action, events, feeling appraisals, response categorisation and the labelling of motor expressions related to face, voice and gestures (Scherer and Moors 2019). For example, when the sentences violate the action and emotion meaning, the incongruent sentences have a more significant impact in terms of the neural time course of the P300 component.

Most of these findings are under the previous studies, which observe that participants found happy words faster than sad words. (Kanske and Kotz 2007, Estes and Verges 2008, Hofmann *et al* 2009, Schacht and Sommer 2009b, Palazova *et al* 2011). According to memory allocation, happy words are more quickly processed than sad words; as a result, pleasant words are easier to remember than unpleasant or harmful words (Kissler *et al* 2009). Likewise, compared to negative event verbs, participants are more precise in handling positive event verbs. The precision of positive event and sad emotion incongruent sentences is less than that of positive action or event and happy emotion congruent sentences because positive action or event words can expand the range of attention and provide distractions for sad words. This observation is persistently correlated with the findings of previous studies on emotions (Siegle *et al* 2002), which exhibited that happy words receive more attention compared to sad words. Indeed, when the task is to find the incongruence between the event or action verbs and the emotions in a sentence, the content of the event word actively interferes with the content of the emotion word. Any emotional prediction is based on the nature of the event or action. When emotional words are combined with event verbs in sentences, they can be actively processed in the early sensory P100 and the late P300 components. For example, the sad emotion interferes with positive events or action verbs in the early P100 component in the parietal regions and the late component of P300 in the occipital areas. Since emotional words are essential to humans existence (Dillon *et al* 2006), they are closely linked to human reproductive and survival behavioural strategies. Here, an event or action provides background cues to improve reproductive and survival systems where emotions are often combined with the tendency of the events or activities.

2.5.1 Processing of emotion and action in the early ERP components

Studies on emotional words have reported an early effect within 100 ms (Van Hooff *et al* 2008, Scott *et al* 2009b). However, an opinion refutes this result, which means that ERP fluctuations related to meaning cannot occur within 200 ms of the onset of a word (Kissler *et al* 2006). Scholars believe that emotional words' early ERP effects (P1 and N1) are controversial in nature (e.g., Herbert *et al* 2008, Kissler *et al* 2009). Contrary to this suggestion, we found that the early congruency effect between events or actions and emotional words occurs relatively early in P1. In the domain of language, the syntactic incorrect or violation always occurs within the time-windows of the positive P600 (500–700 ms) component (Lau *et al* 2006, Tabullo *et al* 2011, van de Meerendonk *et al* 2013), whereas the semantic violation occurs in the N400 component (380–500 ms). Even the lexical ambiguities with the semantic violation in sentences modulate the amplitudes of N400 (Kutas and Hillyard 1984, Kutas and Federmeier 2000, Dillon *et al* 2006, Borovsky *et al* 2012, Lau *et al* 2013).

Our brain shows a very early negative effect, i.e., EPN, when semantic incongruency is exhibited in the sentences. In contrast, the left anterior negativity component (ELAN 100–300 ms) occurs when the syntactic category of the word (noun or verb) is violated in the sentence (Hahne and Friederici 1999). Likewise, this study also supports that ERPs of semantic violation of upcoming emotion words occur much earlier compared to semantic and syntactic violations. The first congruent effect is established due to the 'consequential nature' of a positive or negative event or action verbs, which can automatically and quickly restore the impending valence of ambiguous and uncertain emotional words. Here, event verbs' concept or semantic domain provides a specific valence context for emotional comments that perceive happiness and sadness. These findings and observations are consistent with the theoretical development of the verbal and non-verbal domain of emotion and action embodiment. Language development is always the context of perception of the valence of emotional words (Barrett *et al* 2007). Event or action verbs provide a sense-based perception and memory-based conceptual anchors that contextualise the cues for processing emotive meaning. This is consistent with prior observations on the internal emotional experiences (happiness, sadness), which lies in situations, events and motor actions (Barsalou 2010, Wilson-Mendenhall *et al* 2011). Overall, we claim that emotions are processed along with events or actions words in an unconscious and inherent way (Fazio *et al* 1986).

2.5.2 Processing of emotion and action in the late ERP components

When the expectation of emotional words in the sentence is violated, the long latency and slow-wave of LPP, LPC and P300 show congruent effects between events and emotions. This result is stable with previous findings on the reading of happy and sad words associated with more significant late positive components (LPC) (Schapkin *et al* 2000, Herbert *et al* 2006, 2008). When the task is to perceive independent emotional versus non-emotional words, faces or pictures, these late ERP components correlate with the detailed and explicit processing of the valence dimension of emotions (Citron 2012). In late positive complex words (LPC 450–700 ms), emotional words cause higher amplitudes than non-emotional words (Dillon *et al* 2006). The non-emotional words that are semantically inconsistent cause negative N400 amplitudes (Olichney *et al* 2000, Kutas and Schimitt 2003). Considering the results of these ERP studies, we describe the integrated processing of incongruent emotional words and event verbs that may be different from processing the semantic conflicts of non-emotional words in sentences. This difference may be due to the nature of various experimental stimuli, designs, and tasks. These different experiments plans and studies always determine whether the effect is a significant negative deflection N400 or a positive deflection P300 (Dillon *et al* 2006).

2.5.3 Regions of brain and hemispheric laterality effect on action and emotion

Concerning the prior studies done on emotional pictures, which states that the positive images are computed on the left side whereas the negative images are processed on the right side of the brain (Aftanas *et al* 2001), we observed that in P1, happy words are computed in the left hemispheric side whereas sad words are computed in the right side of the brain. In summary, the laterality effect in P1 supports the behavioural valence hypothesis (BVH) (Silberman and Weingartner 1986, Van Strien and Morpurgo 1992, Jansari *et al* 2000). BVH denotes that the positive emotion is computed in the left-side of the brain, and the negative emotion is computed on the right side of the brain (Davidson 2003). In P3, a different laterality effect is obtained by explicit processing of action and emotion words. Thus, the time course of ERPs plays a significant role to vary the laterality effect of action and emotion words. ERP studies have primarily examined the various regions such as centro-parietal and parietal areas of the brain involved in emotional word processing (Abbassi *et al* 2011, Citron 2012). A study on fMRI found that, in the pre-frontal cortex (PFC), more activation is elicited for negative emotional words than positive emotional words (Kensinger and Schacter 2006). This observation validates the previous finding that the activation is increased in the brain's frontal, temporal and parietal regions (Van Overwalle and Baetens 2009). Further, this chapter supports the view that the limbic system visa insula, which is connected with the superior-temporal cortex covering the temporal, central and centro-parietal regions, is activated during the processing of event or action stimuli to guide the information to the event or action network before processing of emotional stimuli (Augustine 1996, Rizzolatti *et al* 2001).

In the P100 and P300, we observed that centro-parietal regions processed happy emotional words according to previous literature, The late processing of happy emotion-words in the centro-parietal areas has consistently been reported as compared to early processing of happy emotion-words (Kanske and Kotz 2007, Kissler *et al* 2007, Carretié *et al* 2008, Herbert *et al* 2008, Hinojosa *et al* 2010). Scholars believe that at P3 activation is related to the expansion of happy action or emotional words that activates in the central and posterior (temporal, temporo-parietal, central, centro-parietal, parietal and occipital) regions of the brain (Kissler *et al* 2009, Schacht and Sommer 2009b, Bayer *et al* 2010, Sass *et al* 2010). The cortical and subcortical structures and temporal, parietal and parieto-occipital regions regulate the emotional visual stimuli such as face, body, gesture and words (Lestou *et al* 2008, Ferri *et al* 2013).

2.5.4 Theoretical insights from ERP studies

The previous neuroscience result supports the view that when the actions of body parts are intertwined with emotional context, the information is processed in the parietal cortex (Grosbras and Paus 2006, Thompson and Meyer 2007). Similarly, in the non-verbal context, event or action verbs contextualise the perception of emotion words. If there is any mismatch at the semantic level, the incongruent effect is observed in the P100 and P300 components. These results add to the current knowledge and literature in the field of verbal and non-verbal domains. The perception of emotional words (happy, sad and angry) within the context of events or action verbs play a crucial role in perceiving emotions (Barrett *et al* 2007, Barrett and Kensinger 2010). According to this finding, it is proposed that the contextual proposition of emotion in language can be applied to the knowledge or experience of event action words. in sentences. Event or action verbs provide a context to process emotional words. The non-verbal event model of emotion (Barrett *et al* 2007, Barrett 2009a) can be applied to the conceptual domain of event and emotion words, in which event-verbs may navigate the specific condition where the perception of emotion word can take place. Event verb delivers a prior context to clarify the meaning of emotion word and stimulates neural-effect in the perception of emotion-word in sentences.

In line with the Broaden-and-Build Theory, which is aligned with positive emotional stimuli, proposed by Fredrickson (1998, 2001), this chapter presents the processing advantage for happy feelings in P1 and P3. Both positive and negative events and actions have a significant impact on the thought of emotions. An individual's momentary thought-event or action repertoire is enhanced when positive emotion is evoked with positive actions or events (e.g., joy leads to urge to play, interest leads to the urge to discover, love, establish a close relationship, etc). However, the negative emotion is evoked when the thought of negative events or actions repertoire is integrated with a specific event or activity (e.g., expel, attack, escape, etc) that tends to narrow down the attention (Fredrickson 2004). In this sense, the scope of attention, cognition and event or action widens the cognitive processing of positive affect integrating diverse materials (Isen 1990, Borod *et al* 2000). Moreover, the nature of positive emotion usually heightens the dopamine level in the brain (Ashby *et al* 1999). These findings perpetuate that P3 amplitudes are larger when happy words are stimulated than sad ones since happy words have a broader scope of attention than sad ones. Due to the specific positive event or action tendencies, there is a difference in the cognitive resource allocations in more considerable neurocognitive processing for happy and sad words. Scholars suggest that specific action tendencies are associated with emotions (Frijda 1986, Lazarus 1991, Levenson 1994). Ferri *et al* (2013) demonstrate that an action that is embedded in an emotional pragmatic background (agents' facial expression) elicits a higher neural response than action which is embedded in a neutral context in the motor frontal, central, frontocentral, temporal, tempro-parietal and occipital regions of the brain.

2.6 Conclusion

This chapter describes the early and late processing of verbal and non-verbal stimulus of action or event and emotions. The early ERP components such as P100 and EPN are strongly associated with recognising events or actions that are integrated with emotions. However, the late components of LPC, LPP and P300 are linked with the detail elaborating processing of emotional pictures, voices and words. The top-down processing of meaning to a word occurs in the early ERP component, whereas the bottom-up processing that demands words to meaning in detail has happened in the late components of LPC, LPP and P300. Further, the semantic violation between emotional words and voice or prosody occurs in the late N400 component. Most of these ERP components corroborated with the computational and neurocognitive processing of action and emotions exhibit the larger amplitudes in the frontal, frontocentral, central, temporal and centro-parietal and occipital regions of the brain. Moreover, the feeling of written language has a quick and powerful influence on ERP, regulated by the congruent task of event verbs and emotion. Emotional words are processed much earlier than non-emotional words. The detailed and elaborate semantic conflicts involving emotional words and events in sentences are processed in the late components, as indicated by incongruence between actions and objects (P300) and semantic conflicts (N400). Pleasant words have a more tremendous advantage than unpleasant words in terms of processing in the mid-line, temporal region of the brain. These neurocognitive results opened up a new avenue for future studies into the role of expectancy violation with emotion words based on event or action words across languages. Understanding others actions and emotional tendencies display the intentional goals that ultimately facilitate social interactions and adaptive behaviours for our survival (Keltner and Haidt 1999). This chapter will be valuable, adequate, and beneficial to scientists interested in employing the EEG tools and methods to investigate verbal and non-verbal aspects of neurocognitive processing of actions or events and emotions across cultures and languages.

References

Abbassi E, Kahlaoui K, Wilson M A and Joanette Y 2011 Processing the emotions in words: the complementary contributions of the left and right hemispheres *Cogn. Affect. Behav. Neurosci.* **11** 372–85

Aftanas L, Varlamov A, Pavlov S, Makhnev V and Reva N 2001 Event-related synchronization and desynchronization during affective processing: emergence of valence-related time-dependent hemispheric asymmetries in theta and upper alpha band. *Int. J. Neurosci.* **110** 197–219

Alemanno F, Houdayer E, Cursi M, Velikova S, Tettamanti M, Comi G, Cappa S F and Leocani L 2012 Action-related semantic content and negation polarity modulate motor areas during sentence reading: an event-related desynchronization study *Brain Res.* **1484** 39–49

Andreatta M, Fendt M, Mühlberger A, Wieser M J, Imobersteg S, Yarali A, Gerber B and Pauli P 2012 Onset and offset of aversive events establish distinct memories requiring fear and reward networks *Learn. Mem.* **19** 518–26

Ashby F G, Isen A M and Turken A U 1999 A neuropsychological theory of positive affect and its influence on cognition *Psych. Rev.* **106** 529–50

Augustine J R 1996 Circuitry and functional aspects of the insular lobe in primates including humans *Brain Res. Rev.* **22** 229–44

Barrett L F 2009 Variety is the spice of life: a psychological construction approach to understanding variability in emotion *Cogn. Emot.* **23** 1284–306

Barrett L F and Kensinger E A 2010 Context is routinely encoded during emotion perception *Psychol. Sci.* **21** 595–99

Barrett L F, Lindquist K A and Gendron M 2007 Language as context for the perception of emotion *Trends Cogn. Sci.* **11** 327–32

Barsalou L W 2010 Grounded cognition: past, present, and future. topics in cognitive science *Topics Cogn. Sci.* **2** 716–24

Batty M and Taylor M J 2003 Early processing of the six basic facial emotional expressions *Cogn. Brain Res.* **17** 613–20

Bayer M, Sommer W and Schacht A 2010 Reading emotional words within sentences: the impact of arousal and valence on event-related potentials *Int. J. Psychophysiol.* **78** 299–307

Beauchamp M S and Martin A 2007 Grounding object concepts in perception and action: evidence from fMRI studies of tools *Cortex* **43** 461–68

Bedny M, Caramazza A, Pascual-Leone A and Saxe R 2012 Typical neural representations of action verbs develop without vision *Cereb. Cortex* **22** 286–93

Benedek K, Shayn L and Mahzarin R B 2017 Introducing the open affective standardized image set (OASIS) *Behav. Res. Methods* **49** 457–70

Bennett S D, Burnett A N, Siakaluk P D and Pexman P M 2011 Imageability and body–object interaction ratings for 599 multisyllabic nouns *Behav. Res. Method.* **43** 1100–9

Bernat E, Bunce S and Shevrin H 2001 Event-related brain potentials differentiate positive and negative mood adjectives during both supraliminal and subliminal visual processing *Int. J. Psychophysiol.* **42** 11–34

Biemann C, Heyer G, Quasthoff U and Richter M 2007 The Leipzig Corpora Collection - monolingual corpora of standard size *Proc. Corpus Linguistic 2007, Birmingham, UK*

Binkofski F and Buxbaum L J 2013 Two action systems in the human brain *Brain Lang.* **127** 222–9

Blechert J, Sheppes G, Di Tella C, Williams H and Gross J J 2012 See what you think: reappraisal modulates behavioral and neural responses to social stimuli *Psychol. Sci.* **23** 346–53

Borod J C *et al* 2000 Relationships among facial, prosodic, and lexical channels of emotional perceptual processing *Cogn. Emot.* **14** 193–211

Borod J C, Erhan H, Welkowitz J, Obler L, Whalen J and Grunwald I 1994 Facial, prosodic, and lexical emotional perception: assessment in a clinical population *Clin. Neuropsychol.* **8** 348

Borovsky A, Elman J and Kutas M 2012 Once is enough: N400 indexes semantic integration of novel word meaning *Lang. Learn. Dev.* **8** 278–302

Boulenger V, Roy A C, Paulignan Y, Deprez V, Jeannerod M and Nazir T A 2006 Cross-talk between language processes and overt motor behavior in the first 200 msec of processing *J. Cogn. Neurosci.* **18** 1607–15

Bradley M M and Lang P J 1994 Measuring emotion: the self-assessment manikin and the semantic differential *J. Behav. Ther. Exp. Psych.* **25** 49–59

Brunellière A, Auran C and Delrue L 2019 Does the prosodic emphasis of sentential context cause deeper lexical-semantic processing? *Lang. Cogn. Neurosci.* **34** 29–42

Bublatzky F, Gerdes A, White A J, Riemer M and Alpers G W 2014 Social and emotional relevance in face processing: happy faces of future interaction partners enhance the late positive potential *Front. Human Neurosci.* **8** 493

Candidi M, Leone-Fernandez B, Barber H A, Carreiras M and Aglioti S M 2010 Hands on the future: facilitation of cortico-spinal hand-representation when reading the future tense of hand-related action verbs *Eur. J. Neurosci.* **32** 677–83

Carretié L, Hinojosa J A, Albert J, López-Martín S, De La Gándara B S, Igoa J M and Sotillo M 2008 Modulation of ongoing cognitive processes by emotionally intense words *Psychophy.* **45** 188–96

Casiraghi L, Alahmadi A A, Monteverdi A, Palesi F, Castellazzi G, Savini G, Friston K, Gandini Wheeler-Kingshott C A and D'Angelo E 2019 I see your effort: force-related bold effects in an extended action execution–observation network involving the cerebellum *Cereb. Cortex* **29** 1351–68

Chen J X, Jiang D M and Zhang Y N 2019 A hierarchical bidirectional GRU model with attention for EEG-based emotion classification *IEEE Access* **7** 118530–40

Chen Q, Garcea F E, Jacobs R A and Mahon B Z 2018 Abstract representations of object-directed action in the left inferior parietal lobule *Cereb. Cortex* **28** 2162–74

Chen P, Wang G, Ma R, Jing F, Zhang Y, Wang Y, Zhang P, Niu C and Zhang X 2016 Multidimensional assessment of empathic abilities in patients with insular glioma *Cogn. Affect Behav. Neurosci.* **16** 962–75

Citron M M F, Weekes B S and Ferstl E C 2011 Neural correlates of emotion word processing: the interaction between emotional valence and arousal *Psychophysiology* **48** S3

Citron M M F 2012 Neural correlates of written emotion word processing: a review of recent electrophysiological and homodynamic neuroimaging studies *Brain Lang.* **122** 211–26

Conty L, Dezecache G, Hugueville L and Grezes J 2012 Early binding of gaze, gesture, and emotion: neural time course and correlates *J. Neurosci.* **32** 4531–9

Conty L, N'Diaye K, Tijus C and George N 2007 When eye creates the contact! ERP evidence for early dissociation between direct and averted gaze motion processing *Neuropsychologia* **45** 3024–37

Cracco E, Keysers C, Clauwaert A and Brass M 2019 Representing multiple observed actions in the motor system *Cereb. Cortex* **29** 3631–41

Crepaldi D, Berlingeri M, Paulesu E and Luzzatti C 2011 A place for nouns and a place for verbs? A critical review of neurocognitive data on grammatical-class effects *Brain. Lang.* **116** 33–49

Cuthbert B N, Schupp H T, Bradley M M, Birbaumer N and Lang P J 2000 Brain potentials in affective picture processing: covariation with autonomic arousal and affective report *Biol. Psychol.* **52** 95–111

Cuthbert B N, Bradleym M M and Lang P J 1996 Probing picture perception: activation and emotion *Psychophysiology* **33** 103–11

Dailey M, Cottrell G W and Reilly J 2001 *California facial expressions, CAFE. Unpublished digital images* (San Diego, CA: University of California Computer Science and Engineering Department)

Dalla Volta R, Fabbri-Destro M, Gentilucci M and Avanzini P 2014 Spatiotemporal dynamics during processing of abstract and concrete verbs: an ERP study *Neuropsychologia* **61** 163–74

Damasio A 2003 *Looking for Spinoza: Joy Sorrow and the Feeling Brain* (New York: Harcourt Brace)

Davidson R J 2003 Affective neuroscience and psychophysiology: toward a synthesis *Psychophy.* **40** 655

Davis M H, Meunier F and Marslen-Wilson W D 2004 Neural responses to morphological, syntactic, and semantic properties of single words: an fMRI study *Brain Lang.* **89** 439–49

Deen B and McCarthy G 2010 Reading about the actions of others: biological motion imagery and action congruency influence brain activity *Neuropsychologia* **48** 1607–15

Denefrio S, Simmons A, Jha A and Dennis-Tiwary T A 2017 Emotional cue validity effects: the role of neurocognitive responses to emotion *PLoS One* **12** e0179714

Dillon D G, Cooper J J, Grent T, Woldorff M G and LaBar K S 2006 Dissociation of event-related potentials indexing arousal and semantic cohesion during emotional word encoding *Brain Cogn.* **62** 43–57

Eben C, Billieux J and Verbruggen F 2020 Clarifying the role of negative emotions in the origin and control of impulsive actions *Psychol. Belg.* **60** 1

Ekman P 1993 Facial expression and emotion *Am. Psychol.* **48** 384

Ekman P and Friesen W V 1976 Measuring facial movement *Environ. Psychol. Nonverbal Behav.* **1** 56–75

Estes Z and Verges M 2008 Freeze or flee? Negative stimuli elicit selective responding *Cognition* **108** 557–65

Faja S, Dawson G, Aylward E, Wijsman E M and Webb S J 2016 Early event-related potentials to emotional faces differ for adults with autism spectrum disorder and by serotonin transporter genotype *Clin. Neurophysiol.* **127** 2436–47

Fan B, Zhao M, Jin J, Ding H and Ma Q 2018 Rational civil servant interviewers: evidence from an event-related potential study of beauty premiums in Chinese civil servant interviews *Exp. Brain Res.* **236** 3159–68

Fan L, Xu Q, Wang X, Xu F, Yang Y and Lu Z 2017 The automatic activation of emotion words measured using the emotional face-word Stroop task in late Chinese–English bilinguals *Cogn. Emot.* **32** 315–24

Fazio R H, Sanbonmatsu D M, Powell M C and Kardes F R 1986 On the automatic activation of attitudes *J. Pers. Soc. Psychol.* **50** 229–38

Federmeier K D, Kirson D A, Moreno E M and Kutas M 2001 Effects of transient, mild mood states on semantic memory organization and use: an event-related potential investigation in humans *Neurosci. Lett.* **305** 149–52

Fernandino L and Iacoboni M 2010 Are cortical motor maps based on body parts or coordinated actions? Implications for embodied semantics *Brain Lang.* **112** 44–53

Ferré P and Sánchez-Casas R 2014 Affective priming in a lexical decision task: is there an effect of words' concreteness? *Psicologica* **35** 117–38

Ferri F, Stoianov I P, Gianelli C, D'Amico L, Borghi A M and Gallese V 2010 When action meets emotions: how facial displays of emotion influence goal-related behavior *PLoS One* **5** e13126

Fields E C and Kuperberg G R 2012 It's all about you: an ERP study of emotion and self-relevance in discourse *NeuroImage* **62** 562–74

Ferri F, Ebisch S J, Costantini M, Salone A, Arciero G, Mazzola V, Ferro F M, Romani G L and Gallese V 2013 Binding action and emotion in social understanding *PloS One* **8** e54091

Fischler I and Bradley M 2006 Event-related potential studies of language and emotion: words, phrases, and task effects *Prog. Brain Res.* **156** 185–203

Flanagan J R and Johansson R S 2003 Action plans used in action observation *Nature* **424** 769–71

Foti D, Olvet D M, Klein D N and Hajcak G 2010 Reduced electrocortical response to threatening faces in major depressive disorder *Depress. Anxiety* **27** 813–20

Franken I H, Gootjes L and van Strien J W 2009 Automatic processing of emotional words during an emotional Stroop task *Neuroreport* **20** 776–81

Fredrickson B L 2004 The broaden–and–build theory of positive emotions *Phil. Trans. R. Soc. London* B **359** 1367–77

Fredrickson B L 2001 The role of positive emotions in positive psychology: the broaden-and-build theory of positive emotions *Am. Psychol.* **56** 218

Fredrickson B L 1998 What good are positive emotions? *Rev. Gen. Psychol.* **2** 300–19

Friederici A D, Hahne A and Mecklinger A 1996 Temporal structure of syntactic parsing: early and late event-related brain potential effects *J. Exp. Psychol.* **22** 1219

Frijda N H 2010 Impulsive action and motivation *Biol. Psychol.* **84** 570–9

Frijda N H 1986 *The Emotions* (Cambridge: Cambridge University Press)

Frijda N H 2006 *The Laws of Emotion* (New York: Erlbaum)

Frijda N H 1994 Varieties of affect: emotions and episodes, moods, and sentiments *The Nature of Emotion: Fundamental Questions* eds P Ekman and R J Davidson (New York: Oxford University Press) pp 59–67

Frühholz S, Jellinghaus A and Herrmann M 2011 Time course of implicit processing and explicit processing of emotional faces and emotional words *Biol. Psychol.* **87** 265–74

Gallese V and Lakoff G 2005 The brain's concepts: the role of the sensory-motor system in conceptual knowledge *Cogn. Neuropsychol.* **22** 455–79

Gallese V, Fadiga L, Fogassi L and Rizzolatti G 1996 Action recognition in the premotor cortex *Brain* **119** 593–609

Glenberg A M and Kaschak M P 2002 Grounding language in action *Psychon. Bull. Rev.* **9** 558–65

Goldstein L, Pouplier M, Chen L, Saltzman E and Byrd D 2007 Dynamic action units slip in speech production errors *Cognition* **103** 386–412

Gong X, Huang Y X, Wang Y and Luo Y J 2011 Revision of the Chinese facial affective picture system *Chin. Mental Health J.* **25** 40–6

Gootjes L, Coppens L C, Zwaan R A, Franken I H and Van Strien J W 2011 Effects of recent word exposure on emotion-word Stroop interference: an ERP study *Int. J. Psychophysiol.* **79** 356–63

Grèzes J, Erblang M, Vilarem E, Quiquempoix M, Van Beers P, Guillard M, Sauvet F, Mennella R and Rabat A 2021 Impact of total sleep deprivation and related mood changes on approach-avoidance decisions to threat-related facial displays *Sleep* **2021** zsab186

Grèzes J, Armony J L, Rowe J and Passingham R E 2003 Activations related to 'mirror' and 'canonical' neurones in the human brain: an fMRI study *Neuroimage* **18** 928–37

Grosbras M H and Paus T 2006 Brain networks involved in viewing angry hands or faces *Cereb. Cortex* **16** 1087–96

Guex R, Méndez-Bértolo C, Moratti S, Strange B A, Spinelli L, Murray R J, Sander D, Seeck M, Vuilleumier P and Domínguez-Borràs J 2020 Temporal dynamics of amygdala response to emotion-and action-relevance *Sci. Rep.* **10** 1–16

Hagemann J, Straube T and Schulz C 2016 Too bad: bias for angry faces in social anxiety interferes with identity processing *Neuropsychologia* **84** 136–49

Hagoort P 2003 How the brain solves the binding problem for language: a neurocomputational model of syntactic processing *Neuroimage* **20** S18–29

Hagoort P, Indefrey P, Brown C, Herzog H, Steinmetz H and Seitz R J 1999 The neural circuitry involved in the reading of German words and pseudowords: a PET study *J. Cogn. Neurosci.* **11** 383–98

Hahne A and Friederici A D 1999 Electrophysiological evidence for two steps in syntactic analysis: early automatic and late controlled processes *J. Cogn. Neurosci.* **11** 194–205

Hajcak G, MacNamara A and Olvet D M 2010 Event-related potentials, emotion, and emotion regulation: an integrative review *Developmental Neuropsychol.* **35** 129–55

Hajcak G, Weinberg A, MacNamara A and Foti D 2012 ERPs and the study of emotion *Oxford Handbook of Event-Related Potential Components* eds S J Luck and E S Kappenman (New York: Oxford University Press) pp 441–72

Hajcak G, Molnar C, George M S, Bolger K, Koola J and Nahas Z 2007 Emotion facilitates action: a transcranial magnetic stimulation study of motor cortex excitability during picture viewing *Psychophysiology* **44** 91–7

Hauk O, Davis M H, Kherif F and Pulvermueller F 2008 Imagery or meaning? Evidence for a semantic origin of category-specific brain 45 activity in metabolic imaging. *Euro. J. Neurosci.* **27** 1856–66

Hauk O, Johnsrude I and Pulvermüller F 2004 Somatotopic representation of action words in human motor and premotor cortex *Neuron* **41** 301–7

Haxby J V, Hoffman E A and Gobbini M I 2000 The distributed human neural system for face perception *Trends Cogn. Sci.* **4** 223–33

Herbert C, Junghofer M and Kissler J 2008 Event related potentials to emotional adjectives during reading *Psychophysiology* **45** 487–98

Herbert C, Kissler J, Junghofer M, Peyk P and Rockstroh B 2006 Processing of emotional adjectives: evidence from startle EMG and 55 ERPs *Psychophysiology* **43** 197–206

Herbert C, Pauli P and Herbert B M 2010 Self-reference modulates the processing of emotional stimuli in the absence of explicit self-referential appraisal instructions *Soc. Cogn. Affect. Neurosci.* **6** 653–61

Herbert C, Sfärlea A and Blumenthal T 2013 Your emotion or mine: labeling feelings alters emotional face perception—an ERP study on automatic and intentional affect labeling *Frontiers Human Neurosci.* **7** 378

Herrmann M J, Ehlis A C, Muehlberger A and Fallgatter A J 2005 Source localization of early stages of face processing *Brain Topogr.* **18** 77–85

Hepach R and Westermann G 2013 Infants' sensitivity to the congruence of others' emotions and actions *J. Exp. Child Psychol.* **115** 16–29

Hilt P M, Cardellicchio P and D'Ausilio A 2020 The neurophysiology of action perception *Modelling Human Motion* (Cham: Springer) pp 17–32

Hinojosa J A, Méndez-Bértolo C and Pozo M A 2010 Looking at emotional words is not the same as reading emotional words: behavioral and neural correlates *Psychophy.* **47** 748–57

Hirschfeld G, Feldker K and Zwitserlood P 2012 Listening to 'flying ducks': individual differences in sentence–picture verification investigated with ERPs *Psychophysiology* **49** 312–21

Hofmann M J, Kuchinke L, Tamm S, Võ M L and Jacobs A M 2009 Affective processing within 1/10 of a second: high arousal is necessary for early facilitative processing of negative but not positive words *Cogn. Affect. Behav. Neurosci.* **9** 389–97

Holmes E A, Mathews A, Mackintosh B and Dalgleish T 2008 The causal effect of mental imagery on emotion assessed using picture-word cues *Emotion* **8** 395

Isen A M 1990 The influence of positive and negative affect on cognitive organization: some implications for development *Psychological and Biological Approaches to Emotion* ed N Stein, B Leventhal and T Trabasso (Hillsdale, NJ: Erlbaum) pp 75–94

Ishii K, Kobayashi Y and Kitayama S 2010 Interdependence modulates the brain response to word–voice incongruity *Soc. Cognit. Affect. Neurosci.* **5** 307–17

Itier R J and Neath-Tavares K N 2017 Effects of task demands on the early neural processing of fearful and happy facial expressions *Brain Res.* **1663** 38–50

Jansari A, Tranel D and Adolphs R 2000 A valence specific lateral bias for discriminating emotional facial expressions in free field *Cogn. Emot.* **14** 341–53

Jenison R L, Rangel A, Oya H, Kawasaki H and Howard M A 2011 Value encoding in single neurons in the human amygdala during decision making *J. Neurosci.* **31** 331–38

Jetha M K, Zheng X, Schmidt L A and Segalowitz S J 2012 Shyness and the first 100 ms of emotional face processing *Soc. Neurosci.* **7** 74–89

Junghöfer M, Bradley M M, Elbert T R and Lang P J 2001 Fleeting images: a new look at early emotion discrimination *Psychophysiology* **38** 175–8

Kanske P and Kotz S A 2007 Concreteness in emotion words: ERP evidence from a hemi filed study *Brain Res.* **1148** 138–48

Karl C, Hewig J and Osinsky R 2016 Passing faces: sequence-dependent variations in the perceptual processing of emotional faces *Soc. Neurosci.* **11** 531–44

Keltner D and Haidt J 1999 Social functions of emotions at four levels of analysis *Cogn. Emot.* **13** 505–21

Kemmerer D, Rudrauf D, Manzel K and Tranel D 2012 Behavioral patterns and lesion sites associated with impaired processing of lexical and conceptual knowledge of actions *Cortex* **48** 826–48

Kemmerer D and Gonzalez-Castillo J 2010 The two-level theory of verb meaning: an approach to integrating the semantics of action with the mirror neuron system *Brain Lang.* **112** 54–76

Kensinger E A and Schacter D L 2006 Amygdala activity is associated with the successful encoding of item, but not source, information for positive and negative stimuli *J. Neurosci.* **26** 2564–70

Kensinger E A 2007 Negative emotion enhances memory accuracy: behavioral and neuroimaging evidence *Curr. Direct. Psychol. Sci.* **16** 213–18

Kissler J and Herbert C 2012 Emotion, etmnooi, or emotion? Faster lexical access to emotional than to neutral words during reading *Biol. Psychol.* **92** 464–79

Kissler J, Assadollahi R and Herbert C 2006 Emotional and semantic networks in visual word processing: insight from ERP studies *Prog. Brain Res.* **156** 147–83

Kissler J, Herbert C, Winkler I and Junghofer M 2009 Emotion and attention in visual word processing-an ERP study *Biol. Psychol.* **80** 75–83

Kissler J, Herbert C, Peyk P and Junghofer M 2007 Buzzwords: early cortical responses to emotional words during reading *Psychol. Sci.* **18** 475–80

Kiefer M, Schuch S, Schenck W and Fiedler K 2007 Mood states modulate activity in semantic brain areas during emotional word encoding *Cereb. Cortex* **17** 1516–30

Kilner J M, Vargas C, Duval S, Blakemore S J and Sirigu A 2004 Motor activation prior to observation of a predicted movement *Nat. Neurosci.* **7** 1299–301

Kiehl K A, Liddle P F, Smith A M, Mendrek A, Forster B B and Hare R D 1999 Neural pathways involved in the processing of concrete and abstract words *Human Brain Mapp.* **7** 225–33

Klepp A, Niccolai V, Sieksmeyer J, Arnzen S, Indefrey P, Schnitzler A and Biermann-Ruben K 2017 Body-part specific interactions of action verb processing with motor behaviour *Behav. Brain Res.* **328** 149–58

Krolak-Salmon P, Hénaff M A, Vighetto A, Bertrand O and Mauguière F 2004 Early amygdala reaction to fear spreading in occipital, temporal, and frontal cortex: a depth electrode ERP study in human *Neuron* **42** 665–76

Kuchinke L and Mueller C J 2019 Are there similarities between emotional and familiarity-based processing in visual word recognition? *J. Neurolinguistics* **49** 84–92

Kuhnke P, Kiefer M and Hartwigsen G 2020 Task-dependent recruitment of modality-specific and multimodal regions during conceptual processing *Cereb. Cortex* **30** 3938–59

Kurdi B, Lozano S and Banaji M R 2017 Introducing the open affective standardized image set (OASIS) *Behavior Res. Methods* **49** 457–70

Kutas M and Federmeier K D 2000 Electrophysiology reveals semantic memory use in language comprehension *Trends. Cogn. Sci.* **4** 463–70

Kutas M and Hillyard S A 1980 Reading senseless sentences: brain potentials reflect semantic incongruity *Science* **207** 203–5

Kutas M and Hillyard S A 1983 Event-related brain potentials to grammatical errors and semantic anomalies *Mem. Cogn.* **11** 539–50

Kutas M and Federmeier K D 2011 Thirty years and counting: finding meaning in the N400 component of the event-related brain potential (ERP) *Ann. Rev. Psychol.* **62** 621–47

Kutas M and Hillyard S A 1984 Brain potentials during reading reflect word expectancy and semantic association *Nature* **307** 161–3

Kutas M and Schmitt B M 2003 Language in microvolts *Mind, Brain, and Language: Multidisciplinary Perspectives* ed M T Banich and M Mack (Hillsdale, NJ: Lawrence Erlbaum Associates) pp 171–209

Lang P J, Bradley M M and Cuthbert B N 2008 International affective picture system (IAPS): affective ratings of pictures and instruction manual *Technical Report* The Center for Research in Psychophysiology, University of Florida

Lang P J, Bradley M M and Cuthbert B N 1999 Int. Affective Picture System (IAPS): instruction manual and affective ratings The Center for Research in Psychophysiology, University of Florida

Lang P J, Bradley M M and Cuthbert B N 1997 Motivated attention: affect, activation, and action *Attention and Orienting: Sensory and Motivational Processes* ed P J Lang, R F Simons and M Balaban (Hillsdale, NJ: Erlbaum) pp 97–135

Lang P J, Bradley M M and Cuthbert B N 2005 *International Affective Picture System (IAPS): Affective Ratings of Pictures and Instruction Manual* (Gainesville, FL: University of Florida)

Lau E F, Holcomb P J and Kuperberg G R 2013 Dissociating N400 effects of prediction from association in single word contexts *J. Cogn. Neurosci.* **25** 484–502

Lau E F, Phillips C and Poeppel D 2008 A cortical network for semantics: (de)constructing the N400 *Nat. Rev. Neurosci.* **9** 920–33

Lau E, Stroud C, Plesch S and Phillips C 2006 The role of structural prediction in rapid syntactic analysis *Brain Lang.* **98** 74–88

Lazarus R S 1991 Cognition and motivation in emotion *Am. Psychol.* **46** 352

Lazarus R S 1991 *Emotion and Adaptation* (New York: Oxford University Press)

Leite J, Carvalho S, Galdo-Alvarez S, Alves J, Sampaio A and Gonçalves Ó F 2012 Affective picture modulation: valence, arousal, attention allocation and motivational significance *Int. J. Psychophysiol.* **83** 375–81

Leppänen J M, Kauppinen P, Peltola M J and Hietanen J K 2007 Differential electrocortical responses to increasing intensities of fearful and happy emotional expressions *Brain Res.* **1166** 103–9

Lestou V, Pollick F E and Kourtzi Z 2008 Neural substrates for action understanding at different description levels in the human brain *J. Cogn. Neurosci.* **20** 324–41

Levenson R W 1994 Human emotions: a functional view *The Nature of Emotion: Fundamental Questions* ed P Ekman and R J Davidson (New York: Oxford University Press) pp 123–6

Levenson R W, Ekman P and Friesen W V 1990 Voluntary facial action generates emotion-specific autonomic nervous system activity *Psychophysiology* **27** 363–84

Li Y, Zeng J, Shan S and Chen X 2018 Occlusion aware facial expression recognition using CNN with attention mechanism *IEEE Trans. Image Process.* **28** 2439–50

Lingnau A and Petris S 2013 Action understanding within and outside the motor system: the role of task difficulty *Cereb. Cortex* **23** 1342–50

Liu T, Pinheiro A, Zhao Z, Nestor P G, McCarley R W and Niznikiewicz M A 2012 Emotional cues during simultaneous face and voice processing: electrophysiological insights *PLoS One* **7** e31001

Luo W, Feng W, He W, Wang N Y and Luo Y J 2010 Three stages of facial expression processing: ERP study with rapid serial visual presentation *Neuroimage* **49** 1857–67

MacGregor L J, Pulvermüller F, van Casteren M and Shtyrov Y 2012 Ultra-rapid access to words in the brain *Nat. Commun.* **3** 711

MacNamara A, Schmidt J, Zelinsky G J and Hajcak G 2012 Electrocortical and ocular indices of attention to fearful and neutral faces presented under high and low working memory load *Biol. Psychol.* **91** 349–56

Marchewka A, Żurawski Ł, Jednoróg K and Grabowska A 2014 The Nencki affective picture system (NAPS): introduction to a novel, standardized, wide-range, high-quality, realistic picture database *Behavior Res. Methods* **46** 596–610

Martin A and Chao L L 2001 Semantic memory and the brain: structure and processes *Curr. Opin. Neurobiol.* **11** 194–201

Martín-Loeches M 2007 The gate for reading: reflections on the recognition potential *Brain Res. Rev.* **53** 89–97

Mavratzakis A, Herbert C and Walla P 2016 Emotional facial expressions evoke faster orienting responses, but weaker emotional responses at neural and behavioural levels compared to scenes: a simultaneous EEG and facial EMG study *Neuroimage* **124** 931–46

Meeren H K, van Heijnsbergen C C and de Gelder B 2005 Rapid perceptual integration of facial expression and emotional body language *Proc. Natl Acad. Sci.* **102** 16518–23

Mennella R, Vilarem E and Grèzes J 2020 Rapid approach-avoidance responses to emotional displays reflect value-based decisions: neural evidence from an EEG study *Neuroimage* **222** 117253

Moseley R, Carota F, Hauk O, Mohr B and Pulvermüller F 2012 A role for the motor system in binding abstract emotional meaning *Cereb. Cortex* **22** 1634–47

Mühlberger A, Wieser M J, Herrmann M J, Weyers P, Tröger C and Pauli P 2009 Early cortical processing of natural and artificial emotional faces differs between lower and higher socially anxious persons *J. Neural Transm.* **116** 735–46

Müller-Bardorff M, Bruchmann M, Mothes-Lasch M, Zwitserlood P, Schlossmacher I, Hofmann D, Miltner W and Straube T 2018 Early brain responses to affective faces: a simultaneous EEG-fMRI study *Neuroimage* **178** 660–7

Müller B C, Kühn S, van Baaren R B, Dotsch R, Brass M and Dijksterhuis A 2011 Perspective taking eliminates differences in co-representation of out-group members' actions *Exp. Brain Res.* **211** 423–8

Muraki E J, Cortese F, Protzner A B and Pexman P M 2020 Heterogeneity in abstract verbs: an ERP study *Brain Lang.* **211** 104863

Nieuwenhuis S, Aston-Jones G and Cohen J D 2005 Decision making, the P3, and the locus coeruleus—norepinephrine system *Psychol. Bull.* **131** 510

Olichney J M, Van Petten C, Paller K A, Salmon D P, Iragui V J and Kutas M 2000 Word repetition in amnesia: electrophysiological measures of impaired and spared memory *Brain* **123** 1948–63

Olofsson J K and Polich J 2007 Affective visual event-related potentials: arousal, repetition, and time-on-task *Biol. Psychol.* **75** 101–8

Osgood C E, May W H, Miron M S and Miron M S 1975 *Cross-Cultural Universals of Affective Meaning* vol 1 (Chicago, IL: University of Illinois Press)

Osiurak F 2014 Mechanical knowledge, but not manipulation knowledge, might support action prediction *Front. Human Neurosci.* **8** 737

Palazova M, Mantwill K, Sommer W and Schacht A 2011 Are effects of emotion in single words non-lexical? Evidence from event-related brain potentials *Neuropsychologia* **49** 2766–75

Paulmann S and Pell M D 2010 Dynamic emotion processing in Parkinson's disease as a function of channel availability *J. Clin. Exp. Neuropsychol.* **32** 822–35

Paulmann S and Kotz S A 2008 An ERP investigation on the temporal dynamic of emotional prosody and emotional semantics in pseudo- and lexical-sentence context *Brian Lang.* **105** 56–69

Peelen M V, Romagno D and Caramazza A 2012 Independent representations of verbs and actions in left lateral temporal cortex *J. Cogn. Neurosci.* **24** 2096–107

Pugh Z H, Choo S, Leshin J C, Lindquist K A and Nam C S 2021 Emotion depends on context, culture and their interaction: evidence from effective connectivity *Soc. Cogn. Affect. Neurosci.* (https://doi.org/10.1093/scan/nsab092)

Reis D L and Gray J R 2009 Affect and action control *Oxford Handbook of Human Action* (Oxford: Oxford University Press) pp 277–97

Peltola M J, Yrttiaho S and Leppänen J M 2018 Infants' attention bias to faces as an early marker of social development *Develop. Sci.* **21** e12687

Pessoa L and Adolphs R 2010 Emotion processing and the amygdala: from a 'low road' to 'many roads' of evaluating biological significance *Nat. Rev. Neurosci.* **11** 773–82

Petit O, Velasco C and Spence C 2019 Digital sensory marketing: integrating new technologies into multisensory online experience *J. Inter. Market.* **45** 42–61

Phillips M L, Drevets W C, Rauch L S and Lane R 2003 Neurobiology of emotion perception: the neural basis of normal emotion perception *Biol. Psych.* **54** 504–14

Pisu V, Uccelli S, Riggio L and Bruno N 2020 Action preparation in grasping reveals generalization of precision between implicit and explicit motor processes *Neuropsychologia* **141** 107406

Pollick F E, Paterson H M, Bruderlin A and Sanford A J 2001 Perceiving affect from arm movement *Cognition* **82** B51–61

Pollick F E, Lestou V, Ryu J and Cho S B 2002 Estimating the efficiency of recognizing gender and affect from biological motion *Vis. Res.* **42** 2345–55

Portugal L C L *et al* 2020 Interactions between emotion and action in the brain *NeuroImage* **214** 116728

Prével A, Hoofs V and Krebs R M 2021 Effect of non-instructed instrumental contingency of monetary reward and positive affect in a cognitive control task *R. Soc. Open Sci.* **8** 202002

Pulvermüller F 2018 Neural reuse of action perception circuits for language, concepts and communication *Prog. Neurobiol.* **160** 1–44

Pulvermüller F and Fadiga L 2010 Active perception: sensorimotor circuits as a cortical basis for language *Nat. Rev. Neurosci.* **11** 351–60

Pulvermüller F, Shtyrov Y and Ilmoniemi R 2005 Brain signatures of meaning access in action word recognition *J. Cogn. Neurosci.* **17** 884–92

Pulvermüller F 2005 Brain mechanisms linking language and action *Nat. Rev. Neurosci.* **6** 576–82

Pulvermüller F, Härle M and Hummel F 2001 Walking or talking? Behavioral and neurophysiological correlates of action verb processing *Brain Lang.* **78** 143–68

Righart R and De Gelder B 2008 Rapid influence of emotional scenes on encoding of facial expressions: an ERP study *Soc. Cogn. Affect. Neurosci.* **3** 270–8

Rizzolatti G, Fogassi L and Gallese V 2001 Neurophysiological mechanisms underlying the understanding and imitation of action *Nat. Rev. Neurosci.* **2** 661–70

Rizzolatti G and Sinigaglia C 2016 The mirror mechanism: a basic principle of brain function *Nat. Rev. Neurosci.* **17** 757–65

Ruba A L, Meltzoff A N and Repacholi B M 2020 The development of negative event-emotion matching in infancy: implications for theories in affective science. *Affect. Sci.* **1** 4–19

Rueschemeyer S A, Lindemann O, van Rooij D, van Dam W and Bekkering H 2010 Effects of intentional motor actions on embodied language processing *Exp. Psychol.* **57** 260–6

Saarimäki H, Gotsopoulos A, Jääskeläinen I P, Lampinen J, Vuilleumier P, Hari R, Sams M and Nummenmaa L 2016 Discrete neural signatures of basic emotions *Cereb. Cortex* **26** 2563–73

Santos I M, Iglesias J, Olivares E I and Young A W 2008 Differential effects of object-based attention on evoked potentials to fearful and disgusted faces *Neuropsychologia* **46** 1468–79

Sass S M *et al* 2010 Time course of attentional bias in anxiety: emotion and gender specificity *Psychophysiology* **47** 247–59

Sato W, Kochiyama T, Uono S, Matsuda K, Usui K, Usui N, Inoue Y and Toichi M 2017 Bidirectional electric communication between the inferior occipital gyrus and the amygdala during face processing *Human Brain Mapping* **38** 4511–24

Schacht A and Sommer W 2009a Time course and task dependence of emotion effects in word processing *Cogn. Affect. Behav. Neurosci.* **9** 28–43

Schacht A and Sommer W 2009b Emotions in word and face processing: early and late cortical responses *Brain Cogn.* **69** 538–50

Schapkin S A, Gusev A N and Kuhl J 2000 Categorization of unilaterally presented emotion words: an ERP analysis *Acta Neurobiol. Exp.* **60** 17–28

Scherer K R and Moors A 2019 The emotion process: event appraisal and component differentiation *Annu. Rev. Psychol.* **70** 719–45

Schindler S, Tirloni C, Bruchmann M and Straube T 2021 Face and emotional expression processing under continuous perceptual load tasks: an ERP study *Biol. Psychol.* **161** 108056

Schirmer A and Kotz S A 2006 Beyond the right hemispheres: brain mechanisms mediating vocal emotional processing *Trends Cogn. Sci.* **10** 24–30

Schupp H T, Stockburger J, Codispoti M, Junghöfer M, Weike A I and Hamm A O 2007 Selective visual attention to emotion *J. Neurosci.* **27** 1082–9

Schupp H T, Stockburger J, Codispoti M, Junghöfer M, Weike A I and Hamm A O 2006 Stimulus novelty and emotion perception: the near absence of habituation in the visual cortex *Neuroreport* **17** 365–9

Schupp H T, Öhman A, Junghöfer M, Weike A I, Stockburger J and Hamm A O 2004 The facilitated processing of threatening faces: an ERP analysis *Emotion* **4** 189

Schupp H T, Markus J, Weike A I and Hamm A O 2003 Emotional facilitation of sensory processing in the visual cortex *Psychol. Sci.* **14** 7–13

Schupp H T, Junghöfer M, Weike A I and Hamm A O 2004a The selective processing of briefly presented affective pictures: an ERP analysis *Psychophysiology* **41** 441–9

Schupp H T, Öhman A, Junghöfer M, Weike A I, Stockburger J and Hamm A O 2004b The facilitated processing of threatening faces: an ERP analysis *Emotion* **4** 189

Schütz-Bosbach S and Prinz W 2007 Prospective coding in event representation *Cogn. Process.* **8** 93–102

Scott G G 2009a Emotion word processing: evidence from electrophysiology, eye movements and decision making *Doctoral Dissertation* University of Glasgow

Scott G G, O'Donnell J P, Leuthold L and Sereno S C 2009b Early emotion word processing: evidence from event-related potentials *Biol. Psych.* **80** 95–104

Sel A, Forster B and Calvo-Merino B 2014 The emotional homunculus: ERP evidence for independent somatosensory responses during facial emotional processing *J. Neurosci.* **34** 3263–7

Sergerie K, Chochol C and Armony J L 2008 The role of amygdala in emotional processing: a quantitative meta-analysis of functional neuroimaging studies *Neurosci. Biobehav. Rev.* **32** 811–30

Shebani Z and Pulvermüller F 2013 Moving the hands and feet specifically impairs working memory for arm-and leg-related action words *Cortex* **49** 222–31

Sidhu D M, Kwan R, Pexman P M and Siakaluk P D 2014 Effects of relative embodiment in lexical and semantic processing of verbs *Acta Psychol.* **149** 32–9

Siegle G J, Steinhauer S R, Thase M E, Stenger V A and Carter C S 2002 Can't shake that feeling: event-related fMRI assessment of sustained amygdala activity in response to emotional information in depressed individuals *Biol. Psychiatry* **51** 693–707

Silberman E K and Weingartner H 1986 Hemispheric lateralization of functions related to emotion *Brain. Cogn.* **5** 322–53

Sitnikova T, Kuperberg G and Holcomb P J 2003 Semantic integration in videos of real–world events: an electrophysiological investigation *Psychophysiology* **40** 160–4

Smith C A and Kirby L D 2011 The role of appraisal and emotion in coping and adaptation *The Handbook of Stress Science: Biology, Psychology, and Health* (New York: Springer) pp 195–208

Smith E, Weinberg A, Moran T and Hajcak G 2013 Electrocortical responses to NIMSTIM facial expressions of emotion *Int. J. Psychophysiol.* **88** 17–25

Tabullo Á, Sevilla Y, Pasqualetti G, Vernis S, Segura E, Yorio A and Wainselboim A 2011 Expectancy modulates a late positive ERP in an artificial grammar task *Brain Res.* **1373** 131–43

Takehara H, Ishihara S and Iwaki T 2020 Comparison between facilitating and suppressing facial emotional expressions using frontal EEG asymmetry *Front. Behav. Neurosci.* **14** 554147

Tarai S and Srinivasan N 2019 Emotional prosody Stroop effect in Hindi: an event related potential study *Prog. Brain Res.* **247** 193–217

Tettamanti M, Rognoni E, Cafiero R, Costa T, Galati D and Perani D 2012 Distinct pathways of neural coupling for different basic emotions *Neuroimage* **59** 1804–17

Tettamanti M, Manenti R, Della Rosa P A, Falini A, Perani D, Cappa S F and Moro A 2008 Negation in the brain: modulating action representations *Neuroimage* **43** 358–67

Tettamanti M, Buccino G, Saccuman M C, Gallese V, Danna M and Scifo P 2005 Listening to action-related sentences activates fronto-parietal motor circuits *J. Cogn. Neurosci.* **17** 273–81

Thompson R A and Meyer S 2007 Socialization of emotion regulation in the family *Handbook of Emotion Regulation* ed J J Gross (New York: Guilford Press) pp 249–68

Tillotson S M, Siakaluk P D and Pexman P M 2008 Body—object interaction ratings for 1,618 monosyllabic nouns *Behav. Res. Method* **40** 1075–8

Toivonen R, Kivelä M, Saramäki J, Viinikainen M, Vanhatalo M and Sams M 2012 Networks of emotion concepts *PLoS One* **7** e28883

Tortosa M I, Lupiáñez J and Ruz M 2013 Race, emotion and trust: an ERP study *Brain Res.* **1494** 44–55

Ubaldi S, Barchiesi G and Cattaneo L 2015 Bottom-up and top-down visuomotor responses to action observation *Cereb. Cortex* **25** 1032–41

Urgesi C, Maieron M, Avenanti A, Tidoni E, Fabbro F and Aglioti S M 2010 Simulating the future of actions in the human corticospinal system *Cereb. Cortex* **20** 2511–21

van de Meerendonk N, Chwilla D J and Kolk H H 2013 States of indecision in the brain: ERP reflections of syntactic agreement violations versus visual degradation *Neuropsychologia* **51** 1383–96

Van Hooff J C, Dietz K and C. Sharma D H B 2008 Neural correlates of intrusion of emotion words in a modified Stroop task *J. Psychophy.* **67** 23–34

Vanhoutte S, Strobbe G, van Mierlo P, Cosyns M, Batens K, Corthals P, De Letter M, Van Borsel J and Santens P 2015 Early lexico-semantic modulation of motor related areas during action and non-action verb processing *J Neurolinguistics* **34** 65–82

Van Overwalle F and Baetens K 2009 Understanding others' actions and goals by mirror and mentalizing systems: a meta-analysis *Neuroimage* **48** 564–84

Van Strien J W and Morpurgo M 1992 Opposite hemispheric activations as a result of emotionally threatening and non-threatening words *Neuropsy.* **30** 845–8

Vilarem E, Armony J L and Grèzes J 2020 Action opportunities modulate attention allocation under social threat *Emotion* **20** 890

Warriner A B, Kuperman V and Brysbaert M 2013 Norms of valence, arousal, and dominance for 13,915 English lemmas *Behav. Res. Method.* **45** 1191–207

Weinberg A, Hilgard J, Bartholow B D and Hajcak G 2012 Emotional targets: evaluative categorization as a function of context and content *Int. J. Psychophysiol.* **84** 149–54

Weinberg A and Hajcak G 2011 The late positive potential predicts subsequent interference with target processing *J. Cogn. Neurosci.* **23** 2994–3007

Weinberg A and Hajcak G 2010 Beyond good and evil: the time-course of neural activity elicited by specific picture content *Emotion* **10** 767

Weinberg A, Hilgard J, Bartholow B D and Hajcak G 2012 Emotional targets: evaluative categorization as a function of context and content *Int. J. Psychophysiol.* **84** 149–54

West G L, Al-Aidroos N, Susskind J and Pratt J 2011 Emotion and action: the effect of fear on saccadic performance *Exp. Brain Res.* **209** 153–8

Wheeler R E, Davidson R J and Tomarken A J 1993 Frontal brain asymmetry and emotional reactivity: a biological substrate of affective style *Psychophy.* **30** 82–9

Williamson S, Harpur T J and Hare R D 1991 Abnormal processing of affective words by psychopaths *Psychophysiology* **28** 260–73

Willms J L, Shapiro K A, Peelen M V, Pajtas P E, Costa A, Moo L R and Caramazza A 2011 Language-invariant verb processing regions in Spanish–English bilinguals *Neuroimage* **57** 251–61

Wilson-Mendenhall C D, Barrett L F, Simmons W K and Barsalou L W 2011 Grounding emotion in situated conceptualization *Neuropsychologia* **49** 1105–27

Wu C, Zhang J and Yuan Z 2021 Exploring affective priming effect of emotion-label words and emotion-laden words: an event-related potential study *Brain Sci.* **11** 553

Wu C, Zhang J and Yuan Z 2019 An ERP investigation on the second language and emotion perception: the role of emotion word type *Int. J. Biling. Educ. Biling* 1–13

Wu C, Zhang J and Yuan Z 2020 Affective picture processing is modulated by emotion word type in masked priming paradigm: an event-related potential study *J. Cogn. Psychol.* **32** 287–97

Yang Y, Li W, Zhang Q, Zhang L, Cheung T and Xiang Y T 2020 Mental health services for older adults in China during the COVID-19 outbreak *Lancet Psych.* **7** e19

Yang J and Shu H 2012 The role of the premotor cortex and the primary motor cortex in action verb comprehension: evidence from Granger causality analysis *Brain Res. Bull.* **88** 460–6

Yu Q and Kitayama S 2019 Does facial action modulate neural responses of emotion? An examination with the late positive potential (LPP) *Emotion* **21** 442–6

Yoon S, Shim M, Kim H S and Lee S H 2016 Enhanced early posterior negativity to fearful faces in patients with anxiety disorder *Brain Topogr.* **29** 262–72

Zald D H 2003 The human amygdala and the emotional evaluation of sensory stimuli *Brain Res.* **41** 88–123

Zhang D, He W, Wang T, Luo W, Zhu X, Gu R, Li H and Luo Y J 2014 Three stages of emotional word processing: an ERP study with rapid serial visual presentation *Soc. Cogn. Affect Neurosci.* **9** 1897–903

Zhang J, Wu C, Meng Y and Yuan Z 2017 Different neural correlates of emotion-label words and emotion-laden words: an ERP study *Frontiers Human Neurosci.* **11** 455

Zhang Q, Lawson A, Guo C and Jiang Y 2006 Electrophysiological correlates of visual affective priming *Brain Res. Bull.* **71** 316–23

Chapter 3

Blood–brain barrier biomarker for neurodegenerative disorder

Arindam Bit, Nishchay Verma and Shashikanta Tarai

This chapter intends to examine biomarkers for neurodegenerative diseases (NDD), developing a possible interaction between neural and micro-vascular systems. Since different forms of NDD reveal distinct diagnostic symptoms, developing a universal biomarker is a challenging task for neuroscientists. Brain tissue loss, blood–brain–barrier (BBB) breakdown, brain hypo-perfusion, and inflammatory responses predict the onset of neurodegeneration (ND). Studies have explored the implication of therapeutic tools to optimize the BBB for curing NDD without simultaneously intervening in nervous and micro-vascular systems. Dysregulation of microvasculature affecting corpus callosum is a blind pathway to intervene. However, biological markers for ND such as white matter hyper (WMH) intensity and ventricular dilation enhanced cerebrospinal fluid (CSF). Thus, CSF and BBB interaction can be considered as biomarkers for cerebrovascular endothelial cells. In this review, we propose multi-modal diagnostic biomarkers, incorporating therapeutic solutions to combat NDD. Regulatory status of T- and B-cells to protect the infiltration of neural, vascular, and glial cells can be used as a tool for biomarkers. In conjunction with these immune units, expressions of serum antibodies and cytoskeletal proteins can also be used to quantify axonal disintegration during stages of ND. Influential crosstalk between these two classes of biomarkers yields potential molecular biomarkers for universal identification of disease-specific pathologies. Further, the incorporation of nanomaterials has also been demonstrated to be used as effective bilateral biomarkers for the management of NDD.

3.1 Introduction

Biological markers (biomarkers) always define the etiological spectrum of neurological disease considering cellular, biochemical or atomic amendments and estimate

doi:10.1088/978-0-7503-3383-2ch3

the fluid used for cell culture like living stuff, cells, in other words, fluid (Mayeux 2004). Broadly, the biological characteristics, processes, and tools, including pharmacological responses to a disease's therapeutic intervention, have been considered biomarkers (Naylor 2003). We examine these etiological ingredients from the existing literature for developing biomarkers for neurodegenerative diseases. The purpose of this paper is to deliver an integrational approach for developing biomarkers of NDD through a cross-talk between cardiovascular and neural systems. The current literature claims that the neurovascular system regulates blood flow in the brain. This system sends the cardiac outputs to the brain to circulate the blood flow. Reduction in cerebral blood flow damages the neurons and also diminishes the energy substrates of neurons. In our body, 20 percentile of heart productivity is received by the human brain. The brain's functioning is heavily dependent upon the blood flow from the cerebral called cerebral blood flow (CBF) (Girouard and Iadecola 2006). Therefore, it is impossible to derive the functioning of the brain by a normal neuronal-vascular relationship. This is one of the causes of neural degeneration in the normal brain. Neural degeneration enhances neurodegenerative disorders causes, diminishing the thickness of the cerebral endothelial membrane from its original value (0.2 to 0.3 mm) to critical. Reducing the thickness of the cerebral endothelial membrane provide changes in the length of brain capillaries. These effects have also influenced the flow of energy substrates and nutrients towards the BBB. Moreover, withdrawal of this interrelationship between the cardiovascular and the BBB can improve the neurotoxins from the brain.

To measure neural activity, changes in central blood flow are determined in the case of hyperemia. If the upstream arterioles dilate, wide and open, it increases the flow in local vasodilation (Duling *et al* 1987). The vascular diameters of arterioles increase with whisker barrel cortex activation. These vascular arterioles are situated 100 μm apart from the activation site (Cox *et al* 1993, Ngai *et al* 1988, Erinjeri and Woolsey 2002). Straight electrical impulses enlarge the diameter of upstream branches and local vascular diameter of the arteriole in the cerebellum (Ladecola *et al* 1997). Neurotransmission changes blood flow in the brain manifesting a linkage between local somatic activity and central blood flow to coordinate synaptic action potential. This synaptic activity activates astrocytes and neurons to induce vasodilation in arterioles.

3.2 Molecular biomarker of neurological disorder

Histamine performs different kinds of work, such as mediator of inflammation and controller of innate and adaptive immunity. However, the effect of histamine on immune cells present in the brain is still under investigation (Dong *et al* 2014). Microglia sequentially expresses all histamine receptors, including H1R, H2R, H3R, and H4R. Histamine activates microglia, generating proinflammatory interleukin-6 (IL-6) and tumour necrosis factor (TNF-α). Microglia recognizes TNF α and IL6 on histamine receptor expression. ND cells play an essential part in building up a protective immune response and in a succession of damaging inflammation during central nervous system disease conditions (Csuka *et al* 2000, Gao *et al* 2003,

Heppner *et al* 2005, Popovich 2000). Neurotoxins and neurodebris activate microglia gradually, which generates inflammatory mediators such as TNF-α, nitric oxide (NO), IL-6, reactive oxygen species (ROS), and prostagladin E2 (PGE2). These pro-inflammatory mediators are inimical to neurons (Block and Hong 2005, Herrera *et al* 2005). The repression of microglia activation and successive inflammatory response may be a novel strategy to eliminate the damaging impact of microglia (Gao *et al* 2003). As histamine acts as a mediator of inflammation and regulator of the adaptive and innate immunity system, there is significantly less known about its importance in brain microglia. Histamine obstructs microglia migration induced by LPS and secretion of IL-1β via activation of H4R (Ferreira *et al* 2012).

3.2.1 Influence of T and B cells on MS recovery

Because of the interdependence of inflammation, neurodegeneration disease progresses in MS stages apropos clinical course and lesion activity, B-cells and T-cells infiltrates are related to demyelinating lesions. In contrast, plasma infiltrates are marked in a patient with secondary progressive multiple sclerosis (SPMS) (Frischer *et al* 2009). In age-matched control T and B cells, infiltrates decrease to a noticeable level, whereas in neurodegeneration, patients exceeded to an extent in normal controls directing to Alzheimer or vascular disease.

Axonal and neuronal degeneration in MS causes inflammation. Anti-inflammatory or immunomodulatory treatments are moderately effective against progressive disorders (Coles *et al* 1999, Filippi *et al* 2000, 2004, Molyneux *et al* 2000). MRI (magnetic resonance imaging) and spectroscopy are used to study the correlation between inflammation, spinal cord atrophy, and progressive brain (Anderson *et al* 2006, Bielekova *et al* 2005, Filippi and Rocca 2005, Zivadinov and Cox 2007). Maximum axonal loss in NAWM (white matter), discovered by Neuro-pathology. These phenomena cause leading axonal injury from demyelinated lesions (DeLuca *et al* 2006, Evangelou *et al* 2005, Lovas *et al* 2000). Neurodegeneration in MS may be considered the preliminary cause of CNS disease and may occur without inflammation (Trapp and Nave 2008). Nerve cells are protected and are surrounded by myelin sheaths and thus are protected from damage due to MS. In autoimmune diseases, these protective myelin sheaths are damaged, affecting their protection of nerve cells and the spinal cord. Disturbances in visual aids, memory loss, trouble in coordination and balance, thinking are a few symptoms of MS. There is no treatment for MS, but MS therapeutics may help slow down the disease progression and also help in controlling symptoms. To protect different types of lesions, in MS MAGUK controls the correct spatial distribution of claudins. ZO-1 proteins are associated with cytoskeleton by way of peripheral membrane-associated guanylate Kinase (multidomain scaffolding protein) (MAGUK includes ZO1, ZO2, and ZO3) (Hawkins and Davis 2005). Tight junction (TJ) abnormalities are associated with ZO-1 expression of different lesions in MS (Kirk *et al* 2003). BBB leakage, which contributes to disease progression and disease-modifying therapy, is related to endothelial abnormalities (Leech *et al* 2007). Prompt prediction of MS depends on inter-muscular interferon beta-1a, which results in relapsing-remitting multiple sclerosis (RRMS) treating with intramuscular interferon β−1a (IFN β−1a) (Bermel *et al* 2013). Early disease activity is decreased on IM IFN β−1a rather than in placebo disease activity markers. In IFN-β therapy, disease activity contributes to gadolinium-enhancing lesions. Severe EDSS gadolinium increasing lesions and worsening new T2 lesions are predicted by persistent disease activity in the IM IFN-β group.

3.2.2 Autoimmune initiators

The ASIA autoimmune syndrome is implied by adjuvants triggering a range of immune-mediated diseases, which starts stimulating chronic exposure to pristane, aluminium, silicone, tetramethyl pentadecane, and another adjuvants including infectious elements. It also involves the start of adjuvant-induced autoimmunity (Perricone *et al* 2013). These environmental factors or adjuvants induce autoimmunity by themselves. The appearance of vaccine disease ASIA is found in general to have favourable genetic background. Environmental factors play a crucial role in the induction of auto-immunity interactions between genetic susceptibility. Chronic fatigue syndrome (CFS) is linked to sleep disturbance and stressful sleep. This syndrome is identified to be due to the presence of adjuvants showing the same sleepless denominators. Early exposure to adjuvants in ASIA syndrome leads to a chain of immunological and biological events that confirm the development of autoimmune disease.

Aluminium-based compounds (alum) contain the bulk of contemporary adjuvants, which lie under this phenomenon of induced autoimmunity. The precipitation of antigens and insoluble particles of potash alum previous to immunization is superintended for excel antibody response compared to soluble antigen. The depot effect is induced by potash alum, which consolidates the required antigen at the injection site, leading to gradual secretion of antigen-to-antigen representing cells for a prolonged period. T-cells and auto-antibodies in Guillain Barre (GB) patients may react to nerve health components. The chemokine secretion level at the injection site is increased by activated dendritic cells and complementary elements activated by aluminium salts (HogenEsch 2002).

Many neurological demyelinating diseases are associated with vaccination. Rapid immerging ascending and symmetric motor paralysis, along with tendon reflex deprivation, indicates an auto polyradiculoneuropathy. GB patients have autoantibodies to gangliosides, and their T-cells react with nerve components. Vaccines exist for Guillain Barre Syndrome (GBS), rabies, influenza, BCG, toxoid, smallpox, tetanus, rubella, mumps, hepatitis B vaccine, oral poliovirus,and there are recombinant or plasma-derived vaccines and diptheria vaccine. Vaccination, gender, vaccine season, age are the relative risks associated with GBS (Lasky *et al* 1998). It is necessary to develop an innovative clinical trail associated with immune stimulation increasing complex modes of antigen presentation specific proteins, infections, viruses like particles, attenuated viruses, gene delivered immunogens and structured arrays. The properties and function of adjuvants should be studied again (Nabel 2013). There is a causal link between temporal association in vaccination and autoimmune disease, HBV influenza, and others. The preservatives and adjuvant can cause autoimmune disease, but an individual's genetic background is essential in determining the start of autoimmune phenomena. Identifying ASIA has initiated finding the good, bad, or ugly of vaccines in concert with adjuvant that triggers autoimmunity. The advantages of vaccines overcome the risks. However, to make a safer vaccine, more attention should be given. Silicone-based implants are safe for most subjects, identification of pre-existing autoimmune disease and genetic testing has played a vital role as a valuable tool for future risk such as stratification previous to implantation to avoid autoimmune disease. The interrelation between environmental factors and genetic susceptibility gained attention in epigenetics, geoepidemiology, twins' and gender infection use (Selmi *et al* 2012, Fu *et al* 2011).

3.2.3 Endothelial cells and NSCs as biomarkers

Adult neural stem cells (NSCs) subventricular zones lie close to blood vessels and are identified using automated computer-based image quantification and con-focal microscopy (Shen *et al* 2008). Glial fibrillary acidic protein (GFAP) cell expressing stem cell marker and proliferation marker instead of laminin comprise the extracellular matrix surrounding vascular endothelial cells. Apical GFAP occupies the microenvironment mixed within the ependymal layer between blood vessels and ventricles. Stem cells behaviour *in vitro* is regulated by the microenvironment (Fuchs *et al* 2004). Neurons are generated by neural stem cells throughout their life span in instructing neurogenesis hippocampal dentate gyrus (Alvarez-Buylla and Lim 2004). GFAP recident close to the vascular surface is expressed by a network of blood vessels lying within sub ventricular zone (SVZ) and NSCs. Determining the relationships of cells with vasculature, NSCs ependymal markers label the cells generating neurospheres in SVZ, T, and B cells (Capela and Temple 2002). NSCs self-renewal and neurogenesis *in vitro* is triggered by endothelial cells (Shen *et al* 2004). *In vivo*, the proliferation of normal SVZ occurs at the proximity of blood vessels. SVZ progenitor moves away from blood vessels and unexpectedly stimulates proliferation due to disturbance in a6 integrin function. T and B cells are close to the vessels to maintain touch with blood vessels and maintain stem cell properties. Proliferation rate increases due to treatment with an anti-a6 antibody which provides the hemostatic control to the stem cell close to the vessel. Progenitors are still in condition to diffuse signals from vessels and stimulate proliferation. Microglia is a class of glial cells derived from leptomeningeal mesenchymal cells (Bechmann *et al* 2007). The following things occur:

- The path from post-capillary venules to Virchow–Robin spaces.
- Advancement through glia limitans into neurophils. Moment of monocyte. Monocyte was the primary origin for the generation of microglia inside the brain (Bechmann *et al* 2005).

The blood generates monocytes cells infiltration. Monocytes networks reconstruct the microglia and axonal degeneration. High control in the microenvironment is required for neural signalling in CNS, given cells that form the interface between blood and CNS (Abbott *et al* 2010). The arachnoid barrier, blood–CSF barrier, and BBB are significant sites for blood CNS exchange. These barriers are composed of tight junctions, transport barriers, and vesicular mechanisms.

3.2.4 Dysferlin as a biomarker

In cell membrane repair, muscle protein involvement, namely dysferlin and its deficiency, causes muscular dystrophy (Hochmeister *et al* 2006). Dysferlin expresses leaky endothelial cells. In CNS, endothelial cells of circumventricular organs consist of dysferlin. In MS, the reactivity of dysferlin is introduced in endothelial cells, and its expression is related to vascular leakage of sperm protein. In inactive lessons and white matter, dysferlin expression is not found in many blood vessels with perivascular infiltrates. Dysferlin generates in endothelial cells, which in turn stimulates tumour necrosis factor. Thus, Dysferlin reveals BBB disturbance and dissociation in perivascular inflammatory enters and acts as leaky brain vessel marker. In neuropathology, BBB dysfunction is the major challenge.

3.2.5 The adaptability of the tight junction as a biomarker

TJ protein associated with the cytoskeleton alters acute and chronic disease. A cellular membrane was created inside the molecular network of BBB TJ. This cellular membrane stops the carriers of molecules in between blood and the interstitial fluid of blood. Thus, in the molecular organization of BBB TJ, there is formation of a cellular membrane that obstructs the transfer of molecules between blood and blood interstitial fluid. Occludin placed inside the TJ of endothelial cells provides a more extraordinary collision on TJ integrity (Bamforth *et al* 1999). It has also been reported that there is a deposit of occludin in neurons, microglia, and neurons in Alzheimer's disease (AD), vascular and front temporal dementia (Romanitan *et al* 2007), producing up-to-date function of occludin and TJ protein inside parthenogenesis of these dementias. The significant elements of BBB are Claudin-5, 3 and 12 (Nitta *et al* 2003, Wolburg 2006), whereas the existence of claudin-1 is contentious (Lee *et al* 2003).

3.3 Brain blood acting as carrier-mediated transporter

Transfer of nutrients, including hexoses, nucleosides, purines, vitamins, amines, and monocarboxylic acids, is facilitated by carrier-mediated transport in brains (Hawkins *et al* 2006, Deeken and Löscher 2007, Ohtsuki and Terasaki 2007, Simpson *et al* 2007, Spector and Johanson 2007). Glucose provides energy to the brain in order to enhance the carrier-mediated transport system of nutrients and is synchronized by plasma and brain metabolic requirements. The primary energy sources of the brain include GLUT1 glucose transporter, CNT2 adenosine transporter, L1 called the large neutral amino acid carrier, and MCT1 known as a Mono-Carp boxy late transporter 1 (Pardridge 2005). GLUT1 is a member of the sodium independent glucose transporter gene family in BBB. Additionally, raft-dependent endocytosis as receptors and ligands from cytomembrane (Lajoie and Nabi 2007) bound endocytosis of caveolae to regulate transcellular permeability. Smooth plasmalemma vesicle forms a subdomain of cholesterol. Sphingolipid-rich rafts have a high content of caveolin-1; they have regulatory functions for the lipid-based microdomains of BBB, which include transcellular permeability controlling transcytosis, endocytosis, and motioning (Parton and Richards 2003). Receptors of insulin, transferrin, albumin RAGE, ceruloplasmin, HDL, LDL, IL1, and VAMP-2 (vesicle-associated membrane protein-2) make up the caveolar membrane (Wolburg 2006) together with members of tyrosine kinase, members of MAPK pathways, heterotrimeric G proteins, the endothelial NO synthase, and protein kinase C.

3.3.1 Role of astrocytes-BEC in synaptic transmission

Astrocytes communicate with cells that are present between capillary BEC and neurons. Electrolyte metabolism and brain water regulation govern astrocytes and BEC interaction (Abbott *et al* 2006). Modulation of synaptic transmission, brain communication pathway, neuronal firing threshold, and plasticity is led by astrocytes (Nedergaard *et al* 2003, Newman 2003). Astrocyte signals control the neurons involving behavioural responses, neural responses, hormonal responses, and underlying hemostasis (Shimizu *et al* 2007). BBB endothelial cells provide a metabolic barrier to pass through the physical barrier, obstruct neural functions, and express various enzymes that alter endogenous and exogenous molecules (Pardridge 2005). Capillary endothelium, astrocytes, and pericytes express Cytoenzymes on the plasma membrane, including endopeptidases, aminopeptidases, and cholinesterase. In the BBC system, to facilitate the bidirectional transport across the blood barrier, hydrophilic molecules cross the endothelial walls to reach neuronal track (Deane and Zlokovic 2007). TJ dominates the papa-cellular permeability of the brain. Capillary endothelial transport across BBB constitutes ion, caveolae-mediated transport, efflux, receptor, and carrier-mediated transport. Initiation of the ATP-binding cassette transporters is done by these molecules from the brain endothelium (Hermann *et al* 2007). The ATP-dependent efflux transporter p-glycoprotein assist ingested toxic lipophilic metabolites in its rapid elimination (Loscher and Potschka 2005, Hermann *et al* 2007). MRD1a, MDR1 gene and MRD1b genes encodes p-GP.

3.3.2 Role of vasoactive mediators in neurotransmission

Neural activity is governed by potassium ion release on blood flow in a neurovascular vessel, leading to vasoactive mediators. The potassium ion is released during astrocytic spatial buffering and neuronal repolarization (Iadecola *et al* 1997). Activity evoked increases the potassium ion concentration, leading to increased blood flow (Iadecola *et al* 1991, Dreier *et al* 1995, Caesar *et al* 1999). Higher activity inside the neural enhances the hydrogen ions and product of ATP catabolism adenosine (Iliff *et al* 2003, Borden *et al* 2007). Interferons (IFNs) are signalling molecules released by host cells in response to various pathogens that act against the DNA and RNA viruses, tumour cells, and parasites. IFNs, in general, stimulate intracellular and intercellular networks that control the resistance against viral infection and improve innate immunity and tumour cells' survival and death.

Toll-like receptors induce IFNs. The interferon stimulated gene (ISG) IFNs simulate gene functions as an identifying viral infection and resisting via its potent proteins. The mutation or suppression of ISGs may affect the initiation and progression of cancer.

3.4 microRNA-based ND detection biomarkers

For diagnosis and monitoring the progression symptoms in NDD, it is necessary to locate effective biomarkers. NDD has exploited a significant loss of neurons and CNS damage. Therefore, it is essential to diagnose the symptoms early to enhance the effectiveness of disease-modifying therapies. Biomarkers may play a key role in early diagnosis of disease, classification of different subtypes of the disease, keeping track of response of therapeutic agent, and monitoring the progression of the illness (Shi *et al* 2009). The miRNA contributes to biomarker development in blood, saliva, and CSF (Chen *et al* 2008). miRNA comes as a product of apoptosis, active transport of cells through micro-vesicles resident within RISC protein (Etheridge *et al* 2011). miRNA profiling in CNS leads to developing miRNA-based biomarkers and circulating to disease-modifying treatments for ND clinical trials. Thus, miRNA plays an important role in AD diagnosis (Cogswell *et al* 2008). miRNA have a crucial function in brain development and neuronal specification, but their part under ND is still uninvestigated.

A sensitive qRT-PCR is used to identify the deregulation of miRNA expression. The miRNA binding site predictions are used to assess the pathway of miRNA's deregulate expression and interact with miRNA and RNA hybrid methods that construct hypergeometric enrichment (Johnson *et al et al* 1992, Ward *et al* 2008). The miRNA is called microRNA, a non-coding RNA molecule that transforms gene expression and our knowledge of miRNA biogenesis and function (Goodall *et al* 2013). The miRNA expression is considered to be a dysfunction of ALS, HD, PD, and AD. miRNA can target many genetic pathways, and its diversity makes it suitable for biomarker development and therapeutic agents in NDD (Friedman *et al* 2009). miRNA is found in a significant amount in the nervous system to develop neurite outgrowth, neuronal differentiation, dendritic spine morphology, and synaptic plasticity. In recent trends, the dysfunction of miRNAs in NDD has been recognized. miRNA functions in protein expression, molecular biomarkers responsible for identifying specific tissue expression patterns, tissue- disease-specific pathologies, dictating in CSF, plasma, serum, and other body fluids.

Molecular disorders result in a declination of cell surface expression, which causes migraine disease (Kahlig *et al* 2008). migraine is a common paroxysmal disorder that is related to transient motor weakness. Migraine FHM(Familial hemiplegic migraine) with aura symptoms, i.e., visual and speech disturbances (Thomsen *et al* 2003, van den Maagdenberg *et al* 2007). FHM3 (familial hemiplegic migraine type 3) occurs due to mutation in the *SCN1A* gene, which encodes voltage-gated sodium channel NaV1.1. The mutations L263V, L1549Q, and Q1489 identify in migraine disorder. L263V and Q1489K can generate the quantifiable sodium current, whereas L1649Q doesn't develop it. Q1489K exhibits the increase of persistent current, which enhances the slow inactivation and delays recovery from fast and slow inactivation. The functioning of inhibitory neurons is obstructed by loss in sodium channel activity. Relationships between migraines provide common disorders with common molecular mechanisms. Molecular markers showing the accumulation of amyloid-β (Aβ) peptides within the brain's extracellular space centre AD pathogenesis and work as a hallmark for AD diagnosis. Synaptic transmission results in the release of amyloid precursor protein (APP), which is endocytosed by the cell surface into the endosome, which triggers the amyloid-beta secretion into brain interstitial fluid. Aβ levels in ISF are significantly effective by inhibition of clathrin-mediated endocytosis. These data may be helpful in AD pathogenesis and therapeutic interventions (Selkoe 2001). Initial polymerization seed of Aβ is necessary for aggregating Ab, plaques formation and growth are controlled by a pool of Aβ in ISF (Gouras *et al* 2000, Meyer-Luehmann *et al* 2003).

3.4.1 DNA configuration changes independent of alterations of the nucleotide sequence

The process of gene regulation via covalent modification of DNA using RNA editing, including miRNA is called epigenetics. DNA methylation and histone protein tail act as a marker interface between environment and genetics (Herceg *et al* 2011). It has been reported that age-specific epigenetic drift suggests that the onset of age in NDD is altered by DNA methylation. Biomarkers that carry protein to the mitochondria act as AD markers, and these biomarkers signatures are developed through proteomics, metabolomics, and genetics. In AD, the changes in WBC could show a relationship to gene expression in the brain. TOMM40 is identified as a marker that carries protein to mitochondria in AD and reveals AD progression (Roses 2010, Chong *et al* 2013).

Epigenetic rearrangement is significant in motor neuron disorders (Tremolizzo *et al* 2014). The methylation of whole blood is identified as a promising age-onset modifier in ALS. It has been found that the percentage of DNA methylation enhances in ALS patients. As Hcy level decreases in early-onset ALS patients, independent of age, DNA methylation % is considered an epigenetic dysfunction marker in ALS. Dissecting studies of biological determinant complexity in ALS help develop therapeutic strategies. Risk modulating factors, including environment (Chio *et al* 2009, Beghi *et al* 2011) and genetic (Corcia *et al* 2012, Gellera *et al* 2012), may commune initiating various death pathways (Redler and Dokholyan 2012). In neurodegenerative disease, the advancing age acts as a risk factor. Toxicity developed from astrocytes and microglia impart in the progression of motor degeneration and ALS disease progression. The most usual form of inherited ALS is found due to mutated superoxide dimutase-1 (SOD1). To the influence neurovascular unit, the ALS disease confirms the toxicity from microglia, whereas astrocytes contribute to the progression of the disease and motor degeneration (Beers *et al* 2006, Boillée *et al* 2006, Di Giorgio *et al* 2007, Nagai *et al* 2007).

3.5 Protein-based biomarker for the injured brain

BBB prevents the free exchange of molecular movements between blood and brain, containing a firmly wrapped monolayer of brain endothelial cells (BEC) (Ohtsuki and Terasaki 2007). Drugs-related CNS therapeutic solutions modulate molecules <400 Da. Lipid interventions of tiny molecules of biological membranes need molecular excitement via a proper channel or medium within the lipid bilayer. BEC is usually linked with a tight junction (TJ) and adherence junctions (AJ) (Hawkins and Davis 2005). TJ mainly exchanges the low para-cellular penetrability and greater electrical control voltage and resistance within BBB (Bazzoni and Dejana 2004). Considering the autoantibodies of serum against the system of nervous proteins that decrease the sequential progressive relationship between exposures to air emissions and clinical condition are found in CNS injury. Serum autoantibodies have functioned as biomarkers for chemical-oriented CNS damage. The availability of clinical biomarkers for the injury of neurons is indispensable for diagnosing and observing the sequential development and temporal injury progression (Jauch *et al* 2006). Serum biomarkers and cytoskeleton proteins have dramatically enhanced care and treatment for patients suffering from TBI (TBI; Žurek *et al* 2012). The fragments of protein from glial cells and injured neuronal are established in CSF (cerebral spinal fluid), which have very short half-lives due to which they can be considered biomarkers.

3.5.1 Neuron-specific enolase (NSE)-based biomarker

Protein breakdown products (BDPs) are essential for identifying pathological characteristics of TBI. BDPs of the dendritically enhanced microtubule-binding protein Tau and alpha-II spectrin structures correlate with the acuteness of injury in rodent models of TBI. Total brain proteins containing alpha and beta-tubulin that exist in nerve cells are influenced by ND (Abou-Donia *et al* 2013). The nervous system (NS) is linked with the seven proteins group, autoantibodies. The numerous types of nerve cells are characterized by the protein that is caused during their neuronal degeneration. The usage of protein biomarkers grants various advantages for the clinical diagnosis and treatment of mTBI. At first, the biomarker measures the peripheral tissues, including the urine, saliva, and blood, which are nominally cost-effective in analyzing, processing, and treating and are comparatively less invasive. Second, the different levels of a biomarker can certainly indicate and specify brain damage.

Moreover, this helps to determine whether brain imaging is essential for a person who sustains in mTBI. Biomarker estimates the significant injury and detects the change in neurobehavioral dysfunction. This suggests that the damage of the brain is not homogeneously disseminated but instead restricted to certain local regions. Further, the deterioration of specific brain regions brings substantial functional and structural changes that may result from the drastic proliferation or reduction in the different levels of a biomarker.

3.6 Use of synaptic vesicles for the treatment of AD

Synaptic vesicle is adequate to initiate and drive the supply of Aβ from neurons (Cirrito *et al* 2005). Vesicle exocytosis is an original and fundamental mechanism responsible for Aβ fabrication and discharge from neurons. Amyloid precursor protein (APP) is often retrieved and recovered from the cell's exterior through clathrin-mediated endocytosis (Nordstedt *et al* 1993). Synaptic dynamic activity and movement in endocytosis too energies more APP into the endocytic subdivision, increasing the higher production of Aβ. The release of Aβ into the ISF of the brain succeeds the synaptic transmission, which is needed for keeping an intermediate event containing APP endocytosis. This is acquired and captured by analyzing a volume of brain tissue and recording the EEG signals. Aβ is also supported by findings of a pathologic study of AD (Wegiel *et al* 2001). Tau is vital for recognizing the amyloid-induced neurotoxicity (Rapoport *et al* 2002). Fibrillary-amyloid affects neurofibrillary changes only in neurons involving neurofibrillary degeneration that occurs early in the medial temporal structures that represent the toxic effects of amyloid. Molecular mechanisms of different brain areas are responsible for developing NDD (Schmitt 2005), captured through fMRI with more excellent task-specific activity. Brain regions with high basal activity show as more prone to amyloid deposition (Buckner *et al* 2005).

Further, Johnson *et al* (2013) have found that carbon-11 PiB is considered a biomarker of AD, measured using positron emission tomography (PET). Amyloid PET and carbon-11 (C-11)-labelled Pittsburgh compound B (PiB) are developed as the chief elements of AD transformation. Pathologic changes of AD are characterized by the cortical grey matter and the accumulation of neurofibrillary tangles, the loss of synaptic and neuronal loss that yield the atrophy of the cerebrum (Naggara *et al* 2006). Pathologic involvement of atrophy shows the initial atrophy in the hippocampus area of patients suffering from mild AD (Brun *et al* 1986, Hanyu *et al* 1999, Kantarci *et al* 2001). The decreased anisotropy in working memory is bilaterally found in the splenium in early AD (Jack *et al* 2010). MRI measurement of CSF tau shows cerebral atrophy that increases neural injury, which is considered a biomarker. The synaptic dysfunction that decreases the fluorodeoxyglucose uptake on PET is mainly due to the degeneration of neurons. These molecular biomarkers facilitate drug development (Klunk *et al* 2004) to combat NDD, considering cognitive and clinical symptom severity.

3.6.1 Autoantibodies to MBP trajectory

Autoantibodies to MBP, a membrane proteolipid, are shaped by Schwann cells in the PNS and oligodendroglia in the CNS (Jauch *et al* 2006). The axonal degeneration which occurs in both PNS and CNS is primarily induced and motivated by the contact of OPs (Abou-Donia 1981). The proteins related to MAP-2 presented in various somatodendritic compartments on neurons exhibit a high level of autoantibodies. The microtubule linked with tau and MAP-2 promotes microtubules connection, cross bridge neurofilaments, polymerization, and stabilization in axons. Autoantibodies to tubulin are presented in virtually all eukaryotic cells and neurons.

3.6.2 Differentiation of AD from bvFTD

Differentiating the clinical classification of bvFTD from AD can certainly be problematic in the life of patients (Mendez *et al* 1993, Varma *et al* 1999,

Rascovsky *et al* 2007). The accurate diagnostic of bvFTD is essentially a critical projection and prediction (Rascovsky *et al* 2005, Roberson *et al* 2005, Chow *et al* 2006) from the point of view of therapeutics (Swartz *et al* 1997, Moretti *et al* 2003, Du Pasquier *et al* 2003, Lebert *et al* 2004, Huey *et al* 2006) and environmental management of patients. Therefore, various criteria should be fixed to decrease the diagnostic features, eliminate any arbitrary division between core and peripheral features, permit a more excellent elasticity to define diagnostic features, and offer more explicit operational procedures by incorporating different types of genetic and neuroimaging findings and distinguishing between possible and fixed bvFTD (Perry and Miller 2001, Robinson 2001, Talerico and Evans 2001, Merrilees and Miller 2003). Further, AD brains reveal neurofibrillary tangles and amyloid plaques (Heneka *et al* 2010). It also exposes neuro-inflammatory dynamics by connecting astrocytes and activated microglia. This discharge of inflammatory mediators includes various components of cytokines, reactive oxygen species, and chemokines. A systematic infection and inflammation modulate the systematic function of the immune and switch the immune cells to a belligerent pro-inflammatory phenotype that can increase the productive power of cytokine and the damage of neurons (Perry and Teeling 2013).

3.6.3 Epileptogenesis biomarkers and PD

So far, no biomarker has been measured to find different aspects of epileptogenesis. The identification and recognition of dependable biomarkers of epileptogenesis could also be used to formulate cost-effective antiepileptogenic drugs and compounds. Epileptogenesis biomarkers have many users and applications for diagnosing, discovering, and validating the anti-epileptogenic interventions (Pitkänen and Engel 2014). It is observed that Parkinson's disease is developed due to degeneration and deactivation of dopamine generation nerve cells in the brain that impairs the motor system. The depletion of dopamine production that damages the nerves of motor neurons cannot coordinate and control body movement (Braak *et al* 2006). Thus, PD is characterized by difficulty in walking, slow moves (bradykinesia), tremors, poor balance, stiffness, and Parkinson's gait symptoms.

GFAP is a unique filamentous protein transduced by astrocytes (80) after TBI. Ubiquitin carboxy-terminal hydrolase L1 (UCHL1), a small cysteine 25 kDa, develops a C-terminal bond between UCHLI and a polypeptide. This enzyme contains a minimum of 1%–2% of the solvable protein in the brain, connected within neurons and neuroendocrine cells. Metabolites lipids, glycolytic intermediates, and neurotransmitters have revealed some possible biomarkers for recognizing TBI. TBI often changes glucose, lactate, glycerol, glutamate, and pyruvate levels in the CSF microdialysates resulting from the injured brain. Phosphocreatine and creatine levels are reviewed after mTBI that increases different levels and layers of metabolites in white matter persisting for up to a maximum of four months of post-injury. One of the injury biomarkers is N-acetylaspartic acid (NAA) in the brain, which is detectable by using MRS protons. NAA is considered a marker of neuronal integrity that indicates neuronal damage for multiple sclerosis, amyotrophic lateral sclerosis (ALS), TBI, and vascular dementia. MBP is the most critical myelin protein module transduced by oligodendrocytes. The MBP test is used to assess cerebrospinal fluid proteins under neurological conditions where demyelination occurs. The white matter that prolix the axonal injury can release the MBP into the serum and CSF. MBP can cause concern for introducing the BBB, enabling its entry into CNS that derives a biomarker.

3.6.4 Conversion from aMCI to ADB using biomarker

Baseline STAND and CSF biomarkers that are estimated by using single-predictor Cox measure the functions of survivorship. Here the baseline STAND is interlinked with a diminutive form of transformation. STAND and log (tau/ A_1–42) are shown to have a predictive power to observe the alternation from aMCI to AD. When CDR-SB over time by the quartiles of biomarker across diagnostic groups, MRI predicts more decline of CDR-SB than CSF. In this context, cognitive paralysis and dysfunction damage the white matter. In the case of structural evaluation for axial or micro-bleeding legions, no abnormalities were found in proton MRS, sensitive-weighted MRI, DTI, andT1-weighted MRI.

The neurofilament protein (NFP) subunit contains various components of the neuronal cytoskeleton (Fuchs *et al* 1998), including extrinsic or high-molecular-weight (NF-H) protein and medium or low-molecular-weight protein (NF-M) and low-molecular-weight (NF-l). These cells control the axonal calibre, including neurofilaments that affect neuronal function and axonal transport (Tagliaferro *et al* 2006). Tau proteins, which form bundles of microtubules and cellular proteins, are located mainly in the axial compartments of neurons. Tau proteins are more abundant in white matter than grey matter in AD patients with TBI (Liliang *et al* 2010). Astrocyte proteins such as S100 and GFAP raised more crew than the control group. Increased layers and levels of autoantibodies in GFAP are interlinked with gliosis from astrocytes after degradation of the cytoskeleton, cellular disintegration and CNS injury (Kövesdi *et al* 2010). GFAP is considered to be a non-specific biomarker of regions of the brain damage leading to several CNS diseases such as dementia (Eng *et al* 1994), Lyme neuroborreliosis (Dotevall *et al* 1999), neuro-psychiatric disorders (Ahlsén *et al* 1993, Kapural *et al* 2002) and cerebral infarction (Aurell *et al* 1991). Traumatic acute injury extensively destroys the astrocytes while releasing a significant amount of S100B (Arolt *et al* 2003) and associating with neuroprotective capability. The discovery of biomarkers helps evaluate exposure and also may aid in regulating the differences across patients diagnosed with clinical illnesses (Schopfer *et al* 2010, Marsillach *et al* 2011, Liyasova *et al* 2011). Peptide bond checks dipeptides using the L1 amino acid transport system (Zlokovic *et al* 1983). Endothelial cells are functioned to express several transport systems for the development of enkephalins (Zlokovic *et al* 1989), neuroactive peptides, and several cytokines and chemokines (Zlokovic *et al* 1990, Banks 2006).

3.7 Heart failure (HF) and mTBI as a regulatory feature of ND

Chronic heart failure is complemented by some structural damage of the central nervous system (CNS). The loss of tissue leads to injury in a specific brain region

(Woo *et al* 2003), confirming neural and cardiovascular responses (Woo *et al* 2005). Brain injury often subsidizes the various morbidities in HF syndrome patients (Packer *et al* 1992). Further, patients with HF decrease the cerebral blood flow beyond the auto-control and regulatory mechanisms. These types of stress are tempted by numerous factors within the syndrome of HF, chronic activation (Tang *et al* 2005), inflammation (Jankowska *et al* 2006), and hormonal abnormalities. Partition of the injurious is also processed by the blockade of sensitive mechanisms, the regional evaluation of perfusion, the minimization of hypoxic exposure due to sleep-related breathing pathology. To perform non-sedated MRI function on HF subjects is reduced the progressive and developmental nature of the disease. The loss of GM volume in the brain is essential for regulating perception, mood, memory, and sympathetic and parasympathetic dyspnea in the bilateral insular cortices, mid-hippocampus, and the superior frontal gyrus.

Memory deficits, mood disturbances, and autonomic dysfunction also appear in adult heart failure (HF) and pediatric diseases (Menteer *et al* 2010). For example, brain areas that control memory functions deflect, mood disturbances, and autonomic dysfunction damage adult HF patients with HF and associated cerebrovascular disease. In addition, many comorbidities and physiological abnormalities, including various cognitive paralysis and functional impairments, are responsible for chronic heart failure (HF) (Putzke *et al* 1998, Almeida *et al* 2001), depression (Havranek *et al* 1999, Murberg *et al* 1999, Vaccarino *et al* 2001), anxiety (Murberg *et al* 1999, Spurkland *et al* 2001, Jiang *et al* 2004), impulsivity (Laakso *et al* 2001, Wernovsky *et al* 2005), and altered autonomic regulation (Esler *et al* 1997, Massin *et al* 1998, Ohuchi *et al* 2003).

As a neurodegenerative disease, amyotrophic lateral sclerosis (ALS) is classified by cell injury, the damage in the upper part of motor neurons in the cerebral cortex. This also manifests as the death of motor neurons in the lower spinal cord and brainstem (Brockington *et al* 2006). It is triggered by the mutations and modulation of Cu/Zn superoxide dismutase (SOD1) that gains toxic elements during the protein mutation. Several pathogenic mechanisms, including inflammation, neurofilament dysfunction, oxidative stress, mitochondrial, and excitotoxicity, activate the death cell pathway in the late-onset of neurodegeneration. The lower motor neurons and upper motor neurons that express the VEGF and VEGFR2 in the cortex are controlled by anterior horn cells (AHCs) for ALS.

3.7.1 Correlation of energy and hypermia

Energy deficit increases the CBF (Attwell and Laughlin 2001, Shulman *et al* 2004) and the functional aspects of hyperemia. This is required for understanding how the brain demands local energy. It has been observed that inhibitory synapses require much less energy than excitatory synapses (Waldvogel *et al* 2000), which increases glucose in the hippocampal area (Ackermann *et al* 1984, Nudo *et al* 1986). Energy that is produced through the anaerobic metabolism of glucose derives from oxidative metabolism. Brain activation increases glycogen utilization. The activation is maximal at the onset, reducing within time (Prichard *et al* 1991). Even at the beginning of activation, the consumption level of oxygen increases minimally, and then it increases continuously during the progress of activation (Fox *et al* 1986, Mintun *et al* 2002). The gradual decrease and increase in oxygen consumption are manifest in the aerobic metabolism of neurons. NADH is produced by transferring protons and electrons during metabolism (Ido *et al* 2004). Lactic acid, which provides additional electrons and protons, is transmitted to NADH, converting it to NAD (+).

3.8 Nanomaterial-based biomarkers for ND

The spinal cord, including the cellular structure of the brain, obfuscates the treatment procedures of ND. Nanotechnology presents a potential solution to this problem enabling the systematic structural interaction with biological layers at the molecular level. Nanomaterials infuse the BBB, which is a collective complication for CNS to target therapeutic modification of the activity of biological stimuli. Nanoscale materials provide products delivered through the BBB to treat CNS diseases and increase the flow of cerebrospinal fluid (CSF) in the brain. In the case of ND, the nano-engineered molecules are crossed through the BBB, targeting some signaling cells to stimulate cell survival and axon elongation (Srikanth and Kessler 2012).

Nanofiber-based biomarkers and nano scaffolds provide structural and trophic support for endogenous and transplanted cells incorporating gene delivery, imaging capabilities, and bioactivity. Nanoscale suppression of Aβ accumulation and plaque formations are investigated for AD treatment. Using nanotechnology methods, the cell membrane environment promotes the α-helical structure of Aβ and reduces the ability of Aβ to accumulate in plaques (Brambilla *et al* 2011). Nanomicelles are alleviated by adding polyethylene glycol (PEG) (Kohno *et al* 1996). The onset of AD is mainly due to oxidative damage, which drives the antioxidants as possible treatments for this disorder (Nunomura *et al* 2001). These molecular compounds are essential to protect neurons as opposed to the excitotoxicity caused by glutamate receptors. So far, neuroprotection against Aβ toxicity has not yet been demonstrated. Acetylcholine hardly crosses the BBB.

As a nano-carrier for acetylcholine, a single-walled carbon nanotube can cross the BBB. Carbon nanotubes with biocompatible components have been explored based on cytotoxicity by considering nanomaterials. The range of non-cytotoxic involved in the delivery of carbon nanotubes was transmitted only to lysosomes but not to mitochondria. Carbon nanotubes are possible nano supports used in the treatment of ND (Yang *et al* 2010). BBB hybridization was facilitated when poly N-butyl cyanoacrylate (PBCA) nanoparticles were coated with polysorbate-80 in compressed form into uncoated particles (Kim *et al* 2007). The presence of PBCA essentially enhances the delivery distribution of rivastigmine in the brain. The properties of cholinesterase inhibitors are enlarged due to nanocarriers that effectively treat AD (Wilson *et al* 2008).

Further, nanotubes consisting of multiwalled carbon with a considerable nerve growth factor (NGF) show extensive growth in *in vitro* PC12 cells and the dorsal root of ganglion neurons (Matsumoto *et al* 2010). The properties of carbon nanotubes that intensify conductive circuits support the electrical connectivity of neurons (Cellot *et al* 2009). The integration and interaction of cells are enhanced by the carbon nanotubes transplanted into the striatum (Mazzatenta *et al* 2007). This raises the possibility of treatment by using a carbon nanotube via deep brain stimulation. Numerous cell lines are induced by carbon nanotubes that are found in the case of apoptosis and necrosis.

3.8.1 Therapeutic management of AD using nano-carriers

Nanocarriers are often used to aid and target the BBB at the molecular level, efficiently transporting drugs into the brain. Plasma membrane highly expresses a DNA aptamer to target cancer cells, nucleolin, and tumour endothelium (Fogal *et al* 2009, Hovanessian *et al* 2010), increasing the resultant anti-proliferative features of paclitaxel against C6 glioma cells (Guo *et al* 2011). To treat CNS disorder, the BBB, cellular environment, and multiple signalling modalities are taken into consideration. To suppress Aβ oligomerization, nanoscale approaches are used to decrease volatile oxygen species and improve functional aspects of neuronal networks. This is achieved by the application of carbon nanotubes for the treatment of ND. Nanoscale scaffolds rewire the optic nerve and spinal cord. Nanocarriers enable the target of the delivery of chemotherapeutics and therapy of genes, ensuing an embarrassment to the progression of brain tumours. Nanotechnology contains an incredible potential in clinical neuroscience for accomplishing the task of revamping the CNS. The disease related to the CNS has a mutual and collective power of nanoscale involvements and the growth of cells to advance the biological underlying of the processes elaborate in this disorder.

3.9 Conclusion

Amyloid imaging is helpful to predict the future clinical condition of MCI and dementia. Amyloid imaging plays an essential role in classifying patients with cognitive impairment and the clinical status of MCI or dementia (Forsberg *et al* 2008, Okello *et al* 2009, Wolk *et al* 2009, Morris *et al* 2009). The slow rate of decline in memory function suggests that amyloid accumulation may accelerate dementia (Jack *et al* 2010, Villemagne *et al* 2011). The imaging techniques to apply presynaptic dopaminergic and amyloid-beta are observed in AD, DLB, and FTD (Burke *et al* 2011). Stem cell defence is mechanized by scaffold design. Inhibition of glial scar formation promotes demyelination of axons that attempt to regenerate and transplant the stem cell for fostering a tolerant atmosphere for the repair of CNS (Hannila *et al* 2007). Technology related to non-material developments is particularly suitable for developing such multimodal dynamic therapy to combat ND.

References

Abbott N J 2002 Astrocyte–endothelial interactions and blood–brain barrier permeability *J. Anat.* **200** 523–34

Abbott N J, Patabendige A A, Dolman D E, Yusof S R and Begley D J 2010 Structure and function of the blood–brain barrier *Neurobiol. Dis.* **37** 13–25

Abbott N J, Rönnbäck L and Hansson E 2006 Astrocyte–endothelial interactions at the blood–brain barrier *Nature Rev. Neurosci.* **7** 41–53

Abou-Donia M B, Abou-Donia M M, ElMasry E M, Monro J A and Mulder M F 2013 Autoantibodies to nervous system-specific proteins are elevated in sera of flight crew members: biomarkers for nervous system injury *J. Toxicol. Environ. Health* A **76** 363–80

Abou-Donia M B 1981 Organophosphorus ester-induced delayed neurotoxicity *Ann. Rev. Pharmacol. Toxicol.* **21** 511–48

Ackermann R F, Finch D M, Babb T L and Engel J 1984 Increased glucose metabolism during long-duration recurrent inhibition of hippocampal pyramidal cells *J. Neurosci.* **4** 251–64

Ahlsén G, Rosengren L, Belfrage M, Palm A, Haglid K, Hamberger A and Gillberg C 1993 Glial fibrillary acidic protein in the cerebrospinal fluid of children with autism and other neuropsychiatric disorders *Biol. Psych.* **33** 734–43

Allt G and Lawrenson J G 2001 Pericytes: cell biology and pathology *Cell Tissues Organs* **169** 1–11

Almeida O P and Flicker L 2001 The mind of a failing heart: a systematic review of the association between congestive heart failure and cognitive functioning *Intern. Med. J.* **31** 290–5

Almeida A, Almeida J, Bolaños J P and Moncada S 2001 Different responses of astrocytes and neurons to nitric oxide: the role of glycolytically generated ATP in astrocyte protection *Proc. Natl Acad. Sci.* **98** 15294–9

Alvarez-Buylla A and Lim D A 2004 For the long run: maintaining germinal niches in the adult brain *Neuron* **41** 683–6

Anderson V M, Fox N C and Miller D H 2006 Magnetic resonance imaging measures of brain atrophy in multiple sclerosis *J. Magnetic Reson. Imaging: An. Off. J. Int. Soc. Magnetic Reson. Med.* **23** 605–18

Archer H A, Edison P, Brooks D J, Barnes J, Frost C, Yeatman T, Fox N C and Rossor M N 2006 Amyloid load and cerebral atrophy in Alzheimer's disease: an 11C-PIB positron emission tomography study *Ann. Neurol.* **60** 145–7

Armulik A, Abramsson A and Betsholtz C 2005 Endothelial/pericyte interactions *Circ. Res.* **97** 512–23

Arolt V, Peters M, Erfurth A, Wiesmann M, Missler U, Rudolf S, Kirchner H and Rothermundt M 2003 S100B and response to treatment in major depression: a pilot study *Eur. Neuropsychopharmacol.* **13** 235–9

Attwell D and Laughlin S B 2001 An energy budget for signaling in the grey matter of the brain *J. Cereb. Blood Flow. Metab.* **21** 1133–45

Aurell A, Rosengren L E, Karlsson B, Olsson J E, Zbornikova V and Haglid K G 1991 Determination of S-100 and glial fibrillary acidic protein concentrations in cerebrospinal fluid after brain infarction *Stroke* **22** 1254–8

Bacskai B J *et al* 2007 Molecular imaging with Pittsburgh Compound B confirmed at autopsy: a case report *Arch. Neurol.* **64** 431–4

Bailey T L, Rivara C B, Rocher A B and Hof P R 2004 The nature and effects of cortical microvascular pathology in aging and Alzheimer's disease *Neurol. Res.* **26** 573–8

Baker M *et al* 2006 Mutations in progranulin cause tau-negative frontotemporal dementia linked to chromosome 17 *Nature* **442** 916–19

Bamforth S D, Kniesel U, Wolburg H, Engelhardt B and Risau W 1999 A dominant mutant of occludin disrupts tight junction structure and function *J. Cell Sci.* **112** 1879–88

Banks W A 2006 The CNS as a target for peptides and peptide-based drugs *Expert. Opin. Drug. Deliv.* **3** 707–12

Banks J A 2006 Improving race relations in schools: from theory and research to practice *J. Soc. Issues* **62** 607–14

Barkhof F, Calabresi P A, Miller D H and Reingold S C 2009 Imaging outcomes for neuroprotection and repair in multiple sclerosis trials *Nat. Rev. Neurol.* **5** 256–66

Barnes J, Boyes R G, Lewis E B, Schott J M, Frost C, Scahill R I and Fox N C 2007 Automatic calculation of hippocampal atrophy rates using a hippocampal template and the boundary shift integral *Neurobiol. Aging* **28** 1657–63

Bazzoni G and Dejana E 2004 Endothelial cell-to-cell junctions: molecular organization and role in vascular homeostasis *Physiol. Rev.* **84** 869–901

Bechmann I *et al* 2005 Circulating monocytic cells infiltrate layers of anterograde axonal degeneration where they transform into microglia *FASEB J.* **19** 1–19

Bechmann I, Galea I and Perry V H 2007 What is the blood–brain barrier (not)? *Trends Immunol.* **28** 5–11

Beers D R, Henkel J S, Xiao Q, Zhao W, Wang J, Yen A A, Siklos L, McKercher S R and Appel S H 2006 Wild-type microglia extend survival in PU. 1 knockout mice with familial amyotrophic lateral sclerosis *Proc. Natl Acad. Sci.* **103** 16021–6

Beghi E *et al* 2007 The heterogeneity of amyotrophic lateral sclerosis: a possible explanation of treatment failure *Curr. Med. Chem.* **14** 3185–200

Beghi E *et al* 2011 Incidence and predictors of acute symptomatic seizures after stroke *Neurology* **77** 1785–93

Begley D J and Brightman M W 2003 Structural and functional aspects of the blood–brain barrier *Peptide Transp. Deliv. Cent. Nerv. Syst.* 39–78

Bermel R A, You X, Foulds P, Hyde R, Simon J H, Fisher E and Rudick R A 2013 Predictors of long-term outcome in multiple sclerosis patients treated with interferon beta *Ann. Neurol.* **73** 95–103

Bielekova B *et al* 2005 MRI as a marker for disease heterogeneity in multiple sclerosis *Neurology* **65** 1071–6

Block M L and Hong J S 2005 Microglia and inflammation-mediated neurodegeneration: multiple triggers with a common mechanism *Prog. Neurobiol.* **76** 77–98

Boillée S, Yamanaka K, Lobsiger C S, Copeland N G, Jenkins N A, Kassiotis G, Kollias G and Cleveland D W 2006 Onset and progression in inherited ALS determined by motor neurons and microglia *Science* **312** 1389–92

Bonilha L, Rorden C, Halford J J, Eckert M, Appenzeller S, Cendes F and Li L M 2007 Asymmetrical extra-hippocampal grey matter loss related to hippocampal atrophy in patients with medial temporal lobe epilepsy *J. Neurol. Neurosurg. Psych.* **78** 286–94

Bonzano L, Tacchino A, Roccatagliata L, Abbruzzese G, Mancardi G L and Bove M 2008 Callosal contributions to simultaneous bimanual finger movements *J. Neurosci.* **28** 3227–33

Borden E C, Sen G C, Uze G, Silverman R H, Ransohoff R M, Foster G R and Stark G R 2007 Interferons at age 50: past, current and future impact on biomedicine *Nat. Rev. Drug. Discov.* **6** 975–90

Borghammer P, Cumming P, Aanerud J and Gjedde A 2009 Artefactual subcortical hyperperfusion in PET studies normalized to global mean: lessons from Parkinson's disease *Neuroimage* **45** 249–57

Botvinick M M, Braver T S, Barch D M, Carter C S and Cohen J D 2001 Conflict monitoring and cognitive control *Psychol. Rev.* **108** 624

Braak H, Bohl J R, Müller C M, Rüb U, de Vos R A and Del Tredici K 2006 Stanley Fahn Lecture 2005: the staging procedure for the inclusion body pathology associated with sporadic Parkinson's disease reconsidered *Mov. Disord.: Off. J. Mov. Disord. Soc.* **21** 2042–51

Brambilla D L, Droumaguet B, Nicolas J, Hashemi S H, Wu L P, Moghimi S M, Couvreur P and Andrieux K 2011 Nanotechnologies for Alzheimer's disease: diagnosis, therapy, and safety issues *Nanomed. Nanotechnol. Biol. Med.* **7** 521–40

Brink B P, Mork S J, Van Der Valk P and Bo L 2004 Grey matter pathology in multiple sclerosis *Normal-appearing White and Grey Matter Damage in Multiple Sclerosis* (Milano: Springer) pp 101–9

Brockington A, Wharton S B, Fernando M, Gelsthorpe C H, Baxter L, Ince P G, Lewis C E and Shaw P J 2006 Expression of vascular endothelial growth factor and its receptors in the central nervous system in amyotrophic lateral sclerosis *J. Neuropathol. Exp. Neurol.* **65** 26–36

Brown A M, Tekkök S B and Ransom B R 2003 Glycogen regulation and functional role in mouse white matter *J. Physiol.* **549** 501–12

Brun A and Englund E 1986 Brain changes in dementia of Alzheimer's type relevant to new imaging diagnostic methods *Prog. Neuro-Psychopharmacol. Biol. Psych.* **10** 297–308

Buckner R L *et al* 2005 Molecular, structural, and functional characterization of Alzheimer's disease: evidence for a relationship between default activity, amyloid, and memory *J. Neurosci.* **25** 7709–17

Büki A and Povlishock J T 2006 All roads lead to disconnection? Traumatic axonal injury revisited *Acta Neurochir.* **148** 181–94

Burke J F, Albin R L, Koeppe R A, Giordani B, Kilbourn M R, Gilman S and Frey K A 2011 Assessment of mild dementia with amyloid and dopamine terminal positron emission tomography *Brain* **134** 1647–57

Bussière T *et al* 2002 Stereologic assessment of the total cortical volume occupied by amyloid deposits and its relationship with cognitive status in aging and Alzheimer's disease *Neuroscience* **112** 75–91

Cabeza R and Nyberg L 2000 Imaging cognition II: an empirical review of 275 PET and fMRI studies *J. Cognit. Neurosci.* **12** 1–47

Caesar A J 1999 Insect-pathogen synergisms are the foundation of weed biocontrol *Proc. 10th Int. Symp. on Biological Control of Weeds*

Cameron B and Landreth G E 2010 Inflammation, microglia, and Alzheimer's disease *Neurobiol. Dis.* **37** 503–9

Capela A and Temple S 2002 LeX/ssea-1 is expressed by adult mouse CNS stem cells, identifying them as nonependymal *Neuron* **35** 865–75

Cardo L F, Coto E, de Mena L, Ribacoba R, Moris G, Menéndez M and Alvarez V 2013 Profile of microRNAs in the plasma of Parkinson's disease patients and healthy controls *J. Neurol.* **260** 1420–2

Cellot G *et al* 2009 Carbon nanotubes might improve neuronal performance by favouring electrical shortcuts *Nat. Nanotechnol.* **4** 126–33

Chen X *et al* 2008 Characterization of microRNAs in serum: a novel class of biomarkers for diagnosis of cancer and other diseases *Cell Res.* **18** 997–1006

Chestnut B A, Chang Q, Price A, Lesuisse C, Wong M and Martin L J 2011 Epigenetic regulation of motor neuron cell death through DNA methylation *J. Neurosci.* **31** 16619–36

Chetelat G, Desgranges B, De La Sayette V, Viader F, Eustache F and Baron J C 2002 Mapping gray matter loss with voxel-based morphometry in mild cognitive impairment *Neuroreport* **13** 1939–43

Chio A, Logroscino G, Hardiman O, Swingler R, Mitchell D, Beghi E, Traynor B G and Consortium E 2009 Prognostic factors in ALS: a critical review *Amyotroph. Lateral Scler.* **10** 310–23

Chong M S, Goh L K, Lim W S, Chan M, Tay L, Chen G, Feng L, Ng T P, Tan C H and Lee T S 2013 Gene expression profiling of peripheral blood leukocytes shows consistent longitudinal downregulation of TOMM40 and upregulation of KIR2DL5A, PLOD1, and SLC2A8 among fast progressors in early Alzheimer's disease *J. Alzheimer's Dis.* **34** 399–405

Chow T W, Hynan L S and Lipton A M 2006 MMSE scores decline at a greater rate in frontotemporal degeneration than in AD *Dement. Geriatr. Cognit. Disord.* **22** 194–9

Cirrito J R *et al* 2005 Synaptic activity regulates interstitial fluid amyloid-β levels in vivo *Neuron* **48** 913–22

Cirrito J R, Kang J E, Lee J, Stewart F R, Verges D K, Silverio L M, Bu G, Mennerick S and Holtzman D M 2008 Endocytosis is required for synaptic activity-dependent release of amyloid-β vivo *Neuron* **58** 42–51

Cogswell J P *et al* 2008 Identification of miRNA changes in Alzheimer's disease brain and CSF yields putative biomarkers and insights into disease pathways *J. Alzheimer's Dis.* **14** 27–41

Colcombe S J, Kramer A F, Erickson K I, Scalf P, McAuley E, Cohen N J, Webb A, Jerome G J, Marquez D X and Elavsky S 2004 Cardiovascular fitness, cortical plasticity, and aging *Proc. Natl Acad. Sci.* **101** 3316–21

Coles S, Heffernan J and Tawn J 1999 Dependence measures for extreme value analyses *Extremes* **2** 339–65

Corcia P *et al* 2012 Homozygous SMN2 deletion is a protective factor in the Swedish ALS population *Eur. J. Hum. Genet.* **20** 588–91

Cox J L, Chapman G, Murray D and Jones P 1996 Validation of the Edinburgh Postnatal Depression Scale (EPDS) in non-postnatal women *J. Affect. Dis.* **39** 185–9

Croll S D *et al* 2004 VEGF-mediated inflammation precedes angiogenesis in adult brain *Exp. Neurol.* **187** 388–402

Cruts M, Gijselinck I, Van Der Zee J, Engelborghs S, Wils H, Pirici D, Rademakers R, Vandenberghe R, Dermaut B, Martin J J and Van Duijn C 2006 Null mutations in progranulin cause ubiquitin-positive frontotemporal dementia linked to chromosome 17q21 *Nature* **442** 920–4

Csuka E, Hans V H, Ammann E, Trentz O, Kossmann T and Morganti-Kossmann M C 2000 Cell activation and inflammatory response following traumatic axonal injury in the rat *Neuroreport* **11** 2587–90

Davatzikos C, Fan Y, Wu X, Shen D and Resnick S M 2008 Detection of prodromal Alzheimer's disease via pattern classification of magnetic resonance imaging *Neurobiol. Aging* **29** 514–23

De Leon M J *et al* 2004 MRI and CSF studies in the early diagnosis of Alzheimer's disease *J. Intern. Med.* **256** 205–23

Deane R and Zlokovic B V 2007 Role of the blood–brain barrier in the pathogenesis of Alzheimer's disease *Curr. Alzheimer Res.* **4** 191–7

Deeken J F and Löscher W 2007 The blood–brain barrier and cancer: transporters, treatment, and Trojan horses *Clin. Cancer Res.* **13** 1663–74 del Zoppo G J and Milner R 2006 Integrin–matrix interactions in the cerebral microvasculature *Arter. Thromb. Vasc. Biol.* **26** 1966–75

Del Tredici K, Rüb U, De Vos R A, Bohl J R and Braak H 2002 Where does parkinson disease pathology begin in the brain? *J. Neuropathol. Exp. Neurol.* **61** 413–26

DeLuca G C, Williams K, Evangelou N, Ebers G C and Esiri M M 2006 The contribution of demyelination to axonal loss in multiple sclerosis *Brain* **129** 1507–16

Detre J A and Wang J 2002 Technical aspects and utility of fMRI using BOLD and ASL *Clin. Neurophysiol.* **113** 621–34

Devanand D P *et al* 2007 Hippocampal and entorhinal atrophy in mild cognitive impairment: prediction of Alzheimer disease *Neurology* **68** 828–36

Di Giorgio F P, Carrasco M A, Siao M C, Maniatis T and Eggan K 2007 Non–cell autonomous effect of glia on motor neurons in an embryonic stem cell–based ALS model *Nat. Neurosci.* **10** 608–14

Dong H, Zhang W, Zeng X, Hu G, Zhang H, He S and Zhang S 2014 Histamine induces upregulated expression of histamine receptors and increases release of inflammatory mediators from microglia *Mol. Neurobiol.* **49** 1487–500

Dore-Duffy P and Manna J C L 2007 Physiologic angiodynamics in the brain *Antioxid. Redox Signal.* **9** 1363–72

Dotevall L and Hagberg L 1999 Successful oral doxycycline treatment of Lyme disease-associated facial palsy and meningitis *Clin. Infect. Dis.* **28** 569–74

Drake C T and Iadecola C 2007 The role of neuronal signaling in controlling cerebral blood flow *Brain Lang.* **102** 141–52

Draper K and Ponsford J 2008 Cognitive functioning ten years following traumatic brain injury and rehabilitation *Neuropsychology* **22** 618

Dreier J, Bermpohl A and Eichenlaub R 1995 Southern hybridization and PCR for specific detection of phytopathogenic Clavibacter michiganensis subsp. michiganensis *Phytopathology* **85** 462–8

Driscoll I, Davatzikos C, An Y, Wu X, Shen D, Kraut M and Resnick S 2009 Longitudinal pattern of regional brain volume change differentiates normal aging from MCI *Neurology* **72** 1906–13

Duling B R *et al* 1987 Vasomotor control: functional hyperemia and beyond *Federation Proc.* **vol 46** pp 251–63

Dunn B D, Dalgleish T and Lawrence A D 2006 The somatic marker hypothesis: a critical evaluation *Neurosci. Biobehav. Rev.* **30** 239–71

Du Pasquier A, Plitz I, Menocal S and Amatucci G 2003 A comparative study of Li-ion battery, supercapacitor and nonaqueous asymmetric hybrid devices for automotive applications *J. Power Sources* **115** 171–8

Eng L F and Ghirnikar R S 1994 GFAP and astrogliosis *Brain Pathol.* **4** 229–37

Erickson K I *et al* 2011 Exercise training increases size of hippocampus and improves memory *Proc. Natl Acad. Sci.* **108** 3017–22

Erinjeri J P and Woolsey T A 2002 Spatial integration of vascular changes with neural activity in mouse cortex *J. Cereb. Blood Flow. Metab.* **22** 353–60

Esler M, Kaye D, Lambert G, Esler D and Jennings G 1997 Adrenergic nervous system in heart failure *Am. J. Cardiol.* **80** 7L

Etheridge A, Lee I, Hood L, Galas D and Wang K 2011 Extracellular microRNA: a new source of biomarkers *Mutat. Res./Fund. Mol. Mech. M.* **717** 85–90

Evangelou N, DeLuca G C, Owens T and Esiri M M 2005 Pathological study of spinal cord atrophy in multiple sclerosis suggests limited role of local lesions *Brain* **128** 29–34

Fabri M and Polonara G 2013 Functional topography of human corpus callosum: an FMRI mapping study *Neural Plast.* **2013** 251308

Ferreira R, Santos T, Gonçalves J, Baltazar G, Ferreira L, Agasse F and Bernardino L 2012 Histamine modulates microglia function *J. Neuroinflammation* **9** 1–16

Figueroa-Romero C, Hur J, Bender D E, Delaney C E, Cataldo M D, Smith A L, Yung R, Ruden D M, Callaghan B C and Feldman E L 2012 Identification of epigenetically altered genes in sporadic amyotrophic lateral sclerosis *PLoS One* **7** e52672

Filippi M, Iannucci G, Cercignani M, Rocca M A, Pratesi A and Comi G 2000 A quantitative study of water diffusion in multiple sclerosis lesions and normal-appearing white matter using echo-planar imaging *Arch. Neurol.* **57** 1017–21

Filippi M and Rocca M A 2005 MRI evidence for multiple sclerosis as a diffuse disease of the central nervous system *J. Neurol.* **252** v16–24

Firbank M J, Colloby S J, Burn D J, McKeith I G and O'Brien J T 2003 Regional cerebral blood flow in Parkinson's disease with and without dementia *Neuroimage* **20** 1309–19

Fogal V, Sugahara K N, Ruoslahti E and Christian S 2009 Cell surface nucleolin antagonist causes endothelial cell apoptosis and normalization of tumor vasculature *Angiogenesis* **12** 91–100

Forsberg A, Engler H, Almkvist O, Blomquist G, Hagman G, Wall A, Ringheim A, Långström B and Nordberg A 2008 PET imaging of amyloid deposition in patients with mild cognitive impairment *Neurobiol. Aging* **29** 1456–65

Fotenos A F, Snyder A Z, Girton L E, Morris J C and Buckner R L 2005 Normative estimates of cross-sectional and longitudinal brain volume decline in aging and AD *Neurology* **64** 1032–9

Fox M D, Snyder A Z, Vincent J L, Corbetta M, Van Essen D C and Raichle M E 2005 The human brain is intrinsically organized into dynamic, anticorrelated functional networks *Proc. Natl Acad. Sci.* **102** 9673–8

Fox P T and Raichle M E 1986 Focal physiological uncoupling of cerebral blood flow and oxidative metabolism during somatosensory stimulation in human subjects *Proc. Natl Acad. Sci.* **83** 1140–4

Friedman R C, Farh K K H, Burge C B and Bartel D P 2009 Most mammalian mRNAs are conserved targets of microRNAs *Genome Res.* **19** 92–105

Frischer J M, Bramow S, Dal-Bianco A, Lucchinetti C F, Rauschka H, Schmidbauer M, Laursen H, Sorensen P S and Lassmann H 2009 The relation between inflammation and neurodegeneration in multiple sclerosis brains *Brain* **132** 1175–89

Frisoni G B and Caroli A 2007 Neuroimaging outcomes for clinical trials *J. Nutr. Health Aging* **11** 348

Fu S M, Deshmukh U S and Gaskin F 2011 Pathogenesis of systemic lupus erythematosus revisited 2011: end organ resistance to damage, autoantibody initiation and diversification, and HLA-DR *J. Autoimmun.* **37** 104–12

Fuchs E, Tumbar T and Guasch G 2004 Socializing with the neighbors: stem cells and their niche *Cell* **116** 769–78

Fuchs S Y, Adler V, Buschmann T, Wu X and Ronai Z E 1998 Mdm2 association with p53 targets its ubiquitination *Oncogene* **17** 2543–7

Gao H M, Liu B, Zhang W and Hong J S 2003 Novel anti-inflammatory therapy for Parkinson's disease *Trends Pharmacol. Sci.* **24** 395–401

Gellera C, Ticozzi N, Pensato V, Nanetti L, Castucci A, Castellotti B, Lauria G, Taroni F, Silani V and Mariotti C 2012 ATAXIN2 CAG-repeat length in Italian patients with amyotrophic lateral sclerosis: risk factor or variant phenotype? Implication for genetic testing and counseling *Neurobiol. Aging* **33** 1847–e15

Geurts J J and Barkhof F 2008 Grey matter pathology in multiple sclerosis *Lancet Neurol.* **7** 841–51

Ghiso J and Frangione B 2002 Amyloidosis and Alzheimer's disease *Adv. Drug. Delivery Rev.* **54** 1539–51

Giannakopoulos P, Herrmann F R, Bussière T, Bouras C, Kövari E, Perl D P, Morrison J H, Gold G and Hof P R 2003 Tangle and neuron numbers, but not amyloid load, predict cognitive status in Alzheimer's disease *Neurology* **60** 1495–500

Girouard H and Iadecola C 2006 Neurovascular coupling in the normal brain and in hypertension, stroke, and Alzheimer disease *J. Appl. Physiol.* **100** 328–35

Goodall E F, Heath P R, Bandmann O, Kirby J and Shaw P J 2013 Neuronal dark matter: the emerging role of microRNAs in neurodegeneration *Front. Cell. Neurosci.* **7** 178

Gouras G K *et al* 2000 Intraneuronal Aβ42 accumulation in human brain *Am. J. Pathol.* **156** 15–20

Grabe H J, Ahrens N, Rose H J, Kessler C and Freyberger H J 2001 Neurotrophic factor S100beta in major depression *Neuropsychobiology* **44** 88–90

Greenberg D A and Jin K 2005 From angiogenesis to neuropathology *Nature* **438** 954–9

Guo J, Gao X, Su L, Xia H, Gu G, Pang Z, Jiang X, Yao L, Chen J and Chen H 2011 Aptamer-functionalized PEG–PLGA nanoparticles for enhanced anti-glioma drug delivery *Biomaterials* **32** 8010–20

Haass C and Selkoe D J 2007 Soluble protein oligomers in neurodegeneration: lessons from the Alzheimer's amyloid β-peptide *Nat. Rev. Mol. Cell Biol.* **8** 101–12

Hajdu S D, Agmon-Levin N and Shoenfeld Y 2011 Silicone and autoimmunity *Eur. J. Clin. Invest.* **41** 203–11

Hannila S S, Siddiq M M and Filbin M T 2007 Therapeutic approaches to promoting axonal regeneration in the adult mammalian spinal cord *Int. Rev. Neurobiol.* **77** 57–105

Hanyu H *et al* 1999 Diffusion-weighted and magnetization transfer imaging of the corpus callosum in Alzheimer's disease *J. Neurological Sci.* **167** 37–44

Harrison P J 2004 The hippocampus in schizophrenia: a review of the neuropathological evidence and its pathophysiological implications *Psychopharmacology* **174** 151–62

Havranek E P, Ware M G and Lowes B D 1999 Prevalence of depression in congestive heart failure *Am. J. Cardiol.* **84** 348–50

Hawkins B T and Davis T P 2005 The blood–brain barrier/neurovascular unit in health and disease *Pharmacol. Rev.* **57** 173–85

Hawkins P T, Anderson K E, Davidson K and Stephens L R 2006 Signalling through Class I PI3Ks in mammalian cells *Biochem. Soc. Trans.* **34** 647–62

Heckers S and Konradi C 2002 Hippocampal neurons in schizophrenia *J. Neural Transm.* **109** 891–905

Heneka M T, O'Banion M K, Terwel D and Kummer M P 2010 Neuroinflammatory processes in Alzheimer's disease *J. Neural Transm.* **117** 919–47

Henneman W J P, Sluimer J D, Barnes J, Van Der Flier W M, Sluimer I C, Fox N C, Scheltens P, Vrenken H and Barkhof F 2009 Hippocampal atrophy rates in Alzheimer disease: added value over whole brain volume measures *Neurology* **72** 999–1007

Henriksen K *et al* 2013 An enzyme-generated fragment of tau measured in serum shows an inverse correlation to cognitive function *PLoS One* **8** e64990

Heppner F L *et al* 2005 Experimental autoimmune encephalomyelitis repressed by microglial paralysis *Nat. Med.* **11** 146–52

Herceg Z 2016 Epigenetic mechanisms as an interface between the environment and genome *Hypoxia* 3–15

Herceg Z and Vaissière T 2011 Epigenetic mechanisms and cancer: an interface between the environment and the genome *Epigenetics* **6** 804–19

Hermann B P and Heckert L L 2007 Transcriptional regulation of the FSH receptor: new perspectives *Molecular Cellular Endocrinol.* **260** 100–8

Herrera A J, Tomas-Camardiel M, Venero J L, Cano J and Machado A 2005 Inflammatory process as a determinant factor for the degeneration of substantia nigra dopaminergic neurons *J. Neural Transm.* **112** 111–19

Hershey T, Black K J, Carl J L, McGee-Minnich L, Snyder A Z and Perlmutter J S 2003 Long term treatment and disease severity change brain responses to levodopa in Parkinson's disease *J. Neurol. Neurosurg. Psych.* **74** 844–51

Hirano S, Asanuma K, Ma Y, Tang C, Feigin A, Dhawan V, Carbon M and Eidelberg D 2008 Dissociation of metabolic and neurovascular responses to levodopa in the treatment of Parkinson's disease *J. Neurosci.* **28** 4201–9

Hochmeister S *et al* 2006 Dysferlin is a new marker for leaky brain blood vessels in multiple sclerosis *J. Neuropathol. Exp. Neurol.* **65** 855–65

HogenEsch H 2002 Mechanisms of stimulation of the immune response by aluminum adjuvants *Vaccine* **20** S34–9

Hovanessian A G, Soundaramourty C, Khoury D E, Nondier I, Svab J and Krust B 2010 Surface expressed nucleolin is constantly induced in tumor cells to mediate calcium-dependent ligand internalization *PLoS One* **5** e15787

Huey E D, Putnam K T and Grafman J 2006 A systematic review of neurotransmitter deficits and treatments in frontotemporal dementia *Neurology* **66** 17–22

Iadecola C, Zhang F, Casey R, Nagayama M and Ross M E 1997 Delayed reduction of ischemic brain injury and neurological deficits in mice lacking the inducible nitric oxide synthase gene *J. Neurosci.* **17** 9157–64

Iadecola C 2004 Neurovascular regulation in the normal brain and in Alzheimer's disease *Nat. Rev. Neurosci.* **5** 347–60

Iadecola C and Kraig R P 1991 Focal elevations in neocortical interstitial K+ produced by stimulation of the fastigial nucleus in rat *Brain Res.* **563** 273–7

Ido Y, Chang K and Williamson J R 2004 NADH augments blood flow in physiologically activated retina and visual cortex *Proc. Natl Acad. Sci.* **101** 653–8

Iliff J J, D'Ambrosio R, Ngai A C and Winn H R 2003 Adenosine receptors mediate glutamate-evoked arteriolar dilation in the rat cerebral cortex *Am. J. Physiol.—Heart Circ. Physiol* **284** H1631–7

Jack C R Jr, Knopman D S, Jagust W J, Shaw L M, Aisen P S, Weiner M W, Petersen R C and Trojanowski J Q 2010 Hypothetical model of dynamic biomarkers of the Alzheimer's pathological cascade *Lancet Neurol.* **9** 119–28

Jahshan C, Heaton R K, Golshan S and Cadenhead K S 2010 Course of neurocognitive deficits in the prodrome and first episode of schizophrenia *Neuropsychology* **24** 109

Jankowska E A, Ponikowski P, Piepoli M F, Banasiak W, Anker S D and Poole-Wilson P A 2006 Autonomic imbalance and immune activation in chronic heart failure–pathophysiological links *Cardiovasc. Res.* **70** 434–45

Jauch E C, Lindsell C, Broderick J, Fagan S C, Tilley B C and Levine S R 2006 Association of serial biochemical markers with acute ischemic stroke: the National Institute of Neurological

Disorders and Stroke recombinant tissue plasminogen activator stroke study *Stroke* **37** 2508–13

Jia G, Wang H, Yan L, Wang X, Pei R, Yan T, Zhao Y and Guo X 2005 Cytotoxicity of carbon nanomaterials: single-wall nanotube, multi-wall nanotube, and fullerene *Environ. Sci. Technol.* **39** 1378–83

Jiang W *et al* 2004 Prognostic value of anxiety and depression in patients with chronic heart failure *Circulation* **110** 3452–6

Johansen-Berg H and Rushworth M F 2009 Using diffusion imaging to study human connectional anatomy *Annu. Rev. Neurosci.* **32** 75–94

Johnson K A *et al* 2013 Appropriate use criteria for amyloid PET: a report of the Amyloid Imaging Task Force, the Society of Nuclear Medicine and Molecular Imaging, and the Alzheimer's Association *Alzheimer's Dement.* **9** E1–16

Johnson S W and North R A 1992 Opioids excite dopamine neurons by hyperpolarization of local interneurons *J. Neurosci.* **12** 483–8

Johnson N L, Kemp A W and Kotz S 2005 *Univariate Discrete Distributions* vol 444 (New York: Wiley)

Jouvet P *et al* 2000 Branched chain amino acids induce apoptosis in neural cells without mitochondrial membrane depolarization or cytochrome c release: implications for neurological impairment associated with maple syrup urine disease *Mol. Biol. Cell* **11** 1919–32

Kahlig K M, Rhodes T H, Pusch M, Freilinger T, Pereira-Monteiro J M, Ferrari M D, Van Den Maagdenberg A M, Dichgans M and George A L 2008 Divergent sodium channel defects in familial hemiplegic migraine *Proc. Natl Acad. Sci.* **105** 9799–804

Kalus P, Buri C, Slotboom J, Gralla J, Remonda L, Dierks T, Strik W K, Schroth G and Kiefer C 2004 Volumetry and diffusion tensor imaging of hippocampal subregions in schizophrenia *Neuroreport* **15** 867–71

Kantarci K *et al* 2001 Mild cognitive impairment and Alzheimer disease: regional diffusivity of water *Radiology* **219** 101–7

Kanu A, Whitfield J and Leffler C W 2006 Carbon monoxide contributes to hypotension-induced cerebrovascular vasodilation in piglets *Am. J. Physiol.-Heart Circ. Physiol.* **291** H2409–14

Kapural M, Krizanac-Bengez L J, Barnett G, Perl J, Masaryk T, Apollo D, Rasmussen P, Mayberg M R and Janigro D 2002 Serum S-100β as a possible marker of blood–brain barrier disruption *Brain Res.* **940** 102–4

Karas G B, Scheltens P, Rombouts S A, Visser P J, van Schijndel R A, Fox N C and Barkhof F 2004 Global and local gray matter loss in mild cognitive impairment and Alzheimer's disease *Neuroimage* **23** 708–16

Kasama S, Tachibana H, Kawabata K and Yoshikawa H 2005 Cerebral blood flow in Parkinson's disease, dementia with Lewy bodies, and Alzheimer's disease according to three-dimensional stereotactic surface projection imaging *Dement. Geriatr. Cognit. Disord.* **19** 266–75

Khoo S K, Petillo D, Kang U J, Resau J H, Berryhill B, Linder J, Forsgren L, Neuman L A and Tan A C 2012 Plasma-based circulating MicroRNA biomarkers for Parkinson's disease *J. Parkinson's Dis.* **2** 321–31

Kim H R, Andrieux K, Gil S, Taverna M, Chacun H, Desmaële D, Taran F, Georgin D and Couvreur P 2007 Translocation of poly (ethylene glycol-co-hexadecyl) cyanoacrylate nanoparticles into rat brain endothelial cells: role of apolipoproteins in receptor-mediated endocytosis *Biomacromolecules* **8** 793–9

Kim J, Whyte J, Patel S, Avants B, Europa E, Wang J, Slattery J, Gee J C, Coslett H B and Detre J A 2010 Resting cerebral blood flow alterations in chronic traumatic brain injury: an arterial spin labeling perfusion FMRI study *J. Neurotrauma* **27** 1399–411

Kim K *et al* 2007 Recombination signatures distinguish embryonic stem cells derived by parthenogenesis and somatic cell nuclear transfer *Cell Stem Cell* **1** 346–52

Kinnunen K M, Greenwood R, Powell J H, Leech R, Hawkins P C, Bonnelle V, Patel M C, Counsell S J and Sharp D J 2011 White matter damage and cognitive impairment after traumatic brain injury *Brain* **134** 449–63

Kirk J, Plumb J, Mirakhur M and McQuaid S 2003 Tight junctional abnormality in multiple sclerosis white matter affects all calibres of vessel and is associated with blood–brain barrier leakage and active demyelination *J. Pathol.: A J. Pathol. Soc. Gt. Br. Irel.* **201** 319–27

Klunk W E *et al* 2004 Imaging brain amyloid in Alzheimer's disease with Pittsburgh Compound-B *Ann. Neurol.: Off. J. Am. Neurol. Assoc. Child. Neurol. Soc.* **55** 306–19

Kohno H *et al* 1996 Bni1p implicated in cytoskeletal control is a putative target of Rho1p small GTP binding protein in Saccharomyces cerevisiae *EMBO J.* **15** 6060–8

Kövesdi E, Lückl J, Bukovics P, Farkas O, Pál J, Czeiter E, Szellár D, Dóczi T, Komoly S and Büki A 2010 Update on protein biomarkers in traumatic brain injury with emphasis on clinical use in adults and pediatrics *Acta Neurochir.* **152** 1–17

Koyama A, Okereke O I, Yang T, Blacker D, Selkoe D J and Grodstein F 2012 Plasma amyloid-β as a predictor of dementia and cognitive decline: a systematic review and meta-analysis *Arch. Neurol.* **69** 824–31

Krumbholz M *et al* 2005 BAFF is produced by astrocytes and up-regulated in multiple sclerosis lesions and primary central nervous system lymphoma *J. Exp. Med.* **201** 195–200

Kumar-Singh S and Broeckhoven C V 2007 Frontotemporal lobar degeneration: current concepts in the light of recent advances *Brain Pathol.* **17** 104–14

Kuroki N *et al* 2006 Fornix integrity and hippocampal volume in male schizophrenic patients *Biol. Psych.* **60** 22–31

Laakso M P, Vaurio O, Koivisto E, Savolainen L, Eronen M, Aronen H J, Hakola P, Repo E, Soininen H and Tiihonen J 2001 Psychopathy and the posterior hippocampus *Behav. Brain Res.* **118** 187–93

Lajoie P and Nabi I R 2007 Regulation of raft-dependent endocytosis *J. Cell. Mol. Med.* **11** 644–53

Lambert J C *et al* 2013 Genome-wide haplotype association study identifies the FRMD4A gene as a risk locus for Alzheimer's disease *Mol. Psych.* **18** 461–70

Lasky T *et al* 1998 The Guillain–Barré syndrome and the 1992–1993 and 1993–1994 influenza vaccines *New England J. Med.* **339** 1797–802

Lebert F, Stekke W, Hasenbroekx C and Pasquier F 2004 Frontotemporal dementia: a randomised, controlled trial with trazodone *Dement. Geriatr. Cogn. Disord.* **17** 355–9

Lee S W, Kim W J, Choi Y K, Song H S, Son M J, Gelman I H, Kim Y J and Kim K W 2003 SSeCKS regulates angiogenesis and tight junction formation in blood–brain barrier *Nat. Med.* **9** 900–6

Leech S, Kirk J, Plumb J and McQuaid S 2007 Persistent endothelial abnormalities and blood–brain barrier leak in primary and secondary progressive multiple sclerosis *Neuropathol. Appl. Neurobiol.* **33** 86–98

Levin H S 2003 Neuroplasticity following non-penetrating traumatic brain injury *Brain Injury* **17** 665–74

Liepelt I, Reimold M, Maetzler W, Godau J, Reischl G, Gaenslen A, Herbst H and Berg D 2009 Cortical hypometabolism assessed by a metabolic ratio in Parkinson's disease primarily reflects cognitive deterioration—[18F] FDG-PET *Mov. Disord.: Off. J. Mov. Disord. Soc.* **24** 1504–11

Liliang P C, Liang C L, Weng H C, Lu K, Wang K W, Chen H J and Chuang J H 2010 τ proteins in serum predict outcome after severe traumatic brain injury *J. Surg. Res.* **160** 302–7

Lipska B K and Weinberger D R 2002 A neurodevelopmental model of schizophrenia: neonatal disconnection of the hippocampus *Neurotox. Res.* **4** 469–75

Liyasova M, Li B, Schopfer L M, Nachon F, Masson P, Furlong C E and Lockridge O 2011 Exposure to tri-o-cresyl phosphate detected in jet airplane passengers *Toxicol. Appl. Pharmacol.* **256** 337–47

Lo E H, Dalkara T and Moskowitz M A 2003 Mechanisms, challenges and opportunities in stroke *Nat. Rev. Neurosci.* **4** 399–414

Lok J, Gupta P, Guo S, Kim W J, Whalen M J, van Leyen K and Lo E H 2007 Cell–cell signaling in the neurovascular unit *Neurochem. Res.* **32** 2032–45

Löscher W and Potschka H 2005 Drug resistance in brain diseases and the role of drug efflux transporters *Nat. Rev. Neurosci.* **6** 591–602

Lovas G, Szilágyi N, Majtényi K, Palkovits M and Komoly S 2000 Axonal changes in chronic demyelinated cervical spinal cord plaques *Brain* **123** 308–17

MacDonald C L *et al* 2011 Detection of blast-related traumatic brain injury in US military personnel *N. Engl. J. Med.* **364** 2091–100

Machado-Vieira R, Lara D R, Portela L V C, Goncalves C A, Soares J C, Kapczinski F and Souza D O 2002 Elevated serum S100B protein in drug-free bipolar patients during first manic episode: a pilot study *Eur. Neuropsychopharmacol.* **12** 269–72

Magliozzi R, Howell O, Vora A, Serafini B, Nicholas R, Puopolo M and Aloisi F 2007 Meningeal B-cell follicles in secondary progressive multiple sclerosis associate with early onset of disease and severe cortical pathology *Brain* **130** 1089–104

Man S, Ubogu E E and Ransohoff R M 2007 Inflammatory cell migration into the central nervous system: a few new twists on an old tale *Brain Pathol.* **17** 243–50

Margis R, Margis R and Rieder C R 2011 Identification of blood microRNAs associated to Parkinson's disease *J. Biotechnol.* **152** 96–101

Marsillach J, Richter R J, Kim J H, Stevens R C, MacCoss M J, Tomazela D, Suzuki S M, Schopfer L M, Lockridge O and Furlong C E 2011 Biomarkers of organophosphorus (OP) exposures in humans *Neurotoxicology* **32** 656–60

Martins M *et al* 2011 Convergence of miRNA expression profiling, α-synuclein interacton and GWAS in Parkinson's disease *PLoS One* **6** e25443

Massin N, Bohadana A B, Wild P, Hery M, Toamain J P and Hubert G 1998 Respiratory symptoms and bronchial responsiveness in lifeguards exposed to nitrogen trichloride in indoor swimming pools *Occup. Environ. Med.* **55** 258–63

Matsumoto K, Sato C, Naka Y, Whitby R and Shimizu N 2010 Stimulation of neuronal neurite outgrowth using functionalized carbon nanotubes *Nanotechnology* **21** 115101

Mayer A R, Mannell M V, Ling J, Gasparovic C and Yeo R A 2011 Functional connectivity in mild traumatic brain injury *Hum. Brain Mapp.* **32** 1825–35

Mayeux R 2004 Biomarkers: potential uses and limitations *NeuroRx* **1** 182–8

Mazzatenta A, Giugliano M, Campidelli S, Gambazzi L, Businaro L, Markram H, Prato M and Ballerini L 2007 Interfacing neurons with carbon nanotubes: electrical signal transfer and synaptic stimulation in cultured brain circuits *J. Neurosci.* **27** 6931–6

McAllister T W, Flashman L A, McDonald B C and Saykin A J 2006 Mechanisms of working memory dysfunction after mild and moderate TBI: evidence from functional MRI and neurogenetics *J. Neurotrauma* **23** 1450–67

Meinl E, Krumbholz M, Derfuss T, Junker A and Hohlfeld R 2008 Compartmentalization of inflammation in the CNS: a major mechanism driving progressive multiple sclerosis *J. Neurol. Sci.* **274** 42–4

Melzer T R *et al* 2011 Arterial spin labelling reveals an abnormal cerebral perfusion pattern in Parkinson's disease *Brain* **134** 845–55

Mendez M F, Selwood A, Mastri A R and Frey W 1993 Pick's disease versus Alzheimer's disease: a comparison of clinical characteristics *Neurology* **43** 289

Menteer J, Macey P M, Woo M A, Panigrahy A and Harper R M 2010 Central nervous system changes in pediatric heart failure: a volumetric study *Pediatr. Cardiol.* **31** 969–76

Mentis M J, McIntosh A R, Perrine K, Dhawan V, Berlin B, Feigin A, Edwards C, Mattis P and Eidelberg D 2002 Relationships among the metabolic patterns that correlate with mnemonic, visuospatial, and mood symptoms in Parkinson's disease *Am. J. Psych.* **159** 746–54

Merrilees J J and Miller B L 2003 Long-term care of patients with frontotemporal dementia *J. Am. Med. Dir. Assoc.* **4** S162–4

Meyer-Luehmann M *et al* 2003 Extracellular amyloid formation and associated pathology in neural grafts *Nat. Neurosci.* **6** 370–7

Mintun M A, Vlassenko A G, Shulman G L and Snyder A Z 2002 Time-related increase of oxygen utilization in continuously activated human visual cortex *Neuroimage* **16** 531–7

Molyneux P D *et al* 2000 The effect of interferon beta-1b treatment on MRI measures of cerebral atrophy in secondary progressive multiple sclerosis *Brain* **123** 2256–63

Morahan J M, Yu B, Trent R J and Pamphlett R 2009 A genome-wide analysis of brain DNA methylation identifies new candidate genes for sporadic amyotrophic lateral sclerosis *Amyotroph. Lateral Scler.* **10** 418–29

Moretti R, Torre P, Antonello R M, Cazzato G and Bava A 2003 Frontotemporal dementia: paroxetine as a possible treatment of behavior symptoms *Eur. Neurol.* **49** 13–19

Morris J C, Roe C M, Grant E A, Head D, Storandt M, Goate A M, Fagan A M, Holtzman D M and Mintun M A 2009 Pittsburgh compound B imaging and prediction of progression from cognitive normality to symptomatic Alzheimer disease *Arch. Neurol.* **66** 1469–75

Morrison A P *et al* 2012 Early detection and intervention evaluation for people at risk of psychosis: multisite randomised controlled trial *Brit. Med. J.* **344** e2233

Murberg T A, Bru E, Svebak S, Tveterås R and Aarsland T 1999 Depressed mood and subjective health symptoms as predictors of mortality in patients with congestive heart failure: a two-years follow-up study *Int. J. Psych. Med.* **29** 311–26

Nabel G J 2013 Designing tomorrow's vaccines *N. Engl. J. Med.* **368** 551–60

Nagai M, Re D B, Nagata T, Chalazonitis A, Jessell T M, Wichterle H and Przedborski S 2007 Astrocytes expressing ALS-linked mutated SOD1 release factors selectively toxic to motor neurons *Nat. Neurosci.* **10** 615–22

Naggara O, Oppenheim C, Rieu D, Raoux N, Rodrigo S, Dalla Barba G and Meder J F 2006 Diffusion tensor imaging in early Alzheimer's disease *Psych. Res.: Neuroimag.* **146** 243–9

Naylor A R, Cuffe R L, Rothwell P M and Bell P R F 2003 A systematic review of outcomes following staged and synchronous carotid endarterectomy and coronary artery bypass *Eur. J. Vascul. Endovascul. Surg.* **25** 380–9

Nedergaard M, Ransom B and Goldman S A 2003 New roles for astrocytes: redefining the functional architecture of the brain *Trends Neurosci.* **26** 523–30

Newman E A 2003 New roles for astrocytes: regulation of synaptic transmission *Trends Neurosci.* **26** 536–42

Ngai A C, Ko K R, Morii S and Winn H R 1988 Effect of sciatic nerve stimulation on pial arterioles in rats *Am. J. Physiol.-Heart Circulat. Physiol.* **254** H133–9

Nitta T, Hata M, Gotoh S, Seo Y, Sasaki H, Hashimoto N, Furuse M and Tsukita S 2003 Size-selective loosening of the blood–brain barrier in claudin-5-deficient mice *J. Cell Biol.* **161** 653–60

Nobili F *et al* 2009 Amnestic mild cognitive impairment in Parkinson's disease: a brain perfusion SPECT study *Mov. Disord.* **24** 414–21

Nordstedt C, Caporaso G L, Thyberg J, Gandy S E and Greengard P 1993 Identification of the Alzheimer beta/A4 amyloid precursor protein in clathrin-coated vesicles purified from PC12 cells *J. Biolog. Chem.* **268** 608–12

Nudo R J and Masterton R B 1986 Stimulation-induced [14C] 2-deoxyglucose labeling of synaptic activity in the central auditory system *J. Compar. Neurol.* **245** 553–65

Nunomura A *et al* 2001 Oxidative damage is the earliest event in Alzheimer disease *J. Neuropathol. Exp. Neurol.* **60** 759–67

Obeid R and Herrmann W 2006 Mechanisms of homocysteine neurotoxicity in neurodegenerative diseases with special reference to dementia *FEBS Lett.* **580** 2994–3005

Ohtsuki S and Terasaki T 2007 Contribution of carrier-mediated transport systems to the blood–brain barrier as a supporting and protecting interface for the brain; importance for CNS drug discovery and development *Pharm. Res.* **24** 1745–58

Ohuchi H, Takasugi H, Ohashi H, Okada Y, Yamada O, Ono Y, Yagihara T and Echigo S 2003 Stratification of pediatric heart failure on the basis of neurohormonal and cardiac autonomic nervous activities in patients with congenital heart disease *Circulation* **108** 2368–76

Okello A *et al* 2009 Conversion of amyloid positive and negative MCI to AD over 3 years: an 11C-PIB PET study *Neurology* **73** 754–60

Ozmen B, Ozmen D, Parildar Z, Mutaf I, Turgan N and Bayindir O 2006 Impact of renal function or folate status on altered plasma homocysteine levels in hypothyroidism *Endocr. J.* **53** 119–24

Packer M 1992 The neurohormonal hypothesis: a theory to explain the mechanism of disease progression in heart failure *J. Am. Coll. Cardiol.* **20** 248–54

Parton R G and Richards A A 2003 Lipid rafts and caveolae as portals for endocytosis: new insights and common mechanisms *Traffic* **4** 724–38

Pardridge W M 2005 The blood-brain barrier: bottleneck in brain drug development *NeuroRx* **2** 3–14

Patenaude B 2007 Bayesian statistical models of shape and appearance for subcortical brain segmentation *Doctoral Dissertation* University of Oxford

Penadés R, Pujol N, Catalán R, Massana G, Rametti G, García-Rizo C, Bargalló N, Gastó C, Bernardo M and Junqué C 2013 Brain effects of cognitive remediation therapy in schizophrenia: a structural and functional neuroimaging study *Biol. Psych.* **73** 1015–23

Perlstein W M, Cole M A, Demery J A, Seignourel P J, Dixit N K, Larson M J and Briggs R W 2004 Parametric manipulation of working memory load in traumatic brain injury: behavioral and neural correlates *J. Int. Neuropsychol. Soc.* **10** 724–41

Perricone C, Colafrancesco S, Mazor R D, Soriano A, Agmon-Levin N and Shoenfeld Y 2013 Autoimmune/inflammatory syndrome induced by adjuvants (ASIA) 2013: unveiling the pathogenic, clinical and diagnostic aspects *J. Autoimmun.* **47** 1–16

Perry R and Miller B 2001 Behavior and treatment in frontotemporal dementia *Neurology* **56** 11

Perry V H and Teeling J 2013 Microglia and macrophages of the central nervous system: the contribution of microglia priming and systemic inflammation to chronic neurodegeneration *Seminars in Immunopathology* vol 35 (Berlin: Springer) pp 601–12

Petronis A 2010 Epigenetics as a unifying principle in the aetiology of complex traits and diseases *Nature* **465** 721–7

Piepers S *et al* 2009 Randomized sequential trial of valproic acid in amyotrophic lateral sclerosis. *Ann. Neurol.: Off. J. Am. Neurol. Assoc. Child. Neurology Soc.* **66** 227–34

Piorntek J, Winkler L, Wolburg H, Müller S L, Zuleger N, Piehl C, Wiesner B, Krause G and Blasig I E 2008 Formation of tight junction: determinants of homophilic interaction between classic claudins *FASEB J.* **22** 146–58

Pitkänen A and Engel J 2014 Past and present definitions of epileptogenesis and its biomarkers *Neurotherapeutics* **11** 231–41

Pollmann S, Maertens M, von Cramon D Y, Lepsien J and Hugdahl K 2002 Dichotic listening in patients with splenial and nonsplenial callosal lesions *Neuropsychology* **16** 56

Popovich P G 2000 Immunological regulation of neuronal degeneration and regeneration in the injured spinal cord *Prog. Brain Res.* **128** 43–58

Price J L, Ko A I, Wade M J, Tsou S K, McKeel D W and Morris J C 2001 Neuron number in the entorhinal cortex and CA1 in preclinical Alzheimer disease *Arch. Neurol.* **58** 1395–402

Prichard J *et al* 1991 Lactate rise detected by 1H NMR in human visual cortex during physiologic stimulation *Proc. Natl Acad. Sci.* **88** 5829–31

Putzke J D, Williams M A, Rayburn B K, Kirklin J K and Boll T J 1998 The relationship between cardiac function and neuropsychological status among heart transplant candidates *J. Cardiac Failure* **4** 295–303

Qutub A A and Hunt C A 2005 Glucose transport to the brain: a systems model *Brain Res. Rev.* **49** 595–617

Randall C, Mosconi L, De Leon M and Glodzik L 2013 Cerebrospinal fluid biomarkers of Alzheimer's disease in cognitively healthy elderly *Front. Biosci.* **18** 1150

Ransohoff R M, Kivisäkk P and Kidd G 2003 Three or more routes for leukocyte migration into the central nervous system *Nat. Rev. Immunol.* **3** 569–81

Rapoport M, Dawson H N, Binder L I, Vitek M P and Ferreira A 2002 Tau is essential to β-amyloid-induced neurotoxicity *Proc. Natl Acad. Sci.* **99** 6364–9

Rascovsky K *et al* 2005 Rate of progression differs in frontotemporal dementia and Alzheimer disease *Neurology* **65** 397–403

Rascovsky K *et al* 2007 Diagnostic criteria for the behavioral variant of frontotemporal dementia (bvFTD): current limitations and future directions *Alzheimer Disease Assoc. Disorders* **21** S14–8

Ravaglia G, Forti P, Maioli F, Chiappelli M, Montesi F, Tumini E, Mariani E, Licastro F and Patterson C 2007 Blood inflammatory markers and risk of dementia: the Conselice Study of Brain Aging *Neurobiol. Aging* **28** 1810–20

Raz N, Rodrigue K M, Head D, Kennedy K M and Acker J D 2004 Differential aging of the medial temporal lobe: a study of a five-year change *Neurology* **62** 433–8

Redler R L and Dokholyan N V 2012 The complex molecular biology of amyotrophic lateral sclerosis (ALS) *Prog. Mol. Biol. Transl. Sci.* **107** 215–62

Remes A M, Laru L, Tuominen H, Aalto S, Kemppainen N, Mononen H, Någren K, Parkkola R and Rinne J O 2008 Carbon 11–labeled Pittsburgh Compound B positron emission tomographic amyloid imaging in patients with APP locus duplication *Arch. Neurol.* **65** 540–4

Ricker J H, Hillary F G and DeLuca J 2001 Functionally activated brain imaging (O-15 PET and fMRI) in the study of learning and memory after traumatic brain injury *J. Head. Trauma. Rehab.* **16** 191–205

Roberson E D *et al* 2005 Frontotemporal dementia progresses to death faster than Alzheimer disease *Neurology* **65** 719–25

Robinson K M 2001 Rehabilitation applications in caring for patients with Pick's disease and frontotemporal dementias *Neurology* **56** S56–8

Romanitan M O, Popescu B O, Winblad B, Bajenaru O A and Bogdanovic N 2007 Occludin is overexpressed in Alzheimer's disease and vascular dementia *J. Cell. Mol. Med.* **11** 569–79

Rosenblum H, Shoenfeld Y and Amital H 2011 The common immunogenic etiology of chronic fatigue syndrome: from infections to vaccines via adjuvants to the ASIA syndrome *Infect. Dis. Clin.* **25** 851–63

Roses A D 2010 An inherited variable poly-T repeat genotype in TOMM40 in Alzheimer disease *Arch. Neurol.* **67** 536–41

Rovelet-Lecrux A, Hannequin D, Raux G, Le Meur N, Laquerrière A, Vital A, Dumanchin C, Feuillette S, Brice A, Vercelletto M and Dubas F 2006 APP locus duplication causes autosomal dominant early-onset Alzheimer disease with cerebral amyloid angiopathy *Nat. Genet.* **38** 24–6

Rusinek H D, Santi S, Frid D, Tsui W H, Tarshish C Y, Convit A and de Leon M J 2003 Regional brain atrophy rate predicts future cognitive decline: 6-year longitudinal MR imaging study of normal aging *Radiology* **229** 691–6

Sachdev P S 2005 Homocysteine and brain atrophy *Prog. Neuro-Psychopharmacol. Biol. Psych.* **29** 1152–61

Sanchez-Carrion R, Gomez P V, Junque C, Fernandez-Espejo D, Falcon C, Bargallo N, Roig-Rovira T, Ensenat-Cantallops A and Bernabeu M 2008 Frontal hypoactivation on functional magnetic resonance imaging in working memory after severe diffuse traumatic brain injury *J. Neurotrauma* **25** 479–94

Santacruz K *et al* 2005 Tau suppression in a neurodegenerative mouse model improves memory function *Science* **309** 476–81

Scheid R, Preul C, Gruber O, Wiggins C and Von Cramon D Y 2003 Diffuse axonal injury associated with chronic traumatic brain injury: evidence from T2*-weighted gradient-echo imaging at 3 T *Am. J. Neuroradiol.* **24** 1049–56

Schmitt H P 2005 Neuro-modulation, aminergic neuro-disinhibition and neuro-degeneration: draft of a comprehensive theory for Alzheimer disease *Med. Hypotheses* **65** 1106–19

Schopfer L M, Furlong C E and Lockridge O 2010 Development of diagnostics in the search for an explanation of aerotoxic syndrome *Anal. Biochem.* **404** 64–74

Segal S S 2000 Integration of blood flow control to skeletal muscle: key role of feed arteries *Acta Physiol. Scand.* **168** 511–18

Selkoe D J 2001 Clearing the brain's amyloid cobwebs *Neuron* **32** 177–80

Selmi C, Lu Q and Humble M C 2012 Heritability versus the role of the environment in autoimmunity *J. Autoimmun.* **39** 249–52

Seshadri S, Wolf P A, Beiser A S, Selhub J, Au R, Jacques P F, Yoshita M, Rosenberg I H, D'Agostino R B and DeCarli C 2008 Association of plasma total homocysteine levels with subclinical brain injury: cerebral volumes, white matter hyperintensity, and silent brain infarcts at volumetric magnetic resonance imaging in the Framingham Offspring Study *Arch. Neurol.* **65** 642–9

Shaw L M, Korecka M, Clark C M, Lee V M Y and Trojanowski J Q 2007 Biomarkers of neurodegeneration for diagnosis and monitoring therapeutics *Nat. Rev. Drug. Discov.* **6** 295–303

Shen Q *et al* 2004 Endothelial cells stimulate self-renewal and expand neurogenesis of neural stem cells *Science* **304** 1338–40

Shen Q, Wang Y, Kokovay E, Lin G, Chuang S M, Goderie S K, Roysam B and Temple S 2008 Adult SVZ stem cells lie in a vascular niche: a quantitative analysis of niche cell–cell interactions *Cell Stem Cell* **3** 289–300

Shenton M E, Dickey C C, Frumin M and McCarley R W 2001 A review of MRI findings in schizophrenia *Schizophr. Res.* **49** 1–52

Shi M, Caudle W M and Zhang J 2009 Biomarker discovery in neurodegenerative diseases: a proteomic approach *Neurobiol. Dis.* **35** 157–64

Shiiya N, Kunihara T, Miyatake T, Matsuzaki K and Yasuda K 2004 Tau protein in the cerebrospinal fluid is a marker of brain injury after aortic surgery *Ann. Thorac. Surg.* **77** 2034–8

Shimizu H, Watanabe E, Hiyama T Y, Nagakura A, Fujikawa A, Okado H, Yanagawa Y, Obata K and Noda M 2007 Glial Nax channels control lactate signaling to neurons for brain [Na^+] sensing *Neuron* **54** 59–72

Shirani A, Zhao Y, Karim M E, Evans C, Kingwell E, Van Der Kop M L, Oger J, Gustafson P, Petkau J and Tremlett H 2012 Association between use of interferon beta and progression of disability in patients with relapsing-remitting multiple sclerosis *JAMA* **308** 247–56

Shulman R G, Rothman D L, Behar K L and Hyder F 2004 Energetic basis of brain activity: implications for neuroimaging *Trends Neurosci.* **27** 489–95

Simpson I A, Carruthers A and Vannucci S J 2007 Supply and demand in cerebral energy metabolism: the role of nutrient transporters *J. Cereb. Blood Flow. Metab.* **27** 1766–91

Skibinski G *et al* 2005 Mutations in the endosomal ESCRTIII-complex subunit CHMP2B in frontotemporal dementia *Nat. Genet.* **37** 806–8

Sluimer J D, van der Flier W M, Karas G B, Fox N C, Scheltens P, Barkhof F and Vrenken H 2008 Whole-brain atrophy rate and cognitive decline: longitudinal MR study of memory clinic patients *Radiology* **248** 590–8

Smith A D 2002 Imaging the progression of Alzheimer pathology through the brain *Proc. Natl Acad. Sci.* **99** 4135–7

Smith S M *et al* 2009 Correspondence of the brain's functional architecture during activation and rest *Proc. Natl Acad. Sci.* **106** 13040–5

Snyder H M *et al* 2014 Developing novel blood-based biomarkers for Alzheimer's disease *Alzheimer's Dement.* **10** 109–14

Sokoya E M, Burns A R, Setiawan C T, Coleman H A, Parkington H C and Tare M 2006 Evidence for the involvement of myoendothelial gap junctions in EDHF-mediated relaxation in the rat middle cerebral artery *Am. J. Physiol.-Heart Circul. Physiol.* **291** H385–93

Song F *et al* 2012 Plasma apolipoprotein levels are associated with cognitive status and decline in a community cohort of older individuals *PLoS One* **7** e34078

Soreq L, Salomonis N, Bronstein M, Greenberg D S, Israel Z, Bergman H and Soreq H 2013 Small RNA sequencing-microarray analyses in Parkinson leukocytes reveal deep brain stimulation-induced splicing changes that classify brain region transcriptomes *Front. Mol. Neurosci.* **6** 10

Spector R and Johanson C E 2007 Vitamin transport and homeostasis in mammalian brain: focus on Vitamins B and E *J. Neurochem.* **103** 425–38

Spitz G, Maller J J, O'Sullivan R and Ponsford J L 2013 White matter integrity following traumatic brain injury: the association with severity of injury and cognitive functioning *Brain Topogr.* **26** 648–60

Spurkland I, Bjørbaek T and Hagemo P 2001 Psychosocial functioning in children after transplantation of the heart, and heart and lungs *Cardiol. Young* **11** 277–84

Srikanth M and Kessler J A 2012 Nanotechnology—novel therapeutics for CNS disorders *Nat. Rev. Neurol.* **8** 307–18

Stancák A Jr, Lücking C H and Kristeva-Feige R 2000 Lateralization of movement-related potentials and the size of corpus callosum *Neuroreport* **11** 329–32

Swartz K J and MacKinnon R 1997 Mapping the receptor site for hanatoxin, a gating modifier of voltage-dependent K+ channels *Neuron* **18** 675–82

Tagliaferro P, Ramos A J, Onaivi E S, Evrard S G, Lujilde J and Brusco A 2006 Neuronal cytoskeleton and synaptic densities are altered after a chronic treatment with the cannabinoid receptor agonist WIN 55,212-2 *Brain Res.* **1085** 163–76

Talerico K A and Evans L K 2001 Responding to safety issues in frontotemporal dementias *Neurology* **56** S52–5

Tang A C, Liu J Y and Sutherland M T 2005 Recovery of correlated neuronal sources from EEG: the good and bad ways of using SOBI *Neuroimage* **28** 507–19

Thambisetty M, An Y, Kinsey A, Koka D, Saleem M, Güntert A, Kraut M, Ferrucci L, Davatzikos C, Lovestone S and Resnick S M 2012 Plasma clusterin concentration is associated with longitudinal brain atrophy in mild cognitive impairment *Neuroimage* **59** 212–17

Thomsen L L, Olesen J and Russell M B 2003 Increased risk of migraine with typical aura in probands with familial hemiplegic migraine and their relatives *Eur. J. Neurol.* **10** 421–7

Trapp B D and Nave K A 2008 Multiple sclerosis: an immune or neurodegenerative disorder? *Annu. Rev. Neurosci.* **31** 247–69

Tremolizzo L, Rodriguez-Menendez V, Sala G, Di Francesco J C and Ferrarese C 2005 Valproate and HDAC inhibition: a new epigenetic strategy to mitigate phenotypic severity in ALS? *Amyotroph. Lateral Scler.* **6** 185–6

Tremolizzo L *et al* 2014 Whole-blood global DNA methylation is increased in amyotrophic lateral sclerosis independently of age of onset *Amyotroph. Lateral Sclerosis Frontotemp. Degener.* **15** 98–105

Vaccarino V, Kasl S V, Abramson J and Krumholz H M 2001 Depressive symptoms and risk of functional decline and death in patients with heart failure *J. Am. Coll. Cardiol.* **38** 199–205

Varma A R, Snowden J S, Lloyd J J, Talbot P R, Mann D M A and Neary D 1999 Evaluation of the NINCDS-ADRDA criteria in the differentiation of Alzheimer's disease and frontotemporal dementia *J. Neurol., Neurosurg. Psych.* **66** 184–8

Van De Pol L A, Hensel A, van der Flier W M, Visser P J, Pijnenburg Y A, Barkhof F, Gertz H J and Scheltens P 2006 Hippocampal atrophy on MRI in frontotemporal lobar degeneration and Alzheimer's disease *J. Neurol. Neurosurg. Psych.* **77** 439–42 van den Maagdenberg A M, Haan J, Terwindt G M and Ferrari M D 2007 Migraine: gene mutations and functional consequences *Curr. Opin. Neurol.* **20** 299–305

Vemuri P, Wiste H J, Weigand S D, Shaw L M, Trojanowski J Q, Weiner M W, Knopman D S, Petersen R C and Jack C R 2009 MRI and CSF biomarkers in normal, MCI, and AD subjects: predicting future clinical change *Neurology* **73** 294–301

Villemagne V L *et al* 2011 Longitudinal assessment of Aβ and cognition in aging and Alzheimer disease *Ann. Neurol.* **69** 181–92

von Tell D, Armulik A and Betsholtz C 2006 Pericytes and vascular stability *Exp. Cell. Res.* **312** 623–9

Wada K, Arai H, Takanashi M, Fukae J, Oizumi H, Yasuda T, Mizuno Y and Mochizuki H 2006 Expression levels of vascular endothelial growth factor and its receptors in Parkinson's disease *Neuroreport* **17** 705–9

Waldvogel D, van Gelderen P, Muellbacher W, Ziemann U, Immisch I and Hallett M 2000 The relative metabolic demand of inhibition and excitation *Nature* **406** 995–8

Wang S C, Oelze B and Schumacher A 2008 Age-specific epigenetic drift in late-onset Alzheimer's disease *PLoS One* **3** e2698

Ward R D, Holmes B H and O'Hara T D 2008 DNA barcoding discriminates echinoderm species *Molecular Ecology Resources* **8** 1202–11

Watts G D, Wymer J, Kovach M J, Mehta S G, Mumm S, Darvish D, Pestronk A, Whyte M P and Kimonis V E 2004 Inclusion body myopathy associated with Paget disease of bone and frontotemporal dementia is caused by mutant valosin-containing protein *Nat. Genet.* **36** 377–81

Waxman E A and Giasson B I 2008 Specificity and regulation of casein kinase-mediated phosphorylation of α-synuclein *J. Neuropathol. Experiment. Neurol.* **67** 402–16

Wegiel J *et al* 2001 Shift from fibrillar to nonfibrillar Aß deposits in the neocortex of subjects with Alzheimer disease *J. Alzheimer's Dis.* **3** 49–57

Werner C and Engelhard K 2007 Pathophysiology of traumatic brain injury *BJA: Br. J. Anaesth.* **99** 4–9

Wernovsky G, Shillingford A J and Gaynor J W 2005 Central nervous system outcomes in children with complex congenital heart disease *Curr. Opin. Cardiol.* **20** 94–9

White T, Kendi A T K, Lehéricy S, Kendi M, Karatekin C, Guimaraes A, Davenport N, Schulz S C and Lim K O 2007 Disruption of hippocampal connectivity in children and adolescents with schizophrenia—a voxel-based diffusion tensor imaging study *Schizophr. Res.* **90** 302–7

Wilson B, Samanta M K, Santhi K, Kumar K P S, Paramakrishnan N and Suresh B 2008 Poly (n-butylcyanoacrylate) nanoparticles coated with polysorbate 80 for the targeted delivery of rivastigmine into the brain to treat Alzheimer's disease *Brain Res.* **1200** 159–68

Witt S T, Lovejoy D W, Pearlson G D and Stevens M C 2010 Decreased prefrontal cortex activity in mild traumatic brain injury during performance of an auditory oddball task *Brain Imag. Behav.* **4** 232–47

Wolburg H and Lippoldt A 2002 Tight junctions of the blood–brain barrier: development, composition and regulation *Vasc. Pharmacol.* **38** 323–37

Wolburg H, Lippoldt A and Ebnet K 2006 Tight junctions and the blood-brain barrier *Tight Junctions* (Boston, MA: Springer) pp 175–95

Wolf R L and Detre J A 2007 Clinical neuroimaging using arterial spin-labeled perfusion magnetic resonance imaging *Neurotherapeutics* **4** 346–59

Wolk D A *et al* 2009 Amyloid imaging in mild cognitive impairment subtypes *Ann. Neurol.: Off. J. Am. Neurol. Assoc. Child. Neurol. Soc.* **65** 557–68

Woo M A, Macey P M, Keens P T, Kumar R, Fonarow G C, Hamilton M A and Harper R M 2005 Functional abnormalities in brain areas that mediate autonomic nervous system control in advanced heart failure *J. Card. Fail.* **11** 437–46

Woo H A, Chae H Z, Hwang S C, Yang K S, Kang S W, Kim K and Rhee S G 2003 Reversing the inactivation of peroxiredoxins caused by cysteine sulfinic acid formation *Science* **300** 653–6

Wu Z *et al* 2005 Role of the MEOX2 homeobox gene in neurovascular dysfunction in Alzheimer disease *Nat. Med.* **11** 959–65

Yang Z, Zhang Y, Yang Y, Sun L, Han D, Li H and Wang C 2010 Pharmacological and toxicological target organelles and safe use of single-walled carbon nanotubes as drug carriers in treating Alzheimer disease *Nanomed. Nanotechnol. Biol. Med.* **6** 427–41

Young N P, Lucchinetti C F and Weinshenker B G 2008, February Acute disseminated encephalomyelitis: current understanding and controversies *Seminars in Neurology* vol 28 (New York: Thieme Medical Publishers) pp 84–94

Zarei M, Johansen-Berg H, Smith S, Ciccarelli O, Thompson A J and Matthews P M 2006 Functional anatomy of interhemispheric cortical connections in the human brain *J. Anat.* **209** 311–20

Zarow C, Sitzer T E and Chui H C 2008 Understanding hippocampal sclerosis in the elderly: epidemiology, characterization, and diagnostic issues *Curr. Neurol. Neurosci. Rep.* **8** 363–70

Zawia N H, Lahiri D K and Cardozo-Pelaez F 2009 Epigenetics, oxidative stress, and Alzheimer disease *Free. Radic. Biol. Med.* **46** 1241–9

Zhang F F, Cardarelli R, Carroll J, Fulda K G, Kaur M, Gonzalez K, Vishwanatha J K, Santella R M and Morabia A 2011 Significant differences in global genomic DNA methylation by gender and race/ethnicity in peripheral blood *Epigenetics* **6** 623–9

Zhang Y, Brady J M and Smith S 2000, June Hidden Markov random field model for segmentation of brain MR image *Medical Imaging 2000: Image Processing* vol. 3979 (Bellingham, WA: International Society for Optics and Photonics) pp 1126–37

Zivadinov R and Cox J L 2007 Neuroimaging in multiple sclerosis *Int. Rev. Neurobiol.* **79** 449–74

Zlokovic B V, Begley D J and Chain D G 1983 Blood-brain barrier permeability to dipeptides and their constituent amino acids *Brain Res.* **271** 65–71

Zlokovic B V, Mackic J B, Djuricic B and Davson H 1989 Kinetic analysis of leucine-enkephalin cellular uptake at the luminal side of the blood-brain barrier of an *in situ* perfused guinea-pig brain *J. Neurochem.* **53** 1333–40

Zlokovic B V, Hyman S, McComb J G, Lipovac M N, Tang G and Davson H 1990 Kinetics of arginine-vasopressin uptake at the blood-brain barrier *Biochim. Biophys. Acta (BBA)-Biomembranes* **1025** 191–8

Žurek J and Fedora M 2012 The usefulness of S100B, NSE, GFAP, NF-H, secretagogin and Hsp70 as a predictive biomarker of outcome in children with traumatic brain injury *Acta Neurochirurgica* **154** 93–103

Chapter 4

Language degeneration in Alzheimer disease: evidence from neuropsychological, neuropathological and neuroimaging studies

Shashikanta Tarai, Anbu Savekar and Arindam Bit

The growing prevalence of Alzheimer disease (AD) worldwide exacerbates the burdens associated with AD dementia in the elderly population. The mechanisms of prognosis of early AD degeneration bear significance in supporting and enhancing the clinical and neuropathological diagnosis. This chapter incorporates neurocognitive, neuropathology and neuropsychology literature to offer insights into the deficits in structural and functional aspects of brain regions affected by AD. It also provides the association of AD with cognitive decline and language degeneration. It covers 30 studies over the period of the past five years. We examine the implications of bilingualism as a cognitive reserve that will mitigate AD degeneration by delaying functional impairments in specific brain regions. Different types of language impairments are discussed by corroborating the evidence with the underpinnings of irreversible neuronal brain damage due to the progression stages of AD. Thus, in this chapter, we not only elucidate the cognitive degeneration involving decline and impairment of language structure, but we also trace the changes in the brain regions that occur with AD onset and progression.

4.1 Introduction

The increasing global prevalence of dementia amongst the older population is mainly associated with AD, a neurodegenerative disorder. AD features in 75% of all dementia cases, and the AD archetype is characterised by progressive degeneration of the brain, ensuing in atrophy and subsequent death of the individual (González 2014, Prince *et al* 2015, World Health Organization 2019). Dementia is the eventual progression of either AD or any other degenerative disorder in older adults above

doi:10.1088/978-0-7503-3383-2ch4

65. The symptoms of functional abnormalities evident in dementia vary according to dementia and corresponding brain cell deterioration. As a debilitating syndrome in the elderly population, dementia is characterised by loss of memory and cognitive abilities such as the lack of coherence in speech or written language, the loss of recognition, poor executive motor activities or the sensory function or comprehension of the task, the loss of abstract thinking, planning, decision making and inability to perform complex tasks (Jahn 2013, Wiley 2021). The initial symptoms of mild AD are subtle cognitive impairments coupled with episodic memory loss that deteriorates with the disease's gradual progression (Mueller *et al* 2018). The Alzheimer's disorder continuum occurs from mild to moderate, leading to the severe and dementia phase of Alzheimer's disease, eventually resulting in the patient's death. The multifactorial causes of AD besides ageing are mainly genetic, environmental, and lifestyle, which generally associates with the prevalence of hypertension, diabetes, obesity, substance abuse like smoking and drinking and sedentary life (Sahyouni *et al* 2016, Bhatti *et al* 2020, Wiley 2021). Furthermore, cognitive inactivity such as lower levels of education is also recognised as a risk factor (Sahyouni *et al* 2016). The recent AD literature highlights the efficacy of the cognitive reserve paradigm through more excellent cognitive-linguistic skills like bilingualism as a counter-measure to environmental risk factors (Bialystok *et al* 2007, 2014, Gold 2016). The gravity of the existing global scenario is amplified by the widespread prevalence, the alarming increase in cases, the challenges of early diagnosis, the common causal factors attributable to lifestyle and increasing elderly populations (Bhatti *et al* 2020). The burden of diagnosis primarily lies upon neurologists and medical practitioners. Nonetheless, social scientists and researchers are exploring alternative models of early AD detection by studying and exploring AD individuals' interpersonal communication and their functional relations with family members. Synchronising with this approach, this chapter assimilates and analyses literature findings on cognitive degeneration evident as communicative deterioration or impairment underpinned by AD neuronal deterioration in brain regions.

4.1.1 Twentieth-century insights into Alzheimer's disease

In the early part of the 20th century, the German psychiatrist and neuropathologist Dr Alois Alzheimer in 1906 provided significant insights into the neuropathology of AD. The treatment of a 51-year-old patient (Augusta D) exhibiting delusional and psychotic behaviours, intense short term memory loss, predominant language impairment and behavioural changes were extensively studied and documented (Khan 2016, Tellechea *et al* 2018). The patient's brain autopsy's observations and findings correlated the morphological and histological changes with typical neuronal degeneration occurring in AD. In 1906, Dr Alzheimer's description established two neuropathological phenomena in the brain: the presence of amyloid plaques and neurofibrillary tangles (dense bundles of fibrils) that disrupt the neuronal signals in various regions of the brain. However, the debate on the sameness of attributes in presenile and senile dementia remained enmeshed with AD symptoms until the

1970s (Khan 2016). Dr Robert Katzman, in 1976, identified AD as the leading cause of dementia, and his prediction on AD becoming a primary future public health concern for society has currently been validated by health survey reports on AD and dementia (Katzman 1976). The successive neuropathological and neuroimaging studies corroborated the presence of amyloid plaques and neurofibrillary tangles in the brain at autopsy as the gold standard of AD diagnosis (Spires-Jones *et al* 2011, Khan 2016, Sahyouni *et al* 2016, Tellechea *et al* 2018).

The progression of amyloid creates subtle cognitive changes, and further deterioration in cognition corresponds to more considerable amyloid accumulation (Gonzalez 2014). Further investigations on the volume of neurofibrillary tangles in brain autopsy facilitated description of the severity of AD, which is classified in stages I to VI: I and II as mild stages of AD, II–IV corresponding to moderate and stages V and VI corresponding to severe AD. At the same time, the early AD diagnosis is likely to ease prediction of the manifestation, treatment protocols and gathering insights—the multifactorial and heterogeneously complex features of AD challenge developing standard models for early detection. For instance, the literature suggests mild cognitive impairment (MCI) symptoms could be a precursor or prodrome of AD or specific AD symptoms, and other degenerative disorders overlap, thereby increasing the probability of misdiagnosis (Khan 2016). The recent developments and integration of empirical research in neuropathology, neurocognition, neuropsychology and neuroimaging, which explores biomarkers, provide considerable insights into AD pathology to supplement clinical diagnosis and lay pathways to early detection (Mofrad *et al* 2021).

According to the World Health Organization (2019) report on dementia, approximately 50 million elderly people suffer worldwide, and it is further estimated that by the year 2050, some form of dementia will strike 135 million. Globally, AD has affected 55 million, and by 2050, it is likely to increase by 88 million. AD is a devastating, incurable, irreversible neurodegenerative disorder wherein life expectancy diminishes with disease progression. The mean life expectancy is seven years after clinical diagnosis. The cases of AD are currently rising exponentially compared to other terminal illnesses and at an alarming rate. Incidentally, the longer life expectancy renders women vulnerable to AD and dementia (Mebane-Sims 2009, Wiley 2021). Although the incidence of AD development increases with age, statistics reveal disproportionate odds (2:1) where females are more vulnerable to AD than males (Sahyouni *et al* 2016). According to the study reports, more women than men suffer from AD. In fact, out of the elderly in the 71 years age bracket of the older population who had dementia, 2.4 million were women, and only 1 million were men (Mebane-Sims 2009, Wiley 2021). African-Americans' vulnerability towards AD and other forms of dementia is more than whites in the US (Mebane-Sims 2009, Wiley 2021). However, studies suggest the causal factors of AD do not significantly depend on race, although they are most likely to be influenced by other factors like less education and different routinely challenging lifestyles and poor cardio-vascular health contributors (Sahyouni *et al* 2016). Studies suggest that fewer years of education increase the vulnerability and impose a greater likelihood of neuronal degeneration leading to AD. Hence, education as a cognitive reserve is advocated as a preventive strategy to delay the onset of AD and its implications of reducing financial burden. Ample study evidence confirms that AD afflicting the ageing global population is a societal challenge with substantial emotional and economic limitations on families, communities, and health care systems worldwide (Mebane-Sims 2009, Prince *et al* 2015, Sahyouni *et al* 2016, Wiley 2021).

4.1.2 Features and etiology of AD

The AD form of dementia is dichotomised into two distinct types: (i) FAD (familial AD) or early-onset AD (EOAD), and (ii) late-onset AD (LOAD). The etiologic contributors of early and late-onset AD are varied (Sahyouni *et al* 2016). The aetiology of EOAD lies in autosomal dominant family history due to familial AD gene mutation, which develops and emerges earlier than 65 years of age. Although the early onset occurrence is as rare as in less than 5% of the cases; nonetheless, EOAD is an aggressive course of disease (Tellechea *et al* 2018). Gene mutation due to genetics prevails as the key risk factor in the early onset of FAD or EOAD, wherein the amyloid-beta (Aβ) levels in the brain and peripheral tissues are higher than in other individuals without the mutations (Khan 2016). LOAD is genetically complex, multifactorial, heterogeneous, and a sporadic neurodegenerative disorder associated with ageing. It occurs in later years of life, predominantly after 65 years of age and is prevalent in more than 95% of dementia cases. The etiologic contributors are linked not only to the dominant ageing factor and to genetics but also other non-genetic risk factors such as brain injury, vascular disease, hypertension, high cholesterol, atherosclerosis, coronary heart disease, obesity, and diabetes, besides an inactive lifestyle and poor diet (Sahyouni *et al* 2016). The LOAD patients are generally associated with unusual psychiatric and behavioural symptoms (Tellechea *et al* 2018). The amyloid cascade hypothesis explains the development of LOAD, whereby the synaptic loss and neurodegeneration result from a deficit in the clearing of toxic Aβ, which causes an accumulation of toxic Aβ in the brain (Hardy and Selkoe 2002). The gradual degeneration and death of neurons and synapses occur in AD due to the excessive presence of amyloid plaques and neurofibrillary tangles, consequently impacting the cognitive functions correlating to the cognitive decline (Spires-Jones *et al* 2011, Khan 2016, Tellechea *et al* 2018).

4.1.3 AD symptoms—pathological and physiological features

The AD brain autopsy demonstrates prevalent pathological symptoms: synaptic loss, neuroinflammation, neuronal cell death, cortical atrophy and the presence of neurofibrillary tangles and senile plaques (Spires-Jones *et al* 2011, Khan 2016). While the primary incidence of AD degeneration is synaptic dysfunction, as synaptic loss correlates to memory function and cognitive decline. However, the AD progression displays greater functional cognitive deterioration due to increased neuronal death and the formation of neurofibrillary tangles and senile plaques (Khan 2016, Mueller *et al* 2018). Pathophysiology of AD begins long before presenting the clinical symptoms of memory and cognitive deficits (Mueller *et al* 2018). The neuropathological deterioration of a cluster of brain cells associated with memory function correlates to characteristic symptoms of AD's clinical diagnosis, evident as cognitive decline, loss of memory, and learning deficit (Jahn 2013, Tellechea *et al* 2018, Pistono *et al* 2019). The gradual disease progression to the moderate stage is exhibited by confusion, impaired thinking, poor judgement, challenged expressions or communication and disorientation regarding time, location and space. The advanced stage of AD renders the individual incapable of routine self-care like eating, bathing, dressing, disinhibition, inappropriate use of the toilet, incontinence, causing disruption of normal routine activities and needing assistance or caregivers. The final stages of AD correlate to severe conditions of neuronal degeneration, such as total loss of communication ability, failing to recognise loved ones, being bedbound and subsequently death (Mebane-Sims 2009, Wiley 2021).

The insights into AD degeneration which affects and disrupts the lives of suffering individuals, can be gathered by the AD symptoms classified into two: First, by the domains that are affected by the neuronal brain degeneration in the individuals, as shown in table 4.1; Second, based on the symptoms categorised into progression stages of AD (Sahyouni *et al* 2016), as represented in table 4.2.

4.1.4 Biomarkers indicate pathophysiology of the brain in AD

Considering that characteristic pathological features of AD are amyloid Aβ plaques and neurofibrillary tangles (NFTs), the measure of its accumulation is significant to the pathophysiological diagnosis of the AD stage (Spires-Jones *et al* 2011, Ruthirakuhan *et al* 2018, Mofrad *et al* 2021), as shown in figure 4.1. While on the one hand, the prevalent diagnostic biomarkers are post-mortem investigations which indicate the density of Aβ plaques and neurofibrillary tangles (NFT), on the other hand, antemortem investigations also measure Aβ plaques and NFT through an invasive method of cerebrospinal fluid markers (CSF). The biomarkers (CSF—cerebrospinal fluid markers, fMRI—functional magnetic resonance image, PET—positron emission tomography, MRI—magnetic resonance image) reflect the state of the disease through measurable physical, chemical, or anatomical variables (Gonzalez 2014). Neuroimaging techniques of PET and MRI show proximal brain changes with disease progression such as levels of beta-amyloid, Tau, loss of synapses, brain metabolic changes or structural changes. Functional neuroimaging techniques measure brain functions; for instance, fMRI analyses the brain's response to specific stimuli reflected by the stimulus-induced haemodynamic changes in the brain regions. The significance of AD biomarkers is their multiple application for diagnosis and assessment of prognosis and longitudinal tracking, evaluation of therapeutic efficacy, and clinical trials (Khan 2016, Mofrad *et al* 2021). However, the variability of the accuracy of biomarkers fails the diagnostic accuracy in clinical practice for cognitive disorders. Yet, amyloid imaging is regarded as a significant biomarker (González 2014, Khan 2016). The implication of the role of biomarkers in Alzheimer's type of dementia is to confirm the clinical diagnosis of AD by providing information towards early detection of pathophysiologic changes of structural and functional neuronal brain region deterioration and dysfunctions (Khan 2016, Mofrad *et al* 2021).

Table 4.1. The classification of symptoms represents the affected domains in AD.

Physiological	Behavioural	Cognitive	Affective and psychological	Pathological
Deterioration of physical capabilities: Inability to walk, sit, and eventually swallow. Loss of appetite. Decline in muscular coordination. Bladder and bowel incontinence. Changes in sleep patterns. Vulnerability to pneumonia and infection. Disorientation. Loss of balance and coordination. Visuospatial dysfunction–inability to recognise objects or faces.	***Personality or behavioural changes:*** Loss of inhibitions. Social withdrawal. Crying. Irritability. Aggression. Agitation. Mood swings. Wandering/being lost. Restlessness. Suspicion. Impulsiveness. Repetitive behaviours. Incapable of dressing or using the toilet. Need assistance and caregiving for routine activities. No awareness of surroundings.	***Memory and cognitive dysfunction:*** Inability to recall words, addresses, phone numbers, to remember names of new people/information. Forgetfulness. Memory loss. Mental confusion. Lack of concentration and focus. Inability to plan or organise. Decline in thinking, reasoning, making judgements and decisions. Lack of coherence in communicative language (grounding, spatial, temporal and thematic coherence).	***Affective changes:*** Moodiness. Apathy. Agitation. Irritability. Loneliness. ***Psychologicaldecline:*** Delusions. Paranoia. Hallucinations. Depression.	***A pathological decline in the brain:*** Atrophy of brain (shrinking). Degeneration of synapses and neuronal cells. Extracellular amyloid-beta plaque build-up. Intracellular presence of neurofibrillary tangles. Loss of cerebrospinal fluid. Genetical mutation.

Table 4.2. The symptoms are classified according to the various stages of AD.

Early stage (I–II mild stages) **Preclinical/pre-symptomatic phase**	**Middle stage** (II–IV moderate stages) **Predementia phase**	**Late stage** (V–VI severe stages) **Dementia phase**
• Word-finding difficulties • Difficulty remembering names of new people • Difficulty with social and work tasks • Forgetting recently read material • Misplacing valuable objects • Difficulty planning or organising *[Begins in* ***medial temporal lobe*** *(in MCI)]* *Spreads to* ***lateral temporal and parietal lobes***	• Forgetting important events or personal memories • Moodiness or social withdrawal • Inability to recall addresses or telephone numbers • Confusion with dates and locations • Difficulty selecting proper clothing • Bladder and bowel incontinence • Sleep pattern changes • Risk of wandering or being lost • Personality or behavioural changes (suspicion, impulsiveness, delusions, and repetitive behaviours) *Spreads to frontal lobe*	• Need full-time assistance required for activities of daily living • No awareness of recent and past experiences or surroundings • Deterioration of physical capabilities including walking, sitting, and eventually swallowing • Communication problems • Vulnerability to pneumonia and infection *Spreads to occipital lobe*

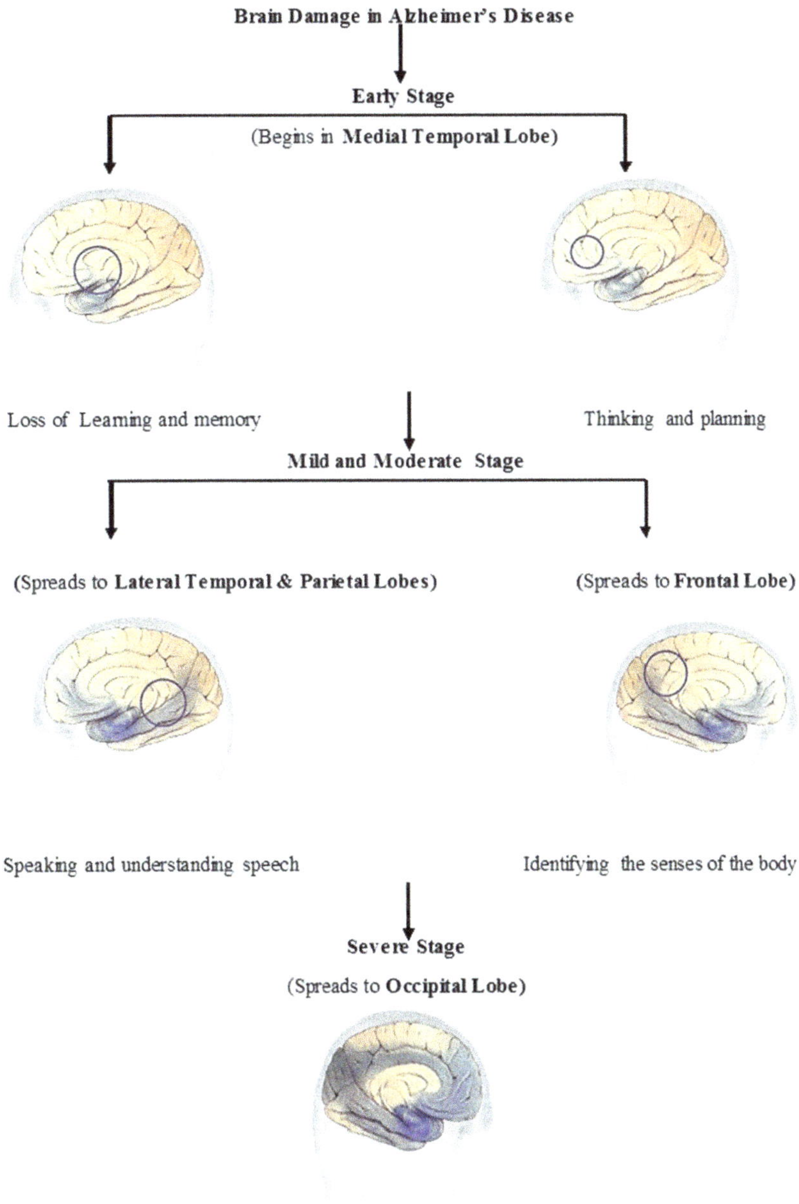

Figure 4.1. The regions of interest (ROI) of the brain are affected by the different stages of AD.

4.1.5 Diagnostic challenges and other degenerative disorders

The diagnostic challenges due to multifactorial causes and heterogeneity of the disease are further amplified by varying symptoms, pathological and clinical complexity. Firstly, AD may be comorbid and prevalent with other old-age neurodegenerative disorders (vascular dementia (VaD), Lewy body disease (LBD),

Parkinson's disease (PD), frontotemporal dementia (FTD), amyotrophic lateral sclerosis (ALS), and tauopathy). For example, an impaired sense of smell is an early symptom of AD and Parkinson and other degenerative diseases (Sahyouni *et al* 2016, Wiley 2021). Further, the symptoms of AD commence mildly and progress slowly, unlike other degenerative disorders. Secondly, gradual progression in AD escapes the attention of close family members who begin to notice symptoms of deterioration when the disease has progressed far into its chronicity. Thirdly, diagnosis is ambiguous for AD due to similarities of symptoms with other disorders such as depression. Given that 30%–40% of AD patients also suffer from depression and have signs of impairment in memory and motor function due to affected cerebellum (Canli *et al* 2004). Therefore, due to the similarities in symptoms, the likelihood of false detection increases, which may incorrectly diagnose individuals with AD or depression. Heterogeneous clinical presentations may cause diagnostic errors, especially in dominant executive or language dysfunctions, and may be mistaken for frontotemporal dementia (FTD). Thus, the absence of a standard diagnostic method makes AD a public health concern worldwide (Khan 2016). The implications of misdiagnosis pose a severe effect on treatment interventions.

Consequently, the detecting of mild and subtle language structure declines in the early stage, which remains primarily unnoticed, undetected and unidentified. Early language assessment, identification of language impairments, and interventions to maintain the natural functional abilities will delay progression to the stage of irreversible brain degeneration (Groves-Wright *et al* 2004). It is estimated that delaying AD through clinical intervention by one year will likely reduce the surging AD cases by 9 million by 2050 (Khan 2016).

4.1.6 Language degeneration: phonology, morphology, syntax and semantics

According to past literature (Emery 2000), a prime symptom of dementia of Alzheimer's type (DAT) was memory impairment, with no attention towards language deterioration. Subsequently, the decline in the language (lexical-semantic impairment) and continued deterioration corresponding to the disease severity was identified as a feature of the early and late-onset disease (Altmann and McClung 2008, Pistono *et al* 2019). In early-onset (EOAD), the disease progression is accelerated, and the language disintegration parallelly follows the accelerated and severe progression. However, the study finding suggests that the memory remains unaffected in the early onset of AD (EOAD) (Tellechea *et al* 2018). Nonetheless, other studies consider language impairments which demonstrate the decline, dysfunctions and degeneration of cognitive, affective, psychological, communicative and behavioural attributes to be the cornerstones of prognosis and diagnosis of AD (Appell *et al* 1982, Ellis 1996, Le *et al* 2011, Mueller *et al* 2018).

Language as a communication process combines encoding and decoding of information (symbols and signs) with a system of rules. Language involves the cognitive functioning to execute, acquire, process, synthesise, store, retrieve, and transmit information (Emery 2000, Robins 2014). Deriving the meaning of information (signs and symbols) creates coherence in communicative language, where sense and understanding of the discourse involve language structures at phonology, morphology, syntax, semantics and pragmatics (Haas 1954, Ellis 1996, Robins 2014). A linguistics study examines language scientifically to establish the relation between sound and meaning. Semiotics in linguistics demonstrates language's hierarchical structure, representing the increasing complexity in language development and processing when interpreting the information (signs and symbols). In other words, the four ranks in language structure, namely: phonology (sounds), morphology (parts of words, words), syntax (sentences, paragraphs) and semantics (expressed meaning). The first rank and the most superficial level is *phonology*. Phonology deals with sound and has no reference to purpose. *Morphology* is the analysis of morphemes or the minor parts of words and words containing meaning. Lexicon is the total cluster of morphemes in a language. There can be two morphological analyses: lexical or vocabulary competence, e.g., confrontation naming, and word-internal morphological analysis, e.g., declension and conjugation involving word-internal changes. Syntax analyses the structure of phrases and sentences, including sentence types, linear word order, differing kinds of clauses, pronomial and prepositional usage, and forms of propositional relations. *Semantics* is the organisation of knowledge and meaning which focus on symbols and their purpose. In the semiotic language hierarchy, semantics is the most complex level as well as the highest rank. The semantic processing or analysis can occur at two levels: firstly, at the word level (morphological), which is simpler to process; secondly, at the sentence level (syntactical), which is complex as it involves larger units such as sentences. These language structures represent the semiotic language model, going from simple to more complex language units, in the hierarchical ranks of phonology, morphology, syntax, semantics (Ellis 1996, Zlatev 2009).

The model of language hierarchy provided a context for the discrete data on language deterioration in DAT (dementia of Alzheimer's type) and adhered to the hierarchical nature of semiotics in language decline (Emery 2000). Interestingly, the study on language decline in the context of the semiotic hierarchy demonstrates the negative relationship between language development sequence and language deterioration. In other words, there is a reversal, i.e., the language forms which are learned last in the sequence of language development deteriorate first, contrary to the anticipation of language deterioration mirroring the learning sequence. The language forms learned last are the most complex in the sequence of language development. Therefore, the final learned complex form becomes the first to be impaired by degeneration in Alzheimer's. The relevance of semiotics in research explorations is demonstrated when the semiotic categories provide a systematic and hierarchical context to scrutinise the nature of language deterioration in AD.

The hierarchical structure of language is evident in linguistic analysis and discourse (Ellis 1996). The brain development linked to language and communicative competence occurs in functionally competent users (Haas 1954, Ellis 1996, Zlatev 2009, Robins 2014). The linguistic evolution correlates to the relationship between grammar and cognitive processing. On the same continuum, two different modes, pre-grammatical and grammatical, exist represented by semantic and structural cohesion. Pre-grammatical is the early stage of language development and linguistic evolution having slow and vocabulary driven processing, is prone to error and is context-dependent (language patterns in children, second language acquisition). Grammatical mode is structural with syntactically complex construction and morphological features acquired later and processed faster with fewer errors (Ellis 1996).

The communicative competence to interact socially and interpersonally includes initiating interaction, sustaining interaction and ending interaction using language effectively. This refers to the coherence of the pragmatics in language structure and measures the thematic relation to previous utterance, topic and maintaining the topic within the discourse (Mueller *et al* 2018). This feature is explored by researchers in the unscripted speeches of prominent public figures or literary texts of writers (Garrard *et al* 2005, Berisha *et al* 2015). Past study on Alzheimer's discourse focused more upon narrative structure than on interactive communication; for instance, Ellis (1996) used a discourse framework to gather insights into the communicative patterns in senile dementia of Alzheimer's type (SDAT). The decline in coherence identified was grounding, temporal, spatial, thematic, and the textual variations of these four types of coherence in Alzheimer's discourse distinguish mild from advanced stages.

Consequently, the absence of coherence in communication was regarded as a diagnosis of SDAT. Study findings reveal (Ellis 1996) that communicative irregularities within the ongoing discourse were linguistic and demonstrate errors semantically rather than syntactically. The discourse responses were syntactically formed yet were pragmatically incoherent in AD patients. In addition, there were communication and cognitive processing difficulties, which showed a divergence between mental reality and linguistic discourse. This kind of AD decline demonstrates the patients' inability to organise information to create meaning and understanding with linguistic forms, which otherwise are used in context with the cognitive reality, to generate coherent language and communication.

4.1.7 Controversial regression hypothesis of language degeneration in AD

According to Ribot's law of regression or reversion, 'in inorganic life, the structures last formed are the first to degenerate while in the biological world, dissolution acts in a contrary direction to evolution, which is—the new perishes before the old and the complex before the simple' (Lust *et al* 2015). The regression or retrogenesis hypothesis (RH) is linked to memory function and maintains that the acquisition in development is reversed in neurodegeneration; in other words, the most recent memory acquisition is lost first while older memories are retained longer in certain conditions of amnesia caused by brain injury. The current study (Jacobs *et al* 2011) on cerebral degeneration supports RH because higher areas of cognitive association indicate traces of functional decline and grey matter atrophy. Converse to this, another study (Westlye *et al* 2010) outcome showed protracted maturation of white matter. While some AD studies on memory appear to support the RH to reveal memory loss with selective retention of older information, there is other evidence in specific pathologies like semantic dementia that demonstrate reversal, wherein most recent events are remembered rather than older ones. The study findings examining RH in the language domain vary or are ambiguous, implying the likelihood of complexity in the empirical study of the RH. Lust *et al* (2015) examined the RH in the domain of language (syntax development in first language acquisition in individuals with MCI (a precursor to AD)), wherein the findings failed to support RH. However, according to the authors, this result fails the validity as a generalisable outcome in studies examining other cognitive memory representations.

While the neuropsychological literature identifies evidence of cognitive and behavioural decline evident as impairments in communication in AD patients, there are no generalisable conclusive models established as diagnostic markers. The literature on language decline in AD patients mostly has varying outcomes due to the heterogeneity of AD symptoms and multifactorial etiologic causes of the degenerative disorder. With advances in technology, neuropathological studies on AD identified and established the structural and functional degeneration in the brain regions due to accumulation of amyloid and neurofibrillary tangles, synaptic loss or neuronal cell death. However, literature tracing the decline of language across stages of AD progression in tandem with the AD progression in neuronal degeneration of brain regions is scarce. Although recent studies are examining language deterioration and cognitive decline in AD, establishing the generalizability of patterns of early language decline corresponding to the anticipated neuronal degeneration in brain regions may provide significant models for early prognosis of AD, its manifestation probability and treatment protocols. Thus, this chapter examines literature across neuropsychological and neuropathological studies to synthesise the findings on the presentation of different hierarchical components of language decline and trace the neuronal brain atrophy in the AD stages. Furthermore, we also examine the literature on the effect of bilingualism on AD brain degeneration which as a cognitive reserve provides an alternative model for delaying AD.

4.2 Methodological insights

This current chapter is a systematic secondary analysis of primary studies on the degenerative decline in AD, which focused on similar research questions regarding neuropsychological and neuropathological changes attributable to AD (Finfgeld 2003, Timulak 2014). This study synthesises findings across time across domains and thematically establishes overall results to underpin the insights and trends related to AD. The current chapter is primarily a qualitative meta-analysis from the approach perspectives of neuropsychology, neurocognition and neuroimaging. First, we focused upon the literature findings in neuropsychology related to the decline of language structure in AD patients and correlate it with the literature findings from neuropathology on neuronal degeneration in brain regions of AD subjects.

The study follows the PRISMA format represented by the flow chart as shown in figure 4.2. The stages include: (1) In the first stage extensive literature survey was conducted to extract relevant literature using keywords. (2) The second stage consisted of reading the title and abstract to eliminate non-relevant and duplicate papers. (3) In the third stage of full-text reading, we applied inclusion and exclusion

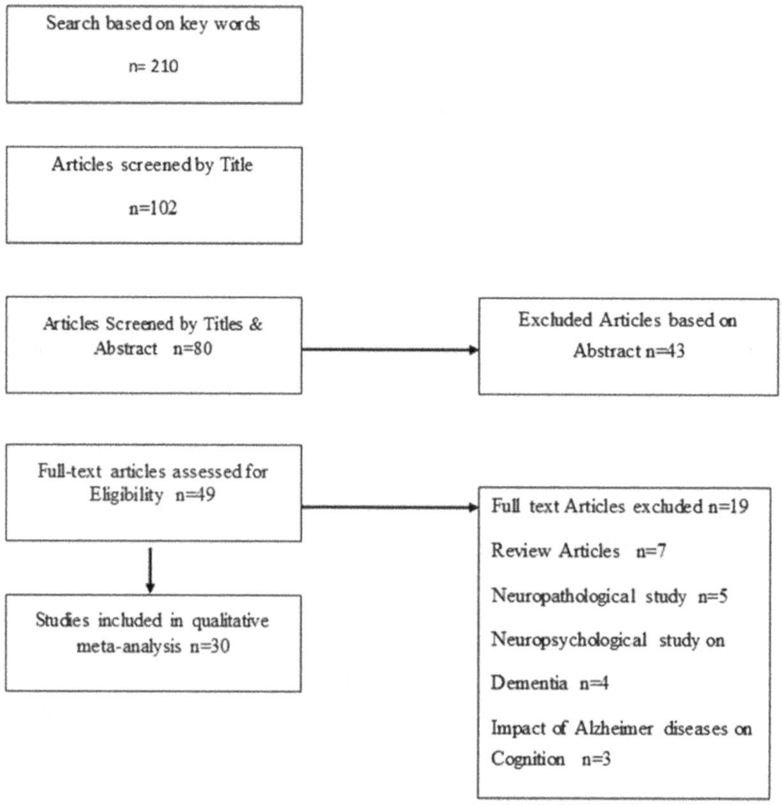

Figure 4.2. The flow chart explains the selection procedures to classify and recognise the research work related to AD.

criteria to identify relevant papers. (4) Next, a systematic matrix of data tabulation was prepared for analysis. (5) Finally, a thorough and close reading of papers and results was done, and findings across chosen literature were established for analysis and discussion.

4.2.1 Selection of literature

A systematic literature survey was conducted by using online electronic databases and search engines. The keywords that were designed to search the electronic database include EEG, AD, behavioural changes, cognitive decline, language impairments, phonological, morphological and syntactic degenerations, the impact of bilingualism, neurological, neuropathological decline, impact and impairment, a biomarker of AD, and the regions of the brain affected by AD.

4.2.2 Inclusion and exclusion criteria for participants

This chapter focuses on AD degeneration regarding decline in language, brain atrophy regions affected due to amyloid deposition that impact cognitive functions to cause language impairment, and the significance of bilingualism as a cognitive reserve in AD. Thus, our inclusion criteria aimed to identify literature relevant to this chapter. The current study considered the following criteria for the selection and analysis of the form. The exclusion parameters followed were to reject identified review articles and duplicate them. Further, we scrutinised papers that did not contain the themes of our study or were articles on dementia, cognitive behaviour and generic neuropathological studies.

To include the research papers in our study, the papers that addressed the following parameters were considered: (a) the survey of AD published is in English; (b) the study employing qualitative or quantitative methods to analyse data; (c) the research papers focused on language decline in AD patients; (d) the study focused on the efficacy of bilingualism in AD patients; (e) the study examined impairment in brain regions caused by AD; (f) the study considered diagnostic tests for identifying the experiment's samples; (g) the participant is an AD patient either suffering from mild, moderate or severe AD; (h) the participant is multilingual, bilingual or monolingual; (i) the age of the participant is above 50 years and identified as probable AD or diagnosed with AD. The total number of published papers chosen for this chapter is 30 (20 neuropsychology and ten neuropathology), wherein 75% (15) are neuropsychology articles, and 80% (8) are neuropathology articles chosen from the last two decades. Tabulation of information and findings of the chosen articles was done to support further result analysis and discussion processes.

4.3 Result

The results of the studies are assimilated to establish our findings categorised as linguistic degeneration observable as neuropsychological and neurocognitive decline and neuropathological degeneration in the brain in AD. Furthermore, the findings across 30 studies are consolidated based on study evidence in structural language decline as in semantic, morphological, syntactical, lexical and the AD degeneration pathophysiology evident through neuroimaging biomarkers corresponding to the affected regions of brain atrophy. Additionally, we look at the effect of bilingualism in AD degeneration in terms of language and pathophysiology.

4.3.1 Neuropsychological degeneration of language structures in AD

This section outlines the findings across studies that illustrate the effects of neuronal degeneration in AD patients exhibiting a neuropsychological decline in language structures. We view the AD patients' deficits in language classified under decline in semantics, syntax, morphology and phonology.

4.3.2 Semantic decline in AD

The decline in the most complex level of language development was assessed in patients with degenerative disorders. The AD patients' ability or impairment in interpreting and analysing the meaning of words and phrases in sentences represents the preservation or deterioration of semantic level in the communicative language. The semantic decline includes syntactic and lexical deficits in the presentations and the processing of communicative language of AD patients. Most studies evaluating language decline used picture description as an assessment tool to analyse the semantic deterioration in AD patients. A comparative study on the early and late stages of SDAT language decline used a picture description task. The subjects of late-stage semantic dementia of Alzheimer's Type (SDAT) responded with significantly fewer observations (actions and objects) on the pictorial themes of 'cookie theft picture' than the subjects of the early stage of SDAT. However, both groups (late and early-stage) of SDAT subjects combined exhibited fewer tasks' observations than the control group (Hier *et al* 1985). Other study results of picture description task-based performance revealed the individuals in a moderate stage of AD performed poorly in both written and verbal assessments as compared to the control group (Groves-Wright *et al* 2004) and those in the mild stage of AD produced less information in the picture description assessment task than the control group (Sajjadi *et al* 2012). At the same time, one study employed interview inputs from caregivers in the AD patients' families to gather information. The caregivers' inputs confirmed that AD patients face difficulty comprehending and communicating their emotions to their caregivers (Komjakraphan and Karuncharernpanit 2021).

Compared with the patients diagnosed with other forms of dementia, the AD patients' performance in cognitive tasks had mixed results across studies. For example, one such experimental study compared patients diagnosed with AD with those having frontal, temporal lobar dementia (FTLD) (Porto *et al* 2008). When compared with FTLD, the AD patients' performance was significantly weaker in tests of verbal and visual episodic memory, immediate verbal memory (logical memory), attention with interference, verbal fluency (semantic and phonemic) and concept formation (Porto *et al* 2008). However, conversely, the results of a longitudinal study showed that the FTD and PPA (semantic dementia, PPA—primary progressive aphasia) subjects had faster language decline than AD patients (Blair *et al* 2007).

4.3.3 Syntactical decline

The assessment of grammatical preservation in sentence processing was done in mild and moderate stage DAT patients with experimental tasks of sentence-picture matching, grammatical sentence judgements, and sentence completion. The language impairment in DAT patients was more prominent than the elderly control group in completing sentences with a single word due to difficulty judging the grammaticality of brief sentences. Furthermore, the patients' errors included grammatical and semantic violations, suggesting significant impairment in syntactic processing (Grossman *et al* 1995). In contrast to Grossman *et al* (1995), another study (Rochon *et al* 1994) suggests a fair amount of syntactical preservation. Rochon *et al*'s (1994) study findings on the early stage of dementia of Alzheimer's type (DAT) examined the responses to different levels of syntax in the sentence-picture matching task. Although the complexity of syntax did not affect performance, the AD patients' performance deteriorated (inability to process meaning) in some functions, as in the case when a sentence had two propositions (complex sentence).

On the other hand, the simple syntax was preserved, and overall semantic was more impaired than syntactic (Rochon *et al* 1994). Findings of a study also revealed AD subjects demonstrated the tendency of phonemic-paraphasia as well as semantic-paraphasia. While issues in moderate stage AD exhibited greater phonemic-paraphasia, which impacted their writing outputs, the subjects with mild AD exhibited more semantic-paraphasia (substitution of words related in meaning for target words such as a *horse* for *zebra*), which impacted their verbal output (Groves-Wright *et al* 2004). A recent study (Can and Kuruoğlu 2018) on syntactic processing demonstrated that patients with early-onset AD used more coordinated sentences only in the Random Speech test and more compound sentences only in the Story Picture Sequencing test to the control group.

4.3.4 Morphological or lexical decline

The AD patients recalled words having higher frequency occurrence far more efficiently than the words with low frequency of occurrence (Barker and Lawson 1968). The early stages of AD are marked by the deficiency in vocabulary and recurrence of words in sentences (Miller and Hague 1975). An autopsy-related study confirmed and proved AD patients significantly differed from MCI patients regarding the proportion of pronouns (Ahmed *et al* 2013). Investigations on the impact of language are written, and verbal features on word fluency revealed inferior performance in both written and verbal production in moderate stage AD than in mild AD and control groups. Moreover, moderate AD showed severe impairment in the written output of word fluency (Groves-Wright *et al* 2004). *Phonological*: The study on initial diagnostic markers for AD (Pastoriza-Dominguez *et al* 2021) examined pauses taken during sentence production, using picture description tasks in AD patients and healthy controls. The results revealed that AD patients in the early stages hold longer breaks in sentences which further impacts their word fluency (Pastoriza-Dominguez *et al* 2021).

Lexical decline in case study: A case study (Garrard *et al* 2005) examined the literary works of the famous British novelist Iris Murdoch (born in 1919, died in 1999) who was diagnosed with AD (wrote her first work '*Under the net*' 1954 and final result '*Jackson's Dilemma*' 1995). The study confirmed a noticeable decline in the vocabulary in her middle stage compared to the initial phase of her creative career, which eventually was corroborated by the destitution of vocabulary in the last book written by her (at 76 years of age). Similarly, the case study on former US President Ronald Reagan (born 1911, died 2004) was diagnosed with AD at 80 years in 1994, six years after relinquishing the post, showed a significant decrease in the number of unique words (non-regular vocabulary) over time and a significant increase in conversational fillers, higher levels of filled and unfilled pauses and non-specific nouns over time (Berisha *et al* 2015). A longitudinal comparative case study finding on three famous writers: Iris Murdoch (diagnosed with AD), Agatha Christie (probable AD) and P D James (healthy control), confirmed the lexical decline is attributable to AD. The literary writings of Iris Murdoch exhibited a significant decrease in the lexicon and the syntactic function of language, and Agatha Christie's scholarly work also revealed traces of similar decline in the later works (Le *et al* 2011).

4.3.5 Lexico-semantic decline in bilinguals

The study findings of highly proficient bilingual AD subjects revealed the decline prevalence in both languages—the dominant and the non-dominant language was similar. However, the performance of bilinguals was better in their dominant language than in their non-dominant language in picture naming task (lexical competence), even though the interaction was not significant between 'group of participants' and 'language dominance' (Costa *et al* 2012). Similarly, a longitudinal study on bilingualism in AD patients corroborated the findings of better performance in the dominant language and similar decline in both languages (Calabria *et al* 2017). The evaluation of highly proficient bilinguals across a cross-sectional study (Costa *et al* 2012) and a longitudinal study (Calabria *et al* 2017) compared to decline in AD and MCI patients and had similar results. Both showed a parallel decline in AD patients for both languages (dominant and non-dominant) when measured for lexico-semantic impairment, where subjects' performance was assessed through picture naming, word translation and word comprehension tasks. The two studies demonstrated AD cognitive decline involving semantic representations and lexical processing as a parallel for both languages, yet the performance was better in the dominant language, specifically in the task involving linguistic competence (picture naming scheme).

A study (Gollan *et al* 2017) of bilingual AD patients and control group focused on the occurrence of intrusion error while reading paragraphs in non-dominant language with switches into dominant language. The results revealed that AD patients elicited more intrusion and produced more within language error than the bilingual control subjects (Gollan *et al* 2017).

4.3.6 Neuropathological degeneration in the brain regions

The degenerative process studied in seven AD patients indicated that the decline occurred only in specific brain regions such as medial temporal (limbic), lateral hemisphere, posterior inferior temporal areas, parieto-occipital lobes, and posterior cingulate gyrus (Brun and Gustafson 1976). In addition, studies traced the changes in the brain caused by the incidence of fibrous tangles (NFT) (abnormal phosphorylated tau protein in the interneurons), which characteristically marks the occurrence of AD. The neuronal changes were found in the entorhinal cortex, which spread to the hippocampus and ultimately led into the brain's isocortex region (Braak *et al* 1993). Further, in Thompson *et al*'s (2003) study, accumulation of NFT mapped the loss of grey matter in the regions of the brain which affects the patients' cognitive capabilities and identified grey matter loss in temporal and limbic cortices leading into frontal and occipital areas of the brain. Furthermore, findings of the neuropsychological and neuropathological study using sigma unit scanner validates that all types of aphasia exhibit the thinning of involving cortical left posterior superior temporal, inferior parietal, medial temporal, and posterior cingulate (Rohrer *et al* 2012).

Zhang *et al*'s (2010) findings showed changes in all AD (mild, moderate and severe) groups in the dissociated functional connectivity between the PCC (posterior cingulate cortex) and a set of regions which included visual cortices bilaterally, inferior temporal cortex, hippocampus, particularly in the medial prefrontal cortex and precuneus or cuneus, as shown in figure 4.3. The disruption of connectivity intensified as the stage of AD progression increased. The regions of interest also exhibit the increased connectivity extending from the left-lateralised frontoparietal areas to bilateral frontoparietal regions (Zhang *et al* 2010, Dai *et al* 2015). Study of the functional connectivity network of the brain revealed that the disruption in the signal connectivity depends upon the range of the connection. The long-range connections (e.g., 100–130 mm) produce more disturbance that specifically marks medial and lateral prefrontal and parietal cortices, insula, and thalamus regions in the brain (Dai *et al* 2015). In line with the earlier study, the multimodal study (Dai *et al* 2019) on functional connectivity network (FCN) and structural connectivity network (SNC) in AD patients and healthy controls (HC) showed pathophysiological disruptions. The FCN and SCN in AD patients had disrupted network integration of overloaded protein cluster tangles due to increased characteristic path length and segregation caused due to decreased intramodular connections in the default mode network, as shown in figure 4.3.

Additionally, only the FCN exhibited a reduced clustering coefficient and reduced rich club connections in AD (Dai *et al* 2019). Thus, although the significant cognitive decline in AD patients is attributed chiefly to the deposition of amyloid, in terms of language, the amyloid burdening is moderately linked with the production of fewer specific words during spontaneous speech. Moreover, amyloid

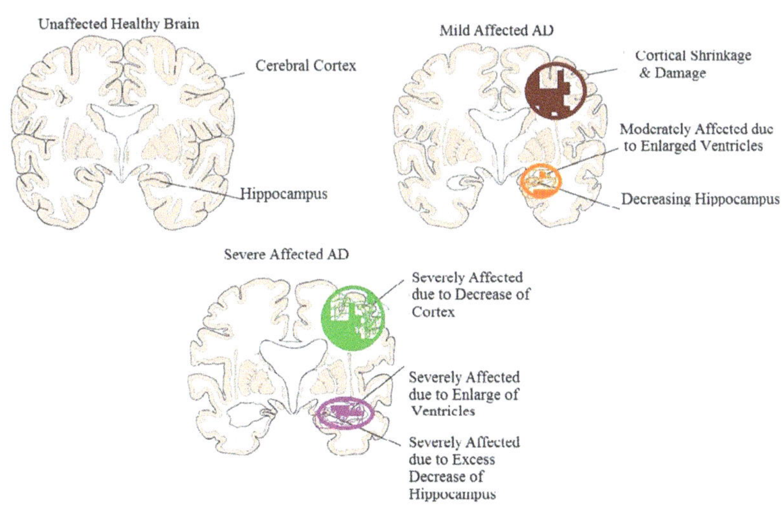

Figure 4.3. The regions of the brain that are affected by AD are classified according to different stages of AD.

burdening does not associate with syntactical and lexical complexities to underpin language decline in fluency or confrontational naming, conversation fillers and type-token ratio (Verfaillie *et al* 2019).

4.3.7 Cognitive reserve association in AD bilinguals and multilinguals

In terms of bilingualism in AD, study evidence suggests bilingualism delays neurodegeneration and generates a cognitive reserve (CR), although it does not prevent AD occurrence and progression. The study on CR in bilinguals demonstrates bilingual AD patients were five years older than monolinguals AD patients (Perani *et al* 2017). The PET scans showed a structural decline in regions responsible for increased connectivity in the executive control: severe cerebral hypometabolism, thereby indicating AD progression in bilinguals. Also, results demonstrated bilingualism increased the metabolism in the orbitofrontal, inferior frontal, and cingulate cortex, thus suggesting brain rewiring, which maintained executive functioning despite effects of neurodegeneration and exhibited delayed AD symptoms. The findings demonstrate that bilinguals show resistance to AD degeneration in delaying the eventual development of AD better than monolinguals. Furthermore, it also corroborates CR and its association with bilingualism (Perani *et al* 2017).

Duncan *et al*'s (2018) study on structural brain differences in terms of cortical thinness and tissue density in monolingual and multilingual AD and MCI patients also examined cognitive reserve (CR) and language and cognitive control (LCC) in AD. Findings revealed higher tissue density in multilingual MCIs than monolingual MCIs; the tissue density in multilingual AD was comparable to monolingual MCI and was lowest in monolingual AD. A steady pattern emerged on cortical thickness between monolingual subjects (MCI and AD) and both multilingual subjects. The multilingual of MCI and AD confirmed the presence of thicker cortex than monolingual subjects. These findings implied that the association of cortical thickness to increased grey matter supports improved memory functioning. Thus, multilingualism is more likely to increase grey matter in LCC areas, delaying cognitive dysfunction due to disease-related atrophy.

Smirnov *et al*'s (2019) findings also confirmed the difference in dominant and non-dominant language correlations in bilingual AD. Smirnov *et al*'s (2019) study outcome suggests temporal cortical thickness (of the entorhinal cortex and middle temporal gyrus) are stimulated by dominant language, and the atrophy therein causes impaired semantic processing to compromise dominant language naming ability. However, the non-dominant language naming correlated to the thickness of the left caudal anterior cingulate cortex (ACC), which continued functioning (for non-dominant language) in AD and but not in MCI in AD patients and consequently maintained the cognitive reserve in bilinguals.

4.4 Discussion

Given that each brain region corresponds to specific cognitive functions, the brain degeneration disrupting the neuronal connections in particular areas will impair corresponding cognitive function, as illustrated in figure 4.4. Thus, a decline in the

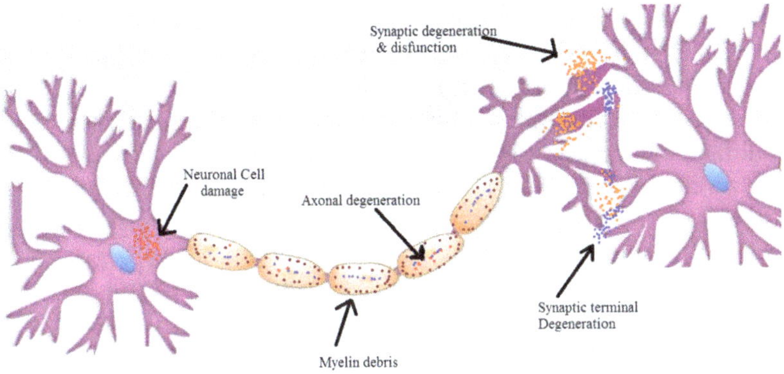

Figure 4.4. Neuronal degeneration occurs due to the progression of AD.

communicative language specifically affecting presentations represents a deficit of specific language structures, indicating the brain regions' irreversible degeneration. Therefore, the biomarkers play the role of verifying the area affected through the neuroimaging evidence (Mofrad *et al* 2021). The brain regions' functional and structural imaging findings provide pathological evidence of deterioration that supports AD progression's clinical diagnosis.

The primary research data of chosen articles from neuropsychology and neuropathology were matrixed into a table with the theme patterns of the research findings. The themes we focused upon were structural language decline based on language hierarchy of semantics, syntax, and morphology-lexicon to gather insights into the significance of language decline and pattern of language degeneration AD. We also examined the theme of brain regions that deteriorate with the progression of AD identified by biomarkers. A further theme of bilingualism as a cognitive reserve and its impact on structural and functional aspects of the brain were analysed to gather insights and understanding.

4.4.1 Neuropsychological and neuropathological representations of AD across studies

Language degeneration with the progression of cognitive impairment in AD is the subject of study since semantic memory and episodic memory are affected in the early stage of AD (Jahn 2013). Although AD has varied effects on people, the common symptom relates to the deficit in remembering new information due to disruption in the brain cells responsible for recent memory. Furthermore, the impaired lexical and semantic retrieval or breakdown of semantic word representation are linked to a deficit of word-finding in AD. Early research primarily focused on assessing memory and executive functions in AD, and subsequent studies examined language deficits such as word retrieval deficits, leading to circumlocutions, non-specific language in early-stage and, comprehension in later stage AD were assessed for cognitive change (Mueller *et al* 2018).

Most of the studies used picture description task for communication assessment (Hier *et al* 1985, Groves-Wright *et al* 2004, Sajjadi *et al* 2012, Ahmed *et al* 2013) as a standardised measure as it does not engage episodic memory or autobiographical memory (Mueller *et al* 2018), to gauge the semantic decline. The picture description task (cookie theft description task) provides information on the AD patients performance based on semantics: (i) information unit—the smallest non-redundant meaningful factor inference; (ii) conciseness—by number of words used to express ideas since circumlocution and repetitions are words—finding related behaviour; (iii) lexical variety—the number of words and unique words, measuring parts of speech with ratio and proportion of noun, pronoun, verb, adjectives; and (iv) quantity of words. The measure of working memory deficit or semantic memory indicates using the language form of complex syntactical structures. Picture description task in terms of syntax and morphology refers to the measure of grammaticality and the lexicons (words) used, which include syntactic complexity, use of words per clause, grammaticality as inappropriate use of tenses, conjunctions, conditionals, subordinate clause and passive voice and syntactic errors in sentences. The measure of language decline following semiotic language hierarchy provides a systematic and structured understanding of the deficit. Studies on AD impact on language deterioration in bilinguals suggest linguistic abilities such as lexical and semantic are affected early, while phonological and morphological processing remain unaffected until the advanced stages of AD (Costa *et al* 2012).

Most neuropsychological studies assessing language decline compared AD with other dementia-related disorders or various stages of AD and MCI to gather evidence and insights into degenerative conditions of dementia (Blair *et al* 2007, Porto *et al* 2008, Sajjadi *et al* 2012, Gollan *et al* 2017). For example, the decline in AD was faster when compared to other degenerative disorders (FTLD) (Porto *et al* 2008); however, in a longitudinal study (Blair *et al* 2007), other dementia forms (FTD, SD, PPA) showed a faster decline. However, other studies compared AD patients with healthy controls. Furthermore, some recent studies simultaneously examined AD deterioration in neuropsychology and neuropathology (Rohrer *et al* 2012, Ahmed *et al* 2013, Duncan *et al* 2018, Dai *et al* 2019, Smirnov *et al* 2019, Verfaillie *et al* 2019).

4.4.2 Neuropsychological decline across studies

The effect of AD on neural regions is associated with cognitive and language impairment, which occur in hierarchical progression (Altmann and McClung 2008). The region of the entorhinal cortex and hippocampus, linked to creating memories, is affected first. Further progression affects adjacent cortical areas of the inferior temporal lobe, temporo-occipital junction and temporoparietal junction, which show loss of knowledge (words), indicating a semantic decline. Consequently, executive functioning and working memory are impaired as the temporoparietal region is linked to the dorsolateral prefrontal cortex. Hence, the deteriorated frontal lobe causes impaired language and cognition (Bright *et al* 2004, Thompson *et al* 2004, Altmann and McClung 2008).

The case study (Garrard *et al* 2005, Le *et al* 2011, Berisha *et al* 2015) analyses were on available discourse samples of well-known figures diagnosed with AD, which were the unscripted speech samples of two former US Presidents and the written literary works of three British authors, to trace language deficits. Although the findings provided information, it was devoid of standardisation that could be extrapolated as a generalisable outcome to other AD patients (Mueller *et al* 2018). Berisha *et al*'s (2015) study compared speeches of former US Presidents Ronald Reagan and G W Bush and found that erstwhile President Ronald Reagan diagnosed with AD exhibited a lower proportion of unique words, higher levels of filled and unfilled pauses. Lexical-semantic decline and loss in memory are indicated by the frequency of breaks (Berisha *et al* 2015, Pistono *et al* 2019, Pastoriza-Dominguez *et al* 2021). Lexical decline and deficits of syntactic functions in language were observed in literary works of Iris Murdoch, which deteriorated with the progression of AD and a similar reduction was observable in the later literary works of Agatha Christie (Garrard *et al* 2005, Le *et al* 2011).

The semantic decline in mild stage AD and syntactical decline in moderate stage AD (Grover-Wright *et al* 2004) confirm the semiotics of language hierarchy wherein semantic rank deteriorates first, subsequently followed by syntactic in the next stage of AD. However, few studies demonstrated a morphological decline in early stages such as vocabulary deficit, recurrence of words in sentences (Miller and Hague 1975), and mostly recall words from a higher frequency of occurrence than words of lower frequency of occurrence (Barker and Lawson 1968). In AD, memory and other cognitive deficits are associated with difficulty in finding words. Fluency remains unaffected until the moderate stage, and the progression to the late stage of AD presents naming difficulty (anomia), comprehension deficits, paraphrastic errors and semantic jargon (Appell *et al* 1982, Murdoch *et al* 1987, Blair *et al* 2007). Given that the prefrontal cortex is damaged in AD patients and decreases functions of syntactical complexity, the decline in syntactic complexity in AD shows impaired linguistic ability in EOAD (Can and Kuruoğlu 2018). The study findings on language preservation and degeneration in DAT (Rochon *et al* 1994, Grossman *et al* 1995) are converse to the complexity (hierarchy) of language structure; within each semiotic rank and across semiotic classes. The sentence comprehension of complex syntactic forms demonstrates significant syntactic and overall semantic processing impairments, while simple syntax remains preserved in Alzheimer patients. Therefore, syntactic preservation-deterioration needs to be approached, perceived and analysed as a fragment of a continuum (Emery 2000, Ahmed *et al* 2013). Studies on AD biomarkers demonstrate the correlation of AD pathology to cognitive functioning, which associates with symptoms of impaired cognitive behaviour in AD patients with their caregivers (Banning *et al* 2020, Komjakraphan and Karuncharernpanit 2021). Although a few studies on language impairment appear to follow the semiotic hierarchy of language, other studies challenge the generalizability of the hierarchy in AD language decline.

4.4.3 Neuropathological deterioration of regions of the brain in AD

Two distinctive features neuropathologically mark AD; first, the extracellular deposition of amyloid plaques begins in the basal regions of the frontal, temporal and occipital lobes and, with the progression of the disease, affect the primary sensory areas. Second, the neurofibrillary tangles primarily affect the transentorhinal region, passing to the limbic system before the neocortex (Khan 2016).

Zhang *et al*'s study showed decreased and increased activities in specific brain regions. While AD-related impairments of functional connectivity were evident in the PCC and areas of visual cortices bilaterally, the inferior temporal cortex, hippocampus, the medial prefrontal cortex, and precuneus increased the connectivity along with disease progression extending from left lateralised frontoparietal and bilateral frontoparietal regions (Zhang *et al* 2010). However, some study findings suggest that the disease affecting brain regions begins first in the temporal and parietal cortex, followed by progression to the cortical areas in the frontal lobe (Gollan *et al* 2017). The brain lesions were identified (Brun and Gustafson 1976), causing cortical degeneration in medial temporal (limbic), lateral hemisphere, posterior inferior temporal areas, parieto-occipital lobes and posterior cingulate gyrus. In addition, studies using neuroimaging techniques show neuronal death in specific brain regions linked to AD, where a reduction in the hippocampus indicates the shrinkage, changes in the volume of brain regions and neuronal loss (West *et al* 1994, Raz 2000, Thompson *et al* 2004, Leong *et al* 2017, Mofrad *et al* 2021).

The accumulation of abnormal levels of NFT associated with brain degeneration involved the entorhinal cortex, hippocampus, isocortex regions and indicated the progression stages of AD decline (Braak *et al* 1993). Furthermore, neuroimaging MRI identified NFT build-up in temporal and limbic cortices, frontal and occipital regions leading to the loss of grey matter in the brain in AD (Thompson *et al* 2003). The accumulation of NFT causes neuronal loss and synaptic decline (Spires *et al* 2011). Dai *et al* (2019, 2015) also confirm disruption in the structural and functional neuronal network due to the accumulation of tangles that affect the grey matter and white matter and abnormal available integration in brain regions (Dai *et al* 2015). The amyloid burdening causes decline with subtle cognitive changes affecting speech fluency, and the further progress towards more considerable amyloid burden corresponds to worsening mental deterioration; although, amyloid deposition does not affect syntactic or lexical complexity (Gonzalez 2014, Verfaillie *et al* 2019).

A study on AD-PPA degeneration showed thinning of cortical regions involving left posterior and superior temporal, inferior parietal, medial temporal, and posterior cingulate in individuals whose presentation included word-finding difficulty and non-fluent spontaneous speech with occasional errors of a phonemic kind but without motor speech impairment (Rohrer *et al* 2012). The temporal lobe is responsible for lexico-semantic processing and conceptual representations; therefore, when affected by AD degeneration, these regions are likely to affect both languages similarly in bilinguals (Costa *et al* 2012, Calabria *et al* 2017).

A neuropathological study used PET to understand the semantic and lexicon processing of both words and pictures in the brain (Bright *et al* 2004). The findings indicate that particular brain areas, i.e., left-frontal and temporal, are activated during the meaning of processing of both image and word language. The robust semantic activation was common to both input modalities in anterior and medial aspects of the left fusiform gyrus, the left parahippocampal and perirhinal cortices, and the left inferior frontal gyrus. The picture processing is likely to show intermediate, pre-semantic stages of visual processing caused due to activation in posterior temporal regions. Though the temporal lobe is involved in processing both words and pictures, their engagement is likely to be determined by the level of specificity at which an object is processed. The findings of neuropathological literature confirm the presence of NFT and amyloid burdening underpin cognitive decline and impairment of language presentation in AD patients. The neuropathological studies demonstrate semantic deterioration; however, the syntactical and morphological impairments are not demarcated.

4.4.4 Neuropsychological implications of cognitive reserve in bilinguals

The lexico-semantic damage in both bilinguals for both languages in word retrieval tasks indicates affected functioning as in impaired language processing. The decline of semantic processing was similar in both languages in highly proficient AD bilinguals, and the performance on task indicating lexical competence was intact for dominant language (Costa *et al* 2012, Calabria *et al* 2017). The lower performance in lexical competence task in the non-dominant language occurs due to impaired lexical retrieval caused by executive control dysfunction rather than semantic memory degradation. The parallel decline in both languages is attributable to both languages being learnt simultaneously in the longitudinal (Calabria *et al* 2017) and cross-sectional study (Costa *et al* 2012). However, Ivanova *et al*'s (2014) study outcome contradicts the findings on parallel language decline. Their results showed differential effects attributed to the non-balanced bilingualism. In other words, the non-dominant language had a poor lexico-semantic connection as it was acquired later in life and also least spoken; consequently, it was most affected. The acquisition age, frequency of use and proficiency of a second language appear to be significant in modulating the pattern of deterioration and the linguistic dominance in presentations (tasks) (Perani *et al* 2003, Perani and Abutalebi 2005). The decline in lexical processing and deterioration in both languages can be explored semiotically to gather insights into each decline in bilinguals. According to the regression hypothesis, the language learnt later will degenerate first and therefore, the dominant language acquired first is far more resistant to cognitive impairment than a language learned second or a non-dominant language.

The cognitive reserve hypothesis explains non-systematic differences correlating the extent of brain damage and functional outcome, wherein mental stimulation serves to enhance cognitive processing and functioning to maintain CR (Stern 2002). Given that, the brain resilience is compromised during the incidence of brain disease; consequently, the disease progression results in irreversible deterioration where no preventive treatment can arrest the damage. Nonetheless, a countermeasure to delay the decline is to increase the neuronal synaptic connections in the brain (see figure 4.4), which creates a more significant presence of neuronal connections to be destroyed than a brain with fewer connections (Sahyouni *et al* 2016). Therefore, the implications of lifestyle factors such as bilingualism are significant in delaying the onset of AD as bilingualism affects the region of LCC (language and cognition control), causing changes such as increased grey matter, which contributes to CR (Bialystok *et al* 2014, Gold 2016). Furthermore, Anderson *et al*'s (2020) analyses on previously established evidence corroborate the contribution of bilingualism towards creating the cognitive reserve. Furthermore, the CR in bilinguals delays AD as it generates neuroplasticity, which makes resistance to the progression of cognitive decline associated with AD compared to monolinguals (Bialsystok *et al* 2007, Zheng *et al* 2018).

The findings across studies on bilingualism and multilingualism in AD individuals demonstrate structural changes that create an alternative functional circuit as in preserved ACC, increased grey matter, cortical thickness and tissue density, all of which serve to resist the effects of advancing AD brain atrophy (Perani *et al* 2017, Duncan *et al* 2018, Smirnov *et al* 2019). These findings confirm previously established evidence that, compared to monolinguals, bilinguals and multilinguals have increased brain matter, grey matter, greater tissue density and thicker cortex leading to executive functioning, language and LCC (Klein *et al* 2014). In addition, studies showed that the age where the incidence of symptoms appeared was 4–5 years later for AD in bilinguals than monolinguals (Alladi *et al* 2013, Perani *et al* 2017). Thus, the current study outcome validates the past established effect that hypothesises bilingualism contributes to building CR, which delays the onset of AD. The benefits associated with neuroplasticity and CR are multi-fold for the AD population (Bialsystok *et al* 2007). The multifactorial lifestyle features such as language (bilingualism, multilingualism), education and demanding occupation induce neurocognitive and neuroplastic changes to provide significant opportunities for socio-cultural and cognitive benefits and have huge CR implications in supporting the AD population (Alladi *et al* 2013, Bialystok *et al* 2014).

4.4.5 Neuropathological evidence of cognitive reserve in bilinguals

The brain structurally reorganising in bilinguals and multilinguals provides scope for delaying AD symptoms and serves as CR (Anderson *et al* 2020). The cognitive reserve in bilinguals is associated with structural changes in brain regions such as cortical thickness, affecting functioning (Duncan *et al* 2018, Smirnov *et al* 2019). Duncan *et al* (2018) correlated increased memory functioning to increased grey matter in LCC and cortical thickness in multilinguals to delay AD-related cognitive dysfunction. Metabolic connectivity in bilinguals increased in orbitofrontal, inferior frontal, and cingulate cortex (Perani *et al* 2017). Grundy *et al* (2017) state that the posterior and subcortical regions are more functional in bilinguals than monolinguals. The increased cortical thickness in the left entorhinal cortex and left middle temporal gyrus associate with impaired semantic performance in the dominant language, which confirms a decline in naming and temporal lobe atrophy occurring in AD. The performance in non-dominant language indicates reliance on the left caudal ACC (anterior cingulate cortex responsible for language switching) in AD (Smirnov *et al* 2019). This implies ACC is functional and devoid of atrophy, regardless of severe atrophy in the inferior frontal gyrus and inferior parietal lobule in AD patients.

Although Altmann and McClung (2008) present the hierarchical model, associating decline in the brain region and language impairments. It is, nonetheless, not a generalisable feature considering in which the AD individuals are affected structurally and functionally in a diverse manner due to varied pathology in the disease progression. Therefore, the presentations of impaired language are exhibited differently depending on the regions' atrophy, which may extend the deterioration or preservation of the brain regions.

4.4.6 Preventive measures and delaying onset of AD

Growing evidence suggests promising developments in recent years wherein scientists are working in the emerging field of AD prevention. The aetiology of Alzheimer's disease is multifactorial, comprising environmental, lifestyle and genetic risk factors. The risk factors for Alzheimer's disease are classified as non-modifiable: being age and individual genetic profiles and modifiable risk factors, which include cognitive inactivity and cardiovascular risk factors (hypertension, diabetes, obesity, physical inactivity and substance abuse). Further, modifiable factors hold the potential to be transfigured into 'cognitive reserve' to provide mental stimulation, to develop more synapses to resist neurodegeneration longer than in individuals with cognitive inactivity and a low level of education. About 35% of the total risk factors of Alzheimer's disease is represented by modifiable risk factors, which can potentially lower AD onset of symptoms by one year (Bhatti *et al* 2020).

Furthermore, study evidence suggests the health of the brain, a highly vascular organ, is closely associated with the heart, blood vessels. Therefore, managing cardiovascular risk factors such as high cholesterol, type 2 diabetes, high blood pressure, and obesity is likely to prevent or delay cognitive decline (Jack 2009, Mebane-Sims 2009, Wiley 2021). Additionally, sustaining cognitive brain health can be done through consistent physical exercise, a low-fat diet, healthy dietary nutrients rich in fruits and vegetables, in addition to a healthy social network, intellectual curiosity and mental stimulation (Sayhouni *et al* 2016, Bhatti *et al* 2020).

The concept of cognitive reserve is pursued through language, education, learning, diet, exercise, lower stress, and occupation to increase resilience to neurological brain damage caused by amyloids in AD (Sahyouni *et al* 2016). The external environmental factors such as education and learning can influence synaptic density and promote the strengthening of existing synaptic connections. Literature suggests that education can delay AD development to a degree since education on cognitive performance before dementia is different in subjects based on primary school education (Jucker *et al* 2006, Sahyouni *et al* 2016). Parallelly, the epidemiological evidence considers bilingualism an instrumental factor in delaying the AD onset process (Perani *et al* 2017, Duncan *et al* 2018, Smirnov *et al* 2019).

4.5 Conclusions

In this chapter, the outcome across studies shows a significant cognitive decline in language processing among Alzheimer's patients, predominantly in the areas of semantic and lexicon aptitude and presentations. The results regarding the patterns and natures of degeneration in language can only be stated in terms of probable hierarchy. The analysis and comparison of decline patterns of the language across most of the studies were found to be idiosyncratic and varied. This conclusion can be explained and approached through Vygotsky's observation. He states that thought and language are mentally represented and developed as two units until two years of age; later, the two units intersect and merge (Vygotsky 1962). In line with this approach and this developmental phenomenon, we suggest that a deeper multi-disciplinary study is required to consolidate the nature of language degeneration in AD, where language and other cognitive declines can be precisely separated and demarcated as per the developmental stages of AD.

References

Ahmed S, Haigh A M F, de Jager C A and Garrard P 2013 Connected speech as a marker of disease progression in autopsy-proven Alzheimer's disease *Brain* **136** 3727–37

Alladi S, Bak T H, Duggirala V, Surampudi B, Shailaja M, Shukla A K, Chaudhuri J R and Kaul S 2013 Bilingualism delays age at onset of dementia, independent of education and immigration status *Neurology* **81** 1938–44

Altmann L J and McClung J S 2008 Effects of semantic impairment on language use in Alzheimer's disease *Seminars in Speech and Language* vol 29 (New York: Thieme Medical Publishers) pp 18–31

Anderson J A, Hawrylewicz K and Grundy J G 2020 Does bilingualism protect against dementia? A meta-analysis *Psychon. Bull. Rev.* **27** 952–65

Appell J, Kertesz A and Fisman M 1982 A study of language functioning in Alzheimer patients *Brain Lang.* **17** 73–91

Banning L C *et al* 2020 The association between biomarkers and neuropsychiatric symptoms across the Alzheimer's disease spectrum *Am. J. Geriatr. Psych.* **28** 735–44

Barker M G and Lawson J S 1968 Nominal aphasia in dementia *Br. J. Psych.* **114** 1351–6

Berisha V, Wang S, LaCross A and Liss J 2015 Tracking discourse complexity preceding Alzheimer's disease diagnosis: a case study comparing the press conferences of Presidents Ronald Reagan and George Herbert Walker Bush *J. Alzheimer's Dis.* **45** 959–63

Bhatti G K, Reddy A P, Reddy P H and Bhatti J S 2020 Lifestyle modifications and nutritional interventions in aging-associated cognitive decline and Alzheimer's disease *Front. Aging Neurosci.* **11** 369

Bialystok E, Craik F I and Freedman M 2007 Bilingualism as a protection against the onset of symptoms of dementia *Neuropsychologia* **45** 459–64

Bialystok E, Craik F I, Binns M A, Ossher L and Freedman M 2014 Effects of bilingualism on the age of onset and progression of MCI and AD: evidence from executive function tests *Neuropsychology* **28** 290

Blair M, Marczinski C A, Davis-Faroque N and Kertesz A 2007 A longitudinal study of language decline in Alzheimer's disease and frontotemporal dementia *J. Int. Neuropsychol. Soc.* **13** 237–45

Braak H, Braak E and Bohl J 1993 Staging of Alzheimer-related cortical destruction *Eur. Neurol.* **33** 403–8

Bright P, Moss H and Tyler L K 2004 Unitary vs multiple semantics: PET studies of word and picture processing *Brain Lang.* **89** 417–32

Brun A and Gustafson L 1976 Distribution of cerebral degeneration in Alzheimer's disease *Arch. Psych. Nervenkr.* **223** 15–33

Calabria M *et al* 2017 Language deterioration in bilingual Alzheimer's disease patients: a longitudinal study *J. Neurolinguistics* **43** 59–74

Can E and Kuruoğlu G 2018 Assessment of syntactic complexity in Alzheimer's disease *3rd Eurasian Conf. on Language and Social Sciences* vol 517

Canli T, Sivers H, Thomason M E, Whitfield-Gabrieli S, Gabrieli J D and Gotlib I H 2004 Brain activation to emotional words in depressed vs healthy subjects *Neuroreport* **15** 2585–8

Costa A *et al* 2012 On the parallel deterioration of lexico-semantic processes in the bilinguals' two languages: evidence from Alzheimer's disease *Neuropsychologia* **50** 740–53

Dai Z, Lin Q, Li T, Wang X, Yuan H, Yu X, He Y and Wang H 2019 Disrupted structural and functional brain networks in Alzheimer's disease *Neurobiol. Aging* **75** 71–82

Dai Z *et al* 2015 Identifying and mapping connectivity patterns of brain network hubs in Alzheimer's disease *Cereb. Cortex* **25** 3723–42

Duncan H D, Nikelski J, Pilon R, Steffener J, Chertkow H and Phillips N A 2018 Structural brain differences between monolingual and multilingual patients with mild cognitive impairment and Alzheimer disease: evidence for cognitive reserve *Neuropsychologia* **109** 270–82

Ellis D G 1996 Coherence patterns in Alzheimer's discourse *Commun. Res.* **23** 472–95

Emery V O B 2000 Language impairment in dementia of the Alzheimer type: a hierarchical decline *Int. J. Psych. Med.* **30** 145–64

Finfgeld D L 2003 Meta-synthesis: the state of the art—so far *Qual. Health Res.* **13** 893–904

Garrard P, Maloney L M, Hodges J R and Patterson K 2005 The effects of very early Alzheimer's disease on the characteristics of writing by a renowned author *Brain* **128** 250–60

Gold B T 2016 Lifelong bilingualism, cognitive reserve and Alzheimer's disease: a review of findings *Linguist. Approaches Biling.* **6** 171–89

Gollan T H, Stasenko A, Li C and Salmon D P 2017 Bilingual language intrusions and other speech errors in Alzheimer's disease *Brain Cogn.* **118** 27–44

González M M 2014 *Atlas of Biomarkers for Alzheimer's Disease* (Berlin: Springer)

Grossman M, Mickanin J, Onishi K and Hughes E 1995 An aspect of sentence processing in Alzheimer's disease: quantifier-noun agreement *Neurology* **45** 85–91

Groves-Wright K, Neils-Strunjas J, Burnett R and O'Neill M J 2004 A comparison of verbal and written language in Alzheimer's disease *J. Commun. Disord.* **37** 109–30

Grundy J G, Anderson J A and Bialystok E 2017 Neural correlates of cognitive processing in monolinguals and bilinguals *Ann. N.Y. Acad. Sci.* **1396** 183

Haas W 1954 On defining linguistic units *Trans. Philol. Soc.* **53** 54–84

Hardy J and Selkoe D J 2002 The amyloid hypothesis of Alzheimer's disease: progress and problems on the road to therapeutics *Science* **297** 353–6

Hier D B, Hagenlocker K and Shindler A G 1985 Language disintegration in dementia: effects of etiology and severity *Brain Lang.* **25** 117–33

Ivanova I, Salmon D P and Gollan T H 2014 Which language declines more? Longitudinal versus cross-sectional decline of picture naming in bilinguals with Alzheimer's disease *J. Int. Neuropsychol. Soc.* **20** 534–46

Jack C 2009 Cerebral and cardiac vascular pathology in Alzheimer's Disease *Current Hypotheses and Research Milestones in Alzheimer's Disease* (Boston, MA: Springer) pp 159–69

Jacobs H I, V, Boxtel M P, Uylings H B, Gronenschild E H, Verhey F R and Jolles J 2011 Atrophy of the parietal lobe in preclinical dementia *Brain Cogn.* **75** 154–63

Jahn H 2013 Memory loss in Alzheimer's disease *Dialogues Clin. Neurosci.* **15** 445

Jucker M, Beyreuther K, Haass C and Nitsch R M (ed) 2006 *Alzheimer: 100 Years and Beyond* (Berlin: Springer)

Katzman R 1976 The prevalence and malignancy of Alzheimer disease: a major killer *Arch. Neurol.* **33** 217–18

Khan T 2016 *Biomarkers in Alzheimer's Disease* (New York: Academic)

Klein D, Mok K, Chen J K and Watkins K E 2014 Age of language learning shapes brain structure: a cortical thickness study of bilingual and monolingual individuals *Brain Lang.* **131** 20–4

Komjakraphan P and Karuncharernpanit S 2021 Experiences of communicating with older adults with Alzheimer's disease: a phenomenological study of family caregivers *Pac. Rim Int. J. Nurs. Res.* **25** 75–86

Le X, Lancashire I, Hirst G and Jokel R 2011 Longitudinal detection of dementia through lexical and syntactic changes in writing: a case study of three British novelists *Lit. Ling. Comput.* **26** 435–61

Leong R L, Lo J C, Sim S K, Zheng H, Tandi J, Zhou J and Chee M W 2017 Longitudinal brain structure and cognitive changes over 8 years in an East Asian cohort *Neuroimage* **147** 852–60

Lust B *et al* 2015 Reversing Ribot: does regression hold in language of prodromal Alzheimer's disease? *Brain Lang.* **143** 1–10

Mebane-Sims I 2009 Alzheimer's disease facts and figures *Alzheimer's Dement. J. Alzheimer's Assoc.* **5** 234–70

Miller E and Hague F 1975 Some characteristics of verbal behaviour in presenile dementia *Psychol. Med.* **5** 255–9

Mofrad S A, Lundervold A, Lundervold A S and Alzheimer's Disease Neuroimaging Initiative 2021 A predictive framework based on brain volume trajectories enabling early detection of Alzheimer's disease *Comput. Med. Imag. Graph.* **90** 101910

Mueller K D, Hermann B, Mecollari J and Turkstra L S 2018 Connected speech and language in mild cognitive impairment and Alzheimer's disease: a review of picture description tasks *J. Clin. Exp. Neuropsychol.* **40** 917–39

Murdoch B E, Chenery H J, Wilks V and Boyle R S 1987 Language disorders in dementia of the Alzheimer type *Brain Lang.* **31** 122–37

Pastoriza-Dominguez P, Torre I G, Dieguez-Vide F, Gomez-Ruiz I, Gelado S, Bello-Lopez J, Avila-Rivera A, Matias-Guiu J, Pytel V and Hernandez-Fernandez A 2021 Speech pause distribution as an early marker for Alzheimer's disease *medRxiv*

Perani D and Abutalebi J 2005 The neural basis of first and second language processing *Curr. Opin. Neurobiol.* **15** 202–6

Perani D, Abutalebi J, Paulesu E, Brambati S, Scifo P, Cappa S F and Fazio F 2003 The role of age of acquisition and language usage in early, high-proficient bilinguals: an fMRI study during verbal fluency *Hum. Brain Mapp.* **19** 170–82

Perani D, Farsad M, Ballarini T, Lubian F, Malpetti M, Fracchetti A, Magnani G, March A and Abutalebi J 2017 The impact of bilingualism on brain reserve and metabolic connectivity in Alzheimer's dementia *Proc. Natl Acad. Sci.* **114** 1690–5

Pistono A, Pariente J, Bézy C, Lemesle B, Le Men J and Jucla M 2019 What happens when nothing happens? An investigation of pauses as a compensatory mechanism in early Alzheimer's disease *Neuropsychologia* **124** 133–43

Porto C S, Bahia V S, Brucki S M D, Caramelli P and Nitrini R 2008 Neuropsychological differences between frontotemporal lobar degeneration and Alzheimer's disease *Dement. Neuropsychol.* **2** 223–7

Prince M J, Wimo A, Guerchet M M, Ali G C, Wu Y T and Prina M 2015 World Alzheimer report 2015-the global impact of dementia: an analysis of prevalence, incidence, cost and trends *Report* (http://www.alz.co.uk/research/world-report-2015)

Raz N 2000 Aging of the brain and its impact on cognitive performance: integration of structural and functional findings *The Handbook of Aging and Cognition* eds F I M Craik and T A Salthouse (Mahwah, NJ: Lawrence Erlbaum Associates Publishers) pp 1–90

Robins R H 2014 *General Linguistics* (London: Routledge)

Rochon E, Waters G S and Caplan D 1994 Sentence comprehension in patients with Alzheimer's disease *Brain Lang.* **46** 329–49

Rohrer J D, Rossor M N and Warren J D 2012 Alzheimer's pathology in primary progressive aphasia *Neurobiol. Aging* **33** 744–52

Ruthirakuhan M, Lanctôt K L, Di Scipio M, Ahmed M and Herrmann N 2018 Biomarkers of agitation and aggression in Alzheimer's disease: a systematic review *Alzheimer's Dement.* **14** 1344–76

Sahyouni R, Verma A and Chen J W 2016 *Alzheimer's Disease Decoded: The History, Present, and Future of Alzheimer's Disease and Dementia* (Singapore: World Scientific)

Sajjadi S A, Patterson K, Tomek M and Nestor P J 2012 Abnormalities of connected speech in semantic dementia vs Alzheimer's disease *Aphasiology* **26** 847–66

Smirnov D S, Stasenko A, Salmon D P, Galasko D, Brewer J B and Gollan T H 2019 Distinct structural correlates of the dominant and non-dominant languages in bilinguals with Alzheimer's disease (AD) *Neuropsychologia* **132** 107131

Spires-Jones T L, Kopeikina K J, Koffie R M, de Calignon A and Hyman B T 2011 Are tangles as toxic as they look? *J. Mol. Neurosci.* **45** 438–44

Stern Y 2002 What is cognitive reserve? Theory and research application of the reserve concept *J. Int. Neuropsychol Soc.* **8** 448–60

Tellechea P, Pujol N, Esteve-Belloch P, Echeveste B, García-Eulate M R, Arbizu J and Riverol M 2018 Early-and late-onset Alzheimer's disease: are they the same entity? *Neurología* **33** 244–53

Thompson P M, Hayashi K M, De Zubicaray G, Janke A L, Rose S E, Semple J, Herman D, Hong M S, Dittmer S S, Doddrell D M and Toga A W 2003 Dynamics of gray matter loss in Alzheimer's disease *J. Neurosci.* **23** 994–1005

Thompson P M *et al* 2004 Mapping hippocampal and ventricular change in Alzheimer disease *Neuroimage* **22** 1754–66

Timulak L 2014 Qualitative meta-analysis *SAGE Handbook Qualitative Data Analysis* (New York: SAGE Publications) p 481

Verfaillie S C *et al* 2019 High amyloid burden is associated with fewer specific words during spontaneous speech in individuals with subjective cognitive decline *Neuropsychologia* **131** 184–92

Vygotsky L S 1962 *Thought and Language* trans E Hanfmann and G Vakar (Cambridge, MA: MIT Press) pp 119–53

West M J, Coleman P D, Flood D G and Troncoso J C 1994 Differences in the pattern of hippocampal neuronal loss in normal ageing and Alzheimer's disease *Lancet* **344** 769–72

Westlye L T, Walhovd K B, Dale A M, Bjørnerud A, Due-Tønnessen P, Engvig A, Grydeland H, Tamnes C K, Østby Y and Fjell A M 2010 Life-span changes of the human brain white matter: diffusion tensor imaging (DTI) and volumetry *Cereb. Cortex* **20** 2055–68

Wiley J 2021 2021 Alzheimer's disease facts and figures *Alzheimer's Dement.* **17** 327–406

World Health Organization 2019 *Risk Reduction of Cognitive Decline and Dementia: WHO Guidelines* (Geneva: World Health Organization)

Zhang H Y, Wang S J, Liu B, Ma Z L, Yang M, Zhang Z J and Teng G J 2010 Resting brain connectivity: changes during the progress of Alzheimer disease *Radiology* **256** 598–606

Zheng Y, Wu Q, Su F, Fang Y, Zeng J and Pei Z 2018 The protective effect of Cantonese/Mandarin bilingualism on the onset of Alzheimer disease *Dement. Geriatr. Cogn. Disord.* **45** 210–19

Zlatev J 2009 The semiotic hierarchy: life, consciousness, signs and language *Cognit. Semiot.* **4** 169–200

Chapter 5

Brain and peripheral sensory motors in presence of social stimuli

Arindam Bit, Bharti Mishra and Shashikanta Tarai

The present chapter assesses the structural of the functional relationship between the morphological variations in the brain's sub-central region and location of enterprise's position in the time of somatotype action based on tongue, larynx, hand, and lips at the distinct level. The structure of the central sulcus is used to foretell the place of operational actuation peaks concerning the motion regarding various effectors within-person. Here is a proper explanation about the sulcus structure, sub-central and nearby opercula cortex (Petrides 2012, 2018), inclusive of inter-independent inconsistency in the morphology of the sulcal region. In this study, two groups of participants have been taken, where in the first study, structural and operational MRI data of motor tasks is obtained from 20 participants, and in the second part, configurational information is received from 30 participants. In addition, also cortical brain surface neuron connection was obtained from 30 participants. Conceivability designs in magnitude and the exterior area were produced, which describe morphological changeability of the inter-independent marked sulcus using Free Surfer's registration. Within the surface probability map, inter-independent inconsistency has been calculated as maxima. Also, the minimum value was estimated for the depth of sulcus in each individual. We can see three sulcal sections from the central regions, which have more depth. Mean cortical expanse and number of vertices covered by surface label were calculated as a scale of measure of sulcal section.

5.1 Motor cortex of the brain, its structural and functional features

During fMRI, the participants were told to repeat lips protuberance or tongue retractions at 1–2 repetitions per second (Eichert *et al* 2020). The breathing format of these participants has been taken into account (inhaling for 1.5 s and exhale

doi:10.1088/978-0-7503-3383-2ch5

for 4 s) using a fixation emblem on the screen. Also, the participants performed a task producing a phonetic unit trail within some specific situations. Participants did one more piece of homework related to phonological and semantic judgments, and this one was done towards a left-hand segment of the left hemisphere in the brain to estimate as a localizer. As a result, the structural motifs and inter-independent inconsistency of the sulcul segment within the central section and sub-central section in the cerebral cortex their connection to enterprise conjured through the motion was studied. A strong relationship in the countenance morphology of sulcul segment in central/sub-central cells and action based on hand, tongue, voice box (larynx) and lips at an independent stage were witnessed. Also, it was evident that morphological inconsistency can describe operational changeability, especially in the sub-central region, having morphological intricacy. Hence, considerable equivalence is present between sulci and operational high markers, which was the same, irrespective of hemisphere except for one area of right hemisphere of the brain, which was the lip cluster. This means the structure-to-junction relationship of a primary motion, including various effectors, had no considerable difference amidst hemisphere. This study's outcome, which explains about structural lineaments of the surface of the brain, proves to be relevant to neurosurgeons for the prevention, diagnosis, surgical treatment, and rehabilitation of disorders that affect any portion of the nervous system, including the brain, spinal cord, central and peripheral nervous system, and cerebrovascular system as well as to guide or 'navigate' within the confines of the skull or vertebral column during surgery. Also, anatomical evidence like this can empower the configuration of operational information for considerable group research.

To summarize, we have witnessed sulcus segments' morphological structure, their inter-independent inconsistencies, and some primary structural features. The function of the larynx while vocal modulation actuates the sub-central area is considered to be very unstable for individual subjects. The inconsistency may describe contradictions within earlier studies on illustration of the interior larynx and methodical association of handedness and discrepancies in the morphology of central and sub-central region of cortex.

5.1.1 Structural and functional connectivity between the bilateral primary motor cortex

A stroke occurs when the blood flow to the brain is restricted or entirely cut off, preventing brain tissue from receiving oxygen and nutrients. It is one of the significant causes of motor disability in adults worldwide (Feigin *et al* 2010). The primary motor cortex (M1) is the most crucial part (Sanes 2010). It primarily harmonizes as well as executes voluntary movements in opposite parts of the body in conjunction with different regions of the sub-cortex. This research aimed to learn more about the anatomical and functional variations that occur between the two sides of the M1 and in the side of the stroke that takes place in the subcortex. To do this, comprehensive neuroimaging (MRI) tests were performed on 24 stroke victims who suffered from a stroke in the sub-cortex of the right hemisphere and 25 healthy controls, keeping specific inclusion criteria in mind. Subjects were told to remain completely motionless and rest for 20 min before the fMRI scanning. The Diffusion Tensor Imaging data were acquired using a single-shot, gradient-recalled echo-planar imaging technique. A single-shot, gradient-recalled echo-planar imaging technique was used to develop resting-state fMRI datasets. The parameters for task-evoked fMRI were the same as for resting-state scanning, except that 100 volumes were collected. All subjects underwent a passive finger-grasping activity during work-induced fMRI imaging.

A qualified experimenter used a 1.0 Hz frequency to perform the job on the index finger and thumb of the left hand. The collected DTI data were processed and analysed with the help of the FMRIB Tools Library and Functional neuro Image software (Li 2015). Statistical parametric mapping software (SPM12) was used to process and analyse the resting-state data. The functional connectivity (FC) of two groups was determined using a two-sample T-test. The fractional anisotropy (FA) of the corpus callosum, the significant anatomical connection between the brain's two hemispheres, was examined among stroke patients and the control group. And it was observed that stroke patients showed a substantial decrease in the FA. Comparison of bilateral corticospinal tract (CST) was also performed within and between the two groups, and a significant reduction in the FA of the suitable CST of the stroke patients was observed compared to the left CST of the stroke patients and bilateral CST in healthy controls. For stroke patients and management, the bilateral CSTs showed no significant differences. The stroke patients with impaired motor pathway who participated in this experiment had lower resting-state functional connectivity (FC) in the two-sided primary motor cortex compared to control participants. Specific brain regions include the left post, pre-central, middle temporal and bilateral para hippocampal gyrus, left inferior parietal, bilateral paracentral lobule, bilateral thalamus, precuneus, and cuneus an increase in activity in stroke patients whose sub cortex was affected in the right hemisphere. There were no areas in stroke patients that exhibited reduced activation when compared to control individuals. There was also a reduction in FA and FC in the two sides of the primary motor cortex in stroke patients. As a result, the bilateral M1s have a reformed brain structure and functional connections between the two hemispheres. Also, it was shown that in stroke victims, a range of motor-related brain areas exhibited increased activity after left-hand movements, which may compensate for the structural and functional impairments in the primary motor cortex region. These locations were more prevalent on the opposite side of the lesion. Elevated activity in the ipsilesional hemisphere suggested that structurally injured areas still had the capacity for functional reconfiguration during motor recovery. Another study revealed that stroke patients' right hemisphere (for right-handed people) might be more significant regarding motor skills. Therefore, stroke patients with damaged right hemispheres were chosen for this study. Recent fMRI investigations in subcortical stroke patients have shown enhanced M1–M1 interconnectivity and a beneficial relationship with the recovery of motor function after therapeutic treatment. Certain limitations of this study included the fact that it did not contain any connections between structural and functional changes and behavioural data from patients. The results need to be confirmed for larger patient groups, and long-term longitudinal investigations should have been conducted that included all phases of stroke.

5.1.2 Somatotopic organization in the motor cortex

The motor cortex is positioned in the forefront of the cerebral cortex, just before the central sulcus, which goes along the side of the brain's hemispheres (Jackson 1958). The motor cortex is categorized into two principal regions: the primary motor cortex, which is found in a gyrus named the precentral gyrus, which is located next to the central sulcus, and the non-primary motor cortex, that is before the primary motor cortex and consists of two areas named the premotor cortex and supplementary motor cortex. Many different regions inside the motor cortex are exceptionally responsive to electrical excitability because it takes less stimulus to induce a similar muscle activity in the primary motor cortex (Penfield and Rasmussen 1950). The PMC is configured so that various sections of the area are linked with motor coordination of the different regions of the body; it exhibits topographical structure comparable to, but less accurate than, that observed in the somatosensory cortex. This somatotopic structure includes various brain areas that govern facial, hand, and leg motions. The scientific data gathered in the latest study indicates that the regulation of multiple parts of the body from M1 also isn't quite as somatotopically organized as the homunculus and simiusculus appear to indicate. Although it is apparent that the depictions of the skull, upper half, and lower half are sequentially and generally distinct, the depictions of shorter body parts are extensively dispersed throughout these critical areas. During reappraisal, statistics from the 1870s to the current day may also be coherent with this widespread arrangement. As a result, the region governing one body component heavily coincides with the region governing nearby parts of the body. For instance, the M1 region that controls the thumb coincides heavily with the regions that govern the rest of the phalanges in the hands. The primary somatosensory cortex has a well-organized somatotopic organization, while the primary visual cortex has a well-organized retinotopicembodiment (Iwamura *et al* 1983, Pons *et al* 1987). Although the proof for M1 inside limb somatotopy is sparse, a more complicated, highly spread structure exists. As a result, M1 is expected to represent essential aspects of a functional organization. The extent of the data processed in M1 might be one such characteristic. A 2-D receptor sheet can be projected isomorphically onto the 2-D cortex in well-structured models. Motions and the muscles that produce them are 3-D, yet they can't be easily projected onto a 2-D cortex. The dimensionality depicted in M1 is considerably more significant than 3 if every muscle with every degree of freedom at the joint and each kinematic or dynamic characteristic of motion is considered a potential dimension. Including in S1, the most distinct and well-structured somatotopic depiction of the various fingers is seen in region 3b, wherein dermal inputs are predominant. In regions 1 and 2, dermal inputs are coupled with inputs from deeper mechanoreceptors in joints and muscles. The somatotopic organization gets increasingly complicated as the number of receptive fields spanning several digits increases, especially in alert animals. M1 is also highly important since evidence has shown that the amount of somatotopic separation in M1 typically mirrors the biomechanical autonomy of various body parts.

5.2 Biochemical pathways of activating brain motor cortex neurons

This study focuses on cellular elements regarding breakdown brain energy, with a specific weightage on metabolic linkages within neurons and astrocytes. The adult brain requires glucose as an energy source. Nonetheless, under some situations, the brain can use alternative blood-derived energy sources, like ketones, in the case of development and deprivation of food or lactate throughout moments of vigorous exercise. The primary activities that promote the brain's high energy requirements include the sustenance and repair of ion gradients depleted due to signalling processes like postsynaptic activity and action adeptness, as well as neurotransmitter absorption and reuse. Among these, potential in the synapse appears to constitute the predominant energy expenditure related to excitability maintenance instead of electrical nerve impulses. Astrocytes are shown to have a specific arrangement of the cells and phenotypical features that allow them to sense their surroundings and respond proactively to changes in their surroundings. An increasing body of evidence indicates that astrocytes play a significant role in neurovascular connectivity or the temporospatial link between functions of neurons and elevated cerebral blood flow (CBF) (another name, functional hyperemia). It was lately discovered that high blood circulation to intrinsically functional brain areas is strongly linked with lactate elevations though adversely associated with CMRO2, implying that under usual physiological circumstances, elevated CBF is influenced by glycolytic metabolism instead of oxidative metabolism (Lin *et al* 2010). Overall, astrocytes are emerging as essential players in the neurovascular unit, acting as bridges between neural impulses and arteries. According to experimental evidence, the level of glucose the astrocytes take in is disproportionally huge when compared with their energy demands. According to the redox switch theory, inhibition of glutamate-induced glucose transport within neurons would create thermodynamically amenable conditions for using lactate as a power source in this type of cell because these mechanisms fight for intracellular NAD (Cerdan *et al* 2006).

Furthermore, research revealing that increasing astrocytic glycogen storage sustains neuronal activity and survival under conditions such as low energy supply, like in the case of deficient blood glucose levels, provided extra proof for glycogen-mediated neuron-glia metabolic linkage. Also, in a mouse in co-culture models, astrocytic glycogen mobilisation is necessary to maintain neuronal activity under intensive stimulation in optic nerve formulation and glutamatergic neurotransmission. In a bead discrimination learning test, pharmacological suppression of glycogenolysis in astrocytes also disrupted memory consolidation in young chickens. It was recently revealed that lactate derived from astrocytic glycogen has a role in developing long-term memory and regulating long-term potentiation (LTP) of synaptic power in the human brain (Suzuki *et al* 2011). This study showed that DAB injection within the hippocampus strongly affected long-term memory configuration in rats during an inhibitory avoidance test. Generally, introducing external lactate can rescue this consequence, but not if the expression of the primary neurological lactate transporter (MCT2) is hindered with anti-sense oligodeoxynucleotides, emphasizing the significance of glycogen-derived lactate transport into neurons for memory formation. Overall, these findings demonstrate that astrocytic glycogen seems more of an urgency reserve; it also serves an essential and integral part in complicated cerebral biological mechanisms, most prominently through the transport of energy molecules in the form of lactate from astrocytes to neurons. A substantial amount of empirical evidence suggests that astrocytes show greater metabolic flexibility when compared to neurons, which means they could effectively alter their energy consumption to different cellular demands.

5.2.1 Blood flow in brain: glial and neuronal control

Cerebral blood circulation is managed through nerve cells and a population of cells with distinctive morphological and functional characteristics that differ within the specific area known as astrocytes. It is essential to understand how nerve cells and astrocytes manage the blood circulation in the cerebral cortex, as neurological computing is energized due to it. Also, it helps to understand the operational scans of the cerebral region and for progressing the management of neuronal abnormalities. As neurotransmitter-led signalling plays a vital part in managing blood flow, this is achieved with the help of astrocytes by utilizing the arterioles and veins. This notion of brain blood flow regulation has helped in the advancement of various latest healing techniques. The human cerebral area constitutes only 2% of body mass, but it utilizes 20% of the energy composed while the body is at rest. Also, this huge energy requirement is essential for normal cerebral operations, with the help of the energy, ion entrance within synaptic, and execution potential (Attwell and Laughlin 2001). The glial and neuronal cells can rupture or die due to insufficient availability of blood glucose in the cerebral cortex, leading to various damage like stroke and bleeding or haemorrhage. The earlier notion was that nerve-related functions induce metabolic activity that triggers growth in blood flow, but a recent study highlighted the fact that neurotransmitter-led glutamate plays a more critical role in brain blood flow regulation with the help of astrocytes. This synaptic discharge of glutamate initiates neuronal *N*-methyld-aspartate receptors causing insertion of Ca^{2+} as well as initiation of NO (nitric oxide), which inflate the vessels (Busija *et al* 2007). It is explained that in the cerebral region, discouragement of nNOS decreases the flow of blood related to neuronal functions (Ma *et al* 1996). Here relatively new concepts of brain energy supply regulation have been discussed as with the help of various brain operational imaging analyses, corrective techniques for variable problems in the central nervous system have become a possibility.

Here the four primary considerations about brain blood circulation are seen: the first is that instead of energy glutamate neurotransmitters, second is that astrocytes perform a significant part of blood flow regulation, third is that oxygen assemblage leads the crucial signalling passages connected, fourth is that regulation of blood circulation happens at the stages of arterioles and capillary. The above-mentioned advancement helps us enhance the knowledge about the power source of neural enumeration and provides various possibilities for treating brain blood flow-related abnormalities. Hence recognizing the signaling passageways which mediate the brain blood circulation gives alternatives for corrective manoeuvring these passageways. This is rather direct for neurotransmitter-led signaling passageways, which rely on various enzymes and receptors which can be blocked at the stages of astrocyte mGluRs. Therefore, with the help of various passageways managing the blood circulation, even slight therapeutic altercation in the flow of blood flow in various situations or particular brain regions is possible. Also, with the help of recent diagnostic techniques of brain blood circulation measurement, even the slightest alteration in CBF is noticeable, and hence the therapeutic measures can even be taken before neuronal abnormalities occur. Also, the significance of capillary pericytes in long term blood flow reduction due to ischaemia has been evident in recent studies as few pericytes show constriction at the beginning of ischaemia. This constriction in Pericytepost ischaemia can be reduced with the help of oxidative or nitrosative stress; hence providing infusing antioxidants on tPA can prove a significant complementary measure.

5.2.2 Neuron–glia metabolic plasticity

Understanding the molecular and cellular characteristics of the brain's energy consumption pattern is extremely important not just for better understanding brain physiology but also for understanding the mechanisms of various neuronal and pathological disorders. The brain has relatively high energy demands despite it occupying only 2% of the body mass. One of several key fundamentals of the brain's physical structures would be that metabolism and circulation are inextricably linked to activities in the brain. Furthermore, a strong link between neural activity and glucose metabolism has been demonstrated. Astrocytes play an important role in linking synaptic activity to glucose consumption via molecular processes involving the sequential engagement of astrocyte-specific glutamate transporters and sodium–potassium ATPase. Glycolysis activation in astrocytes and mono-carboxylate transporter-mediated lactate exchange from astrocytes to neurons has also been discovered. According to the studies, glucose metabolism is related to neural action moderated by glutamate via biochemical mechanisms that are mainly, if not totally, reliant on the couple's astrocytes' function. When examining metabolic activity in activation versus baseline, it is found that the elevation in metabolic response during 'activation' is relatively minimal compared to the 'baseline' activity. The baseline activity represents about 90% of the brain's metabolism and varies under various physiological and pathological conditions. It was found that during activation, oxygen uptake does not increase according to glucose consumption or blood flow. As a result, upon activation, the oxygen supply to the active region increases (due to higher arterial supply), but oxygen consumption increases just a little. It means that the fractional oxygen evacuation is lower, implying that the 'oxygen extraction fraction' (OEF) would decrease upon activation (Gusnard *et al* 2001, Raichle *et al* 2001). It was also observed that in the course of a certain job, along with the instigation of certain regions, deactivation of some areas also took place. Various brain imaging investigations revealed that there are two operating modes with different time durations. The first is the activation mode, which is only there for a short period of time. This mode requires only a small amount of energy, around 10% of baseline activity. The second is the persistent baseline activity mode, which numerically makes up the bulk of brain energy consumption and may dip spontaneously during modality-specific activations and may be connected with a 'post-processing of information' mode. One view of the role of baseline activity is that this mode represents, at least to an extent, continuing synaptic plasticity processes. In different terms, persistent task-independent activity associated with high baseline metabolic action may indicate synaptic plasticity processes connected to the post-processing of input data rather than just 'neuronal noise'. Given the tight relationship between synaptic activity and energy metabolism, it is likely that the processes behind synaptic plasticity are also represented at the energy metabolism level, resulting in related metabolic changes that may be referred to as 'metabolic plasticity'. While we're on the subject of metabolic plasticity, some studies have found that energy consumption decreases in slow-wave sleep (SWS) and increases during REM sleep, according to brain regions (Franzini *et al* 1992). The glycogen production also rises during SWS, increasing by 50%–70% compared to the prior waking period. Sleep deprivation has been demonstrated in recent research to alter several genes encoding proteins associated with energy metabolism. According to the 'homeostatic regulation of sleep fits the brain energy restoration' theory, adenosine, an inhibiting neurotransmitter, could connect sleep governance and energy metabolism. Another theory is that control of the expression of genes encoding enzymes engaged in glycogen metabolism may occur throughout the sleep-waking cycle. Furthermore, the findings of the tests revealed that extended wakefulness causes a double rise in PTG mRNA. Additionally, a rise in glycogen synthase activity implies that the elevation in protein targeting to glycogen seems to have a functional purpose (PTG). It has also been discovered that the hippocampus is engaged in the encoding, storage, and recovery of spatial memory in rodents. The glucose usage was tracked at various stages of a recognized spatial learning challenge, the eight-arm radial maze. The findings revealed that metabolic requirement changes through space and time in the regions involved in the activity, particularly in the hippocampus, during the distinct learning periods. During the training and recall stages, various patterns of metabolic activity were identified. More areas of the CA1 and CA3 were metabolically activated as learning continued, going from the rear and intermediary levels to the frontal level. Furthermore, during recollection, enhanced metabolic action was exclusively detected in the frontal regions of the dentate gyrus.

5.3 Structure and function of the cognitive brain

Despite comparable heredity estimates, schizophrenia and bipolar disorder (SZ and BD) were recognised as distinct disorders, and the subsequent emergence of these schizoaffective disturbances as a fusion of both highlights difficulties with the distinction between the two (Cardno *et al* 1999). This review investigated 24 research findings, including 13 studies of people in the schizophrenia range, eight studies of people with maniac depression, and five investigations of people with schizophrenia and maniac depression. This study examined the data from the scientific literature that used unsupervised clustering approaches to identify subgroups of cognition in grown-up schizophrenic patients, schizoaffective disorder, or bipolar disorder. The quality of each of those studies was assessed using the 'Strengthening the Reporting of Observational Studies in Epidemiology (STROBE)' statement, and they were considered acceptable quality when 70% of the criteria were met (Von Elm *et al* 2007). Single cross-disorder research (that also contributed to research findings of SZ and BD) revealed a three-cluster answer. It demonstrated inter-indicative clustering method was preferential in lowering cognitive heterogeneousness among SZ and BD cases; the subordinate mental type was found in these diseases independently. Four more studies that employed unsupervised clustering algorithms on cognitive information for mixtures of samples of schizophrenia and mood disorder patients all gave a four-cluster result. The occurrence of a cognitive severe dysfunction subtype where disparities of cognitive functioning had a medium to colossal impact on comparison with healthy controls (HCs) was a trait shared by all of the reported solutions.

The cross-disorder solutions consistently showed the over-estimation of BD samples identified having intellectively allocated cognition and the discourse over-estimation of SZ cases in the subtypes with severe cognitive shortfall. This was in accordance with the conventional correlations of cognitive function between these disorders directly. There was also some indication in SZ that the smaller the research, the more subtypes were found, and other methodological variations in statistical techniques and sample characteristics may have impacted outcomes among studies. In addition, irrespective of diagnosis, participants with the most extreme cognitive problems commonly seemed to have the maximum brain abnormalities, symptoms, lower academic background and employment, and high drug dosages in comparison with participants with specific cognitive decline or intellectually spared cognitive capabilities. These cognitive batteries used in the 13-schizophrenia research and the eight BD studies were quite consistent. Cross-disorder studies, on the other hand, had a wider range of cognitive domains evaluated; however, the quantity of clusters found didn't seem to be linked to the quantity or type of cognitive domains evaluated. Notably, the most accuracy in analytical techniques was seen in BD research. Seven of the eight studies employed hierarchical cluster analysis (HCA), and one of these generated a three-cluster answer; a single BD study had alternative latent class analysis (LCA) methodologies that generated a four-cluster result (Bora *et al* 2016). With the exception of just two experiments that provided a two-cluster solution and employed an underrated 'Grade of Membership' approach, the research results among SZ patients did not show a comparable pattern based on the technique used. Three out of five cross-disorder studies utilised k-means cluster analysis, which all produced a four-cluster solution, so did the use of LCA, whereas the only study that produced a three-cluster solution employed HCA (comparable to findings for BD). This review revealed the existence of a serious cognitive impairment subtype (portraying a more significant percentage of schizophrenia spectrum disease instances than mood disorders), which also may be the most beneficial target for future research into genetic dangers and neuropathology in these situations. It also emphasised the importance and potential risks of information motivated strategy to cognitive classification inside and around the psychosis range, along with new studies pointing to the efficacy of integrating cognitive and imaging modalities.

5.3.1 Dynamic changes in cognition and brain structure of developing brain

The intelligence quotient (IQ) has long been employed in clinical psychology. A popular test for measuring psychometric intelligence in children is the Wechsler Intelligence Scale for children (WISC). This scale is used in the context of medical, scientific, and academic contexts in some capacity. When it comes to the full-scale IQ (FSIQ), two composite ratings of verbal intelligence, operational intelligence, and four-factor index scores, this tool offers exceptional psychometric characteristics (VC: verbal comprehension, PO: perceptual organization, FD: freedom from distractibility, and PS: processing speed) (Kaufman *et al* 1993). This research aimed to look at the link between the shape of the brain and subordinate cognitive type in normally developing growing children huge specimens. Cognitive pattern subcategories were expected to arise depending on the outcome level, such as (commonplace or above/below-commonplace) and outcome designs. Participants in the study were 298 healthy Japanese children aged 5.6–18.4 years who had brain MRI scans. On the exact day of the scan, qualified examiners administered the WISC-III to measure a person's innate intellect. Three IQ results (FSIQ, VIQ, and PIQ) and four element indexes (VC, PO, FD, and PS) were derived from the raw data for each subject. Socioeconomic status was also determined using three questions linked to an inquiry about yearly family income, and the other two were related to the highest academic degree of both parents.

SPSS version 20 was used to analyse behavioural data. A scanner was used to acquire all images. Voxel-based morphometry was used to examine the 3D T1-weighted MRI datasets. The statistical parametric mapping programme (SPM8) implemented in Matlab was used to pre-process structural data. Each individual's T1-weighted structural pictures were divided into six tissues. SPM8 was used to perform statistical analysis on the imaging data. The WISC-III factor index scores were used in the cluster analysis to identify six distinct kinds of cognitive processes.

C1, C2, and C4 all performed about as well as they could have in these tests. C1 had a higher VIQ than PIQ and a highest VC score than either of the other candidates. C2 and C4 had the factor index score flipped; C2 had higher PO and PS scores, while C4 had higher VC and FD values. C3, C5, and C6 all have IQs and factor indices that are below average. C5 had a more excellent FD rating than C6, while C6 had a greater PS rating.

In the right middle temporal gyrus, C3 had a higher amount of grey matter, whereas C2 and C4 had a smaller volume of grey matter. Furthermore, the right middle temporal gyrus cluster included posterior regions, such as the superior temporal gyrus. Cognitive processes and the prefrontal and parietal areas, on the other hand, did not show any meaningful relationships. The larger the right central temporal gyrus was in C3, the less the VIQ, PIQ, and component index scores were in WISC compared to the rest of the subtypes. The grey matter size declines with age in the various cerebral areas, according to a previous study. Between the ages of 10 and 12, for example, the temporal cortex reaches its maximum size. Compared with children of different subordinate types, C3 children appeared underdeveloped, agreeing with the predictions (Taki *et al* 2011). Compared to other subtypes, C2 and C4 youngsters had smaller right middle temporal lobe volumes and higher VIQ and PIQ scores, indicating that their brains were more developed. Another study found a link between the extent of disparity and the depth of the anterior and posterior cortices, such as the medial prefrontal, superior temporal, and occipital cortices. These data suggest that these sites mostly explain the variation in the magnitude of the VIQ versus PIQ difference. Right central temporal gyrus is hence critical for cognitive growth (Margolis *et al* 2013). One of the study's shortcomings was that brain regions traditionally thought to have a strong connection with cognitive ability, like frontal and parietal gyri, have not been significantly related to mental processes. It was also revealed that there was no subtype with superior performance. Finally, we can state that this research revealed individual differences in cognitive functions and brain architecture among otherwise healthy children.

5.3.2 Posterior AD-type pathology

'Posterior shift' of Alzheimer's disease (AD) neuro-pathological alterations result in a condition dominated by high-level visual impairments, which is clinically described as posterior cortical atrophy (PCA). The purpose of the study was to investigate if information directed analysis (cluster analysis) established solely on neuropsychiatric observations resulted in the establishment of different patient groups. Particularly, if was feasible to detect patients with vision-spatial abnormalities reliable with the supposition that PCA is a 'dorsal stream' ailment if there have been subordinate groups of patients with a range of deficits within the high-level visual field, in addition to patients with usual impaired memory (Benson *et al* 1988). Twenty-three PCA patients were enrolled using the specified criteria (Mendez 2002, McMonagle 2006). PCA patients were evaluated for the first time, complaining of visual impairment, spatial disorientation, memory problems, and depression. Twenty PCA patients had part or all of Gerstmann's disorder, 18 had Balint's disorder, seven had been neglected, while one had aphasia. Eight PCA patients developed the illness before old age. After being selected using conventional criteria, 16 individuals with DAT were also recruited in the research in 2009. The subjects were exposed to a thorough neuropsychological assessment. Twenty-six tests were selected to explore memory, perception and visuospatial areas, cognitive abilities, language, and math, and they were used as variables in subsequent analyses. A ranked aggregate cluster estimation was done on the acquired factor scores based on statistical recommendations. Cluster estimation is a categorization method of producing similar groups from complex data sets. Also, the objective of this study was to discover the number of times groups could be distinguished solely depending on the performance of the screening batteries.

A hierarchical cluster analysis was performed, with the squared Euclidean distance as a propinquity measure and Ward's minimal variance agglomerative method. ANOVA was used to evaluate variables across clusters. The Fisher LSD method was used for post hoc analyses. Cluster analysis revealed four cognitive dysfunctions in the visuospatial/visuoperceptual, memory, perceptual/calculation, and linguistic domains. DAT and PCA, the two main characteristics of AD pathogenesis, were assigned to clusters 1 and 2. The visuospatial deficit was seen in cluster 1, which comprises a very homogenous mass of PCA subjects, demonstrating that PCA is predominantly a dorsal stream disorder, although the findings tend to corroborate that sensory problems can occur concurrently. The results also suggest that subtypes of AD could have selective visuoperceptual and linguistic deficits. The presence of visuoperceptual deficiency as a primary feature in PCA has been documented, but the development of a sequence driven by linguistic dysfunction has been less predicted given the selection criterion that was used. This most recent study shows that linguistic impairment is a crucial element of AD pathogenesis, even when it doesn't appear as a medically significant aphasic condition. Memory loss was related to hypoperfusion in the left temporoparietal and frontal areas, supporting earlier studies; visuospatial and perceptual deficits were linked with a predominant right parietal hypoperfusion, supporting prior reports. Six of the seven PCA patients with left side disregard were included in this cluster, indicating that neglect is common in neurodegenerative diseases with the uneven engagement of the two hemispheres. The right posterior hypo-perfusion in this cluster was also consistent with the sensory dysfunction manifested mainly by difficulties with face perception. When the deficits were limited to low-level sensing and computing, the participation of the suitable posterior regions was confirmed (cluster 3). Ultimately, hypoperfusion was bilateral temporoparietal and left frontal when the prominent characteristic was linguistic deficit (fluency, reading, and naming). While bitemporal participation is constant with a potential issue with object recognition when confronted with name tasks, the reading deficit might be accounted for by parietal dysfunction. Although dyslexia could be perceptual, it is also possible that participants in cluster 4 had an ogopenic-type disease, with the sub-lexical deficit being among the significant symptoms. In conclusion, a purely data-driven study based on neuropsychological results in the sample of patients would demonstrate that PCA is primarily a dorsal stream condition different from conventional amnestic AD.

5.4 Structure and function of peripheral sensory motors

The peripheral nervous system (PNS) is a term used to describe nerves that are not located in the central nervous system. Peripheral nerves, spinal nerves and neuromuscular connections are all included in this system. The PNS consists of amotor and sensory neurons with their cell bodies in the spinal cord and axons that communicate with a remote target organ. Injuries to peripheral nerves are prevalent in many types of upper limb trauma (Kouyoumdjian 2006). A thorough grasp of neuronal morphology, physiopathology, and medical presentation is required to perform the procedure with peripheral nerve damage (Siemionow *et al* 2009). The peripheral nerve anatomy and blood flow are two essential elements in interpreting surgical procedures and therapy after surgery. By keeping a firm knowledge of these crucial regions, the physiotherapist can optimize the benefits of treatments. In addition, it is critical to comprehend advances in operative repair and growth improvement (Brushart 1991). In situations when a significant injury in muscles and skeletons can hide deeper, severe nerve damage, physiotherapists can become the catalyst for medical assistance. A thorough grasp of the complications connected with peripheral nerve damage, particularly the prolonged onset of symptoms, would enable one to contact prospective specialists at the appropriate time. The physiotherapist is crucial in assessing the amount of Sunderland fourth, fifth, and sixth-degree wounds and their qualification to return.

Furthermore, physiotherapists must speak for patients regarding therapeutic strategies that could improve or optimize tissue repair. The involvement of the physiotherapist in the rehabilitation of functionality after the operation is crucial. It is critical to stop anchoring the surgically restored nerve, although ischemia and extreme lengthening should be prevented. Motion to preserve the nerve's lengthwise extension and glide will reduce the production of damaged tissue, which may sometimes lead to tethered and supermini-posed strain damage. As a result, a monitored reprogram is necessary, with the proviso that sufferers must receive significant instruction to avoid jeopardizing range soon in the rehabilitation procedure. Continuous passive motion (CPM) is a widely used tool; however, it should be constantly supervised for overuse that might be harmful. As per the investigation, the optimum surgical therapy for severe neuronal damage is still direct nerve restoration with epineural micro-articulation (Lundborg 2000). Whenever a tension-free coaptation in a well-vascularized bed can be established, epineural healing is performed.

Alternative procedures comprise grouped fasciculate repair, involving intraneural incision and direct fascicular group fitting and stitching. There are other techniques to use healthy donor nerves to circumvent damaged peripheral nerve connections. This is suggested in wounds to the extremely nearby nerves or those who do not have a proximal nerve stump, such as cervical nerve root avulsions. The two primary areas of research efforts to improve recovery following nerve restoration are ways to increase neurogenesis and techniques that reduce environmental aggravation. For example, enhancing axonal outgrowth from the distal nerve stump (growth factors; electrical excitation of the proximal stump); giving a supportive atmosphere for axons to pass a co-optation (improved conduits; thermal and non-thermal laser; nerve adhesive); postponing or modifying Wallerian deterioration (axon merging); as well as shrinking the denervation (electrical excitation of the motor target). Since the introduction of microsurgical repair procedures well over 50 years ago, functional recovery following peripheral nerve restoration has steadily increased. Despite this, many individuals, especially those with proximal nerve damage, have partial healing and long-term impairment. There are still several unfulfilled goals in peripheral nerve operations, notably: (1) reliable diagnostics for assessing nerve damage in the primary setting; (2) tissue-engineered nerve channels that meet or surpass nerve grafts; and (3) clinical techniques of targeted stabilization till re-innervation. The better outcomes come from direct nerve restoration, and nerve autografts are still considered the premium quality therapy for nerve voids. In tiny gaps, conduits have a minor role.

5.4.1 The sensory neuron of touch

Sensory neurons transform a particular stimulus with the help of their receptors which reside beneath the cuticle on the perimeter of the skeletal structure. Somatotype network decrypts a broad extent of tactile stimuli and hence provides us with the conspicuous capability of identifying objects, distinguishing the constituents, giving feedback of sensations and social transaction. To better understand the environment, the somatotype system performs three major roles: proprioceptive, exteroceptive and interoceptive. An immediate step for identifying innoxious sensations can be intimation about the sensible exterior neurons known as low-threshold mechanoreceptors (LTMRs). This study focuses on the unique mechanisms of LTMRs subtypes and their structural sense of auxiliary and primary axonal estimates. In spinal structure, the physiology of the nervous system examples about intricate external force posing on the skin and how this tactile message is responded to and sent to the brain has been studied in this research (Basbaum *et al* 2009, Smith and Lewin 2009, Todd 2010). Structures about the cell of principle sensible neuron reside within the dorsal base/root of ganglia (DRG) and sensible cranial ganglia. In DRG, one axonal branch of neuron incorporates into the periphery while the other probes into the spine and generates synapses. In extrareceptive somatotype structure deciphering the harmful is most important; hence, most dorsal ganglia neuronal networks are attuned with heat processing and encrypting noxious stimuli. It can be said that understanding benign and malicious touch impression depends upon particular sensile neurons classified as low threshold mechanoreceptors (LTMRs) reacting to harmless benign external stimuli and high-threshold mechanoreceptors (HTMRs) responding to dangerous external stimuli. According to the structure and size of the cell, its axonal length, myelination level, and conduction velocity, all the cutaneous sensory neurons are characterized as Aβ, Aδ, or C. Here C-type neurons are most bounteous and smallest in size, having un-myelinated axons. Also, they are the slowest in terms of conduction velocity (0.2–2 m s^{-1}). At the same time, Aδ and Aβ have large body sizes with heavily myelinated processes and rapid conduction velocities (Aδ 5 to 30 m s^{-1} and Aβs 60 to 100 m s^{-1}).

Hence LTMRs are triggered feeble, benign mechanical pressure probing the skin can be actuated due to hot or cold sensation and their sprouting arrangements with constant external stimulus may be varying from slow adapting (SA) to intermediate adapting (IA) to rapidly adapting (RA). Also, LTMRs end-organ associating patterns are essential, such as combining with glabrous (non-hairy) or hairy skin as hair plays a crucial role in regulating body temperature. The HTMRs are a considerable division of sensible neurons which are properly activated dangerous/

threat external stimulus. The above study signifies the LTMR functions that mutually excerpts and encrypts every aspect of touch-related incentives. Also, in a study amalgamation with physiological documentation within the skin in combination with physiological recordings in the skin–nerve organization, mouse transgenic tools have facilitated the explanation of LTMRs with the help of their morphological and anatomical attributes (Seal *et al* 2009, Li *et al* 2011). Touch and pain are complexly associated, and the study of pain regulating mechanisms explain basic principles of primary touch sensation; hence pain pathways are highlighted due to their relationship with the processing of innocuous touch information, as shown in figure 5.1. Here, psychophysical and neurophysiological research has concluded an intricate image about the peripheral neural pathways involved in tactile perception.

5.4.2 Ageing and peripheral nerve regeneration

Ageing is a natural phenomenon, but it has severe implications for the human mind and body, especially in the PNS; it severely impacts structural and operational aspects of PNS. This loss and abnormality in both nerve fibre, un-myelinated and myelinated, is recorded in older subjects. This loss and abnormality in old age are estimated to be because of a reduction in P0, PMP22 and MBP, essential myelin proteins. Also, a decrease in myelin thickness was visible in auxiliary nerves of elderly animals due to a reduction in observed protein mRNA, a crucial myelin protein. This study aims to understand the impact of agedness on the operational and structural state of PNS and its ability to rejuvenate the nerve after any trauma. In older nerves, enfeeblement in axons is commonly visible due to the lessening of axonal transfer of cytoskeletal proteins. Other impacts of agedness are reduced nerve conveyance velocity, muscle power, autonomous reactions, sensory discernments and endoneurial blood circulation. Alterations in the PNS's intended body parts

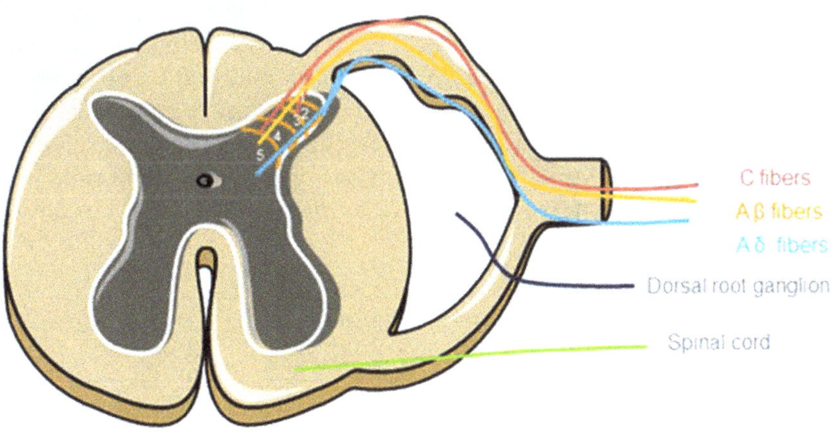

Figure 5.1. Structures and connection of primary nerve fibres Aβ and Aδ (LMTR) organization of primary fibres protruding from spinal cord dorsal horn.

with decline in function, such as motor dysfunctions, have been noticed with agedness as a periodical reduction in muscle power (Einsiedel and Luff 1992, Greig *et al* 1993) and of motor coordination (Potvin *et al* 1980). A study showed that the highest tetanic force induced through medial gastrocnemius muscle was lessened in elder animals accompanyied by increased heat and touch vibration limits (Einsiedel and Luff 1992). These changes in neuronal, Schwann cell, axonal structures can be due to a reduction in post-injury nerve rejuvenation because of ageing. It is seen that in animals, Wallerian degradation is delayed post-trauma due to agedness. In the older subjects, the interactivity within Schwan cell and axons takes more time; also, the tropic and tropic factor's secretion is lower. Axonal rejuvenation and density of axons tend to get reduced in older animals. A degradation of terminal and collateral germination of rejuvenated fibres is noticed due to ageing.

Along with the hindrances in physical activity and motor function, neurological abnormalities and postural flexion are also visible in the older population, approximately 50% (Drachman and Long 1994). Neuropsychological estimation depicts dampening of the central nervous system, slowing new data acquisition, and processing and dampening of fluid intelligence are also associated with ageing (Katzmanand 1983). Due to morphological and functional degradation due to ageing, progressive loss of nerve causes operational impairment in the central nervous structure. Disruption in the autonomous system is related to disruption in cardiovascular functions (i.e., change in heartbeat per second); deep breathing decreases in the older population compared to younger populations (Collins *et al* 1980, Kennedy *et al* 1989, Low 1997). Also, this degradation is combined with phenotypic alterations in the soma of axonal neurons, including protuberance and relocation in the nucleus and advancement in nucleolus diameter. This loss of motor, sensory and autonomous functioning caused by nerve trauma may be addressed by rejuvenating the axons properly by reinnervation of indicated organs. Hence four stages, i.e., Wallerian degradation and chromatolysis, axonal regeneration, showed reinnervation, and axonal maturation are methods of neuronal rejuvenation or reinstitution (Verdú *et al* 1998). The operational importance of renewal lies in replacing the distal nerve section impairment during disintegration, permitting the innervation of indicated organs and the respective operation restitution of those organs, as shown in figure 5.2. Hence this study provides significant knowledge about various aspects of nerve damage and regeneration which is crucial for target organ functioning.

5.5 Biochemical and physiological relationship between motor cortex and cognitive brain

The purpose of this section is to investigate the relationship between brain chemistry and size in the principal motor cortex and the performance of pattern of limb movements made during locomotion in older adults with slight cognitive decline whilst trying to perform a task. Recent imaging investigations have revealed that the primary motor cortex is essential in the regulating system of movement. Twenty

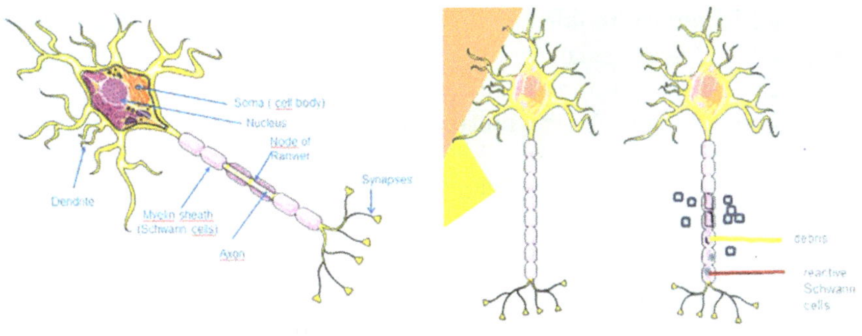

A B

Figure 5.2. (A) Depicts the structure of a healthy neuronal network, (B) illustrates the myelinated fibre and its demyelination with the distal shattering of axon and myelin sheaths with distal segment reactive Schwann cells (rSC) as degenerating debris.

patients with moderate cognitive problems aged 76 years were recruited for this investigation. Their gait was assessed for single and dual tasks using established procedures, and the alteration of gait velocity and stride time changeability were computed and analysed in different task conditions, respectively. Under specific settings, the patients' MRI spectra were also obtained. By sectioning volumetric 3D scans with the FreeSurfer software programme, the grey matter cubic content of the primary motor cortex and a variety of additional control areas of interest were determined (Fischl *et al* 2001). As a covariate, cognitive performance was assessed using the Montreal Cognitive Assessment, a 30-point exam that evaluates various areas of cognition (Nasreddine *et al* 2005). The individuals' attributes were summed using medians, and statistical evaluation was carried out using the SPSS programme. The Chi-square test was performed for assessments between participants depending on median results of metabolite ratios within the primary motor cortex. In addition, the Wilcoxon test was employed to evaluate gait metrics between tasks, and the Pearson correlation matrix was used to determine which gait measures in both studies were explicitly related to metabolite ratios in the primary motor cortex.

Bivariate and SWMH-adjusted partial Pearson correlations were also used to explore the relationships between gait measures in tasks and primary motor cortex volumes and other places of focus. To analyse the link between low N-acetyl creatine and high creatine (independent variables) and gait velocity and sweep time variability while single and dual tasking (dependent variables) after adjusting for various factors. Every model was submitted to its examination. Fourth, the risk variance of aberrant metabolite proportions in the primary motor cortex and the magnitude of the impact of reduced volume in the primary motor cortex were evaluated for individuals who already had significant gait problems during dual-tasking versus those who already had considerable gait problems during dual-tasking who didn't. The findings revealed that the metabolite ratios and size of the primary motor cortex were connected to gait in both single and dual-task circumstances. Slower gait velocity was also associated with greater choline/creatine levels and a reduced primary motor cortex volume. In contrast, more significant stride time variability was associated with reduced N-acetyl creatine levels and, to a limited extent, a reduced primary motor cortex magnitude. Mitigated gait velocity and increased stride time changeability were significant predictors of loss in mobility and stumbles. Moreover, those with poor gaits while dual-tasking were more probable to have aberrant metabolite ratios in the primary motor cortex. Additionally, those who lowered their gait velocity while doing a dual task had a higher (nearly double) probability of having a smaller primary motor cortex volume. This study shows that the primary motor cortex is essential not only in gait but also in establishing a regular walking style when cognitive demands are high. Another research recruited 67 patients at risk of pre-dementia and reported that an adjusted Tinetti scale correlated strongly with N-acetyl aspartate/creatine concentrations in the basal ganglia (Salem *et al* 2008). The current study, of course, has its limitations. To begin with, instead of measuring exact concentrations, the metabolite concentrations were normalised to creatine. Furthermore, the H-MRS data were gathered from a particular region of interest established on an *a priori* hypothesis and validated by the current volumetric analysis. Finally, since the study is cross-sectional, causal conclusions are restricted. An anticipated investigation of the 'Gait and Brain Study' cohort in the upcoming years should look at metabolite alterations in the primary motor cortex and other regions of interest over time to determine whether they have any prognostic score of gait degradation.

5.5.1 Cortical non-pyramidal cells: molecular diversity

This study aim was to look into the anatomical and metabolic characteristics of non-pyramidal cells in the neocortex of the rat. Based on preliminary research, non-pyramidal branches were labelled as fast-spiking (FS) due to their high discharge frequency in the absence of accommodation (McCormick *et al* 1985). However, recent research has demonstrated that these branches contain a wide range of inherent blasting characteristics and accommodate frequency. New-born Wistar rats (16–22 days) were severely sedated with xylazine and ketamine then subsequently decapitated for this study. After slice preparation, whole-cell recordings were done, followed by cytoplasm harvest and RT. Then, Multiplex PCR was performed in two steps followed by southern blot analysis, RNA isolation and intracellular labelling by biocytin injections. Immuno-cytochemical staining was then combined with biocytin labelling. Electrophysiological analysis and statistical analysis followed next. At the single-cell level, the RT-mPCR was designed to detect mRNAs containing three CaBPs and four neuropeptides simultaneously. In this approach, two sets of PCR expansion have been performed after RT. The seven markers were co-amplified in the initial PCR by mixing of respective primer pairs of each. The findings of the original PCR were then used as a standard for seven subsequent expansions, with a specific primer combination. The seven distinct mRNAs were identified, each of which produced one PCR segment of the length predicted by their RNA trail. The RT-mPCR's sensitiveness and selectivity were next evaluated at the single-cell level on cerebellar Purkinje cells. These cells were estimated by their position and form in acute parasagittal cerebellar dissects. CB and PV transcripts were found in the molecular study of a single Purkinje cell. These mRNA classes have been detected in nine of the ten Purkinje cells studied; in one cell, CR mRNAs have been detected, while the other was transcripts. Only CB mRNAs were found in the remaining cell. Overall, the findings of these control studies demonstrated the single-cell RT-sensitivity mPCRs and specificity. From stage V, eight, and stage II–III, ten pyramidal cells were used as controls. Although one layer V pyramidal cell had SS, the other has CCK, and the end one has NPY mRNAs, most layer V pyramidal cells did not display any of the seven indicators. There were no markers in four pyramidal cells examined of layers II–III. The following mRNA expression patterns were discovered in the six surviving layers II–III pyramidal cells: CB–CCK–SS, CB–CCK, CCK, and SS. The data reveals that most FS branch accumulation expresses PV and that 50% of these neurons exhibit CB and neuropeptide mRNA. The RSNP cell group had a far more complex pattern of biochemical marker expression.

Contrary to the biochemical variety of RSNP cells and FS cells, CR and VIP mRNAs were continuously co-expressed by a small subset of IS interneurons. These cells are bipolar in shape and contain transcripts for both GABA and acetylcholine synthesis enzymes. Controls on electrophysiologically characterised pyramidal cells as well as glial cells in neocortical slices further confirmed the amplification method's particularity. These controls support the applicability of this RT-mPCR technique to examine the patterns of mRNAs encoding CB, PV, CR, NPY, VIP, SS, and CCK in single non-pyramidal cells is supported. When looking for the co-articulation of two CaBP mRNA species (CB–PV or CR–CB), several were, but the co-articulation about PV and CR was not even once observed, which is in line with immunohistochemical studies. Among the physiological cell types, RSNP cells have been by far the most prevalent (Kubota *et al* 1994). Further molecular research on IS neurons found that GAD and ChAT mRNAs were co-expressed. It has been suggested that VIP-expressing bipolar neurons may comprise both ChAT and GAD because of the comparative proportions of VIPimmuno-reactive bipolar neurons that exhibit ChAT or GAD in the neocortex (Peters and Harriman 1988). The present research strongly backs up this theory and shows that these cells can now be recognised electro-physiologically based on their erratic blasting patterns.

5.5.2 Influence of fast and slow experience in the primary motor cortex

Acquiring any motor skill and mastering it requires time and practice. This paper tries to show that a modest training session may prove adequate for improving performance which takes longer to manifest. It offers a brief overview of two aspects of skill acquisition—precision and total duration of learning—that, as suggested, might put crucial limitations on the neural core and groundwork of adult skill enhancement. Recent findings have indicated that: (i) the procuration and detainment of physical skills in the adult human brain could lead to considerable expertise reorganisation in particular motor-cortical portrayals; and (ii) these representative alterations take place in phases and have a discrete-time course. When it comes to characteristics of skill learning, it can be said that learning can be substantially influenced by essential physical attributes of the stimulus given while training a perceptual task or by aspects such as the locations, trajectories, and sequence of trajectories experienced by specific effector organs during motor training (Fiorentini and Berardi 1981). The paper also discusses declarative and procedural memory, and it was highlighted that declarative learning can occur quickly and even after a single encounter.

On the other hand, procedural learning is slower and frequently takes numerous repetitions, generally spread out across multiple training sessions, to develop. According to studies, enhanced perceptual performance often produces in two separate steps: number one, a rapid amid-module development which could be influenced by a restricted number of trials on a timeframe of minutes (fast learning), and second, gradually growing, iterative efficiency amplifications that are provoked by training and yet take a while to become efficient in (slow learning) (Karni and Sagi 1993). Twelve youngsters (seven female and five male; all right-hand dominant) participated within those studies to validate the paper's primary hypothesis. Participants were asked that they press the two five-element sets of finger-to-thumb opposing motions illustrated in the instructions using their non-preferred hand and without visual input. The experiment was recorded and analysed. The results showed that in terms of speediness and exactness, the two sequences performed identically at first. On the other hand, training led to a substantial increase in both speediness and exactness for the learned sequence.

Furthermore, with no extra training the next day, a substantial improvement in both speediness and exactness was seen for the taught sequence only compared to the instantaneous performance level after training. It has been demonstrated that not all learning occurs concurrently with practice in a sequential finger opposition task. A very few rapid resistance motions provided sufficient training not just to boost results throughout the workout but also to start substantial new improvements that impact the performance the following day; seemingly, several improvements need time for gaining efficiency and begin to progress after motor training has been completed. Developing an additional skill is characterised by a simultaneous improvement in efficiency and agility (Hallet *et al* 1996). Altogether, the data indicate that human muscle memory increases well after a practice session and is transformed into a long-term imprint over time. Additionally, these findings reveal an important similarity in terms of timing among motor and sensory learning, which could mean motor skill practising mirrors the time constants of fundamental neuronal processes for memory repository that are shared across cortical depictions in the adult mind. Incorporating human imaging data with behavioural measures to track the impact of training over the duration has revealed three considerable details about the neurological underpinnings of skill training in the adult brain. For instance, training can activate mental abilities that last for hours after the session is over. And while numerous brain regions may play a role in early phases in acquiring an additional skill, a key cornerstone for mastery is the availability of a differentiated depiction of the experience characteristics that are crucial to do the task. Finally, the advancement of motor skills takes a bit of time and has two phases that are analogous to the phases of learning perceptual skills. A swift growth point occurs early on (fast learning), continuing steadily after practice iterative performance gain (slow learning).

5.6 Biochemical and physiological relationship between peripheral neurons and cognitive brain

This study aimed to look at the evidence using meta-analytic metrics that support the presence of a distinct potential stimulate or workout limit where the brain's performance gains were maximized. The study was confined to a review of cognitive performance speed instead of covering both precision and agility. Because it was discovered in a previous study that precision was the variable that was reliant on others and did not show a substantial gain in productivity (McMorris *et al* 2011), some researchers have shown limits of nor-epinephrine (NE) along with epinephrine (Epi), or the levels where the plasma level of NE and Epi begin to grow exponentially in response to exercise, may cause enhanced cognitive speed. The term catecholamines are used for NE and Epi here. The measurement of catecholamine threshold (TCATS) is quite invasive in nature. Therefore, measurements of other quantities like ventilator threshold (VT) and lactate threshold (TLA) was done as these are highly correlated with (TCATS) (Yamamoto *et al* 1991). A literature search was conducted using PsycArticles, PsycINFO, PubMed, SportsDISCUS, and Web of Knowledge. Whenever averages and standard deviations were provided, results for reaction time measurements have been estimated using Cohen's d formula. Every single d was then translated to the bias-corrected standardised mean difference, Hedges' g, using the correction factor J, and this has been utilised to compute an average effect size using the random-effects model. The Q test for homogeneity findings was measured and presented as τ2, an exact variance measure, whereas Q is a relative variance level. The Orwin's37Fail-safe N was computed. In the subgroup analysis, the results obtained for each group were examined using a Z-test upon the variances having a random-effects specimen, having independent predictions of τ^2 for each sub-group. The proportion of variance explained by the moderator variable was calculated using R2.

The data indisputably back up the researchers' choice of acute exercise at one or more thresholds to produce increased cognitive speed. However, the notion that medium-strength workouts exhibited a substantial intermediate, average impact size questions the degree to which thresholds represent an actuation point. More significantly, both mean impact measures don't vary statistically. To explain how intense workouts influence intellect, some researchers have proposed that it is due to heightened arousal, which is caused by increased levels of both the neurotransmitters DA and NE. Blood catecholamine levels start rising after 30 min of below-threshold activity. If the exercise lasts more than or equal to 45 min, the hypothalamic-pituitary-adrenal pivot is engaged. This increases the synthesis and secretion of corticotrophin-releasing factor (CRF) and adrenocorticotrophic hormone (ACTH) in the central nervous system, as well as cortisol in the peripheral nervous system (Brandenberger *et al* 1980).

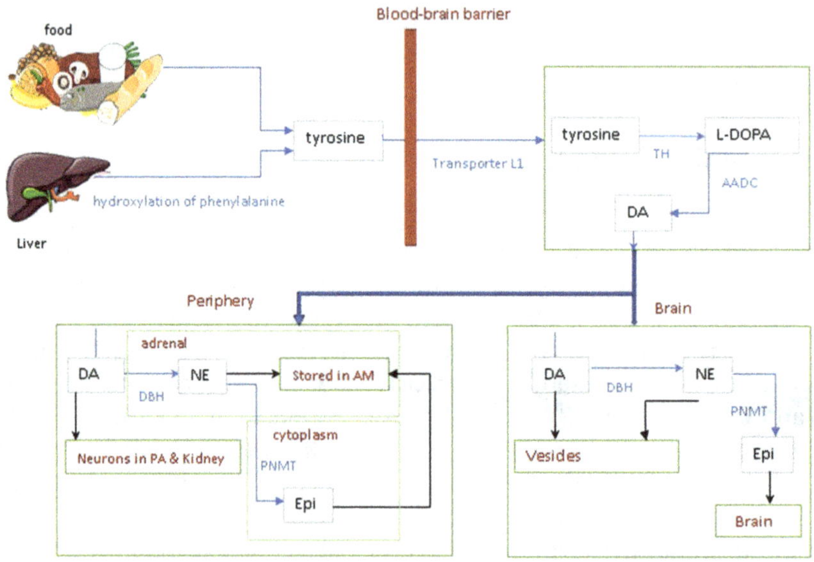

Figure 5.3. Catecholamine synthesis and release. TH = tyrosine hydroxylase; L-DOPA = L-3,4-dihydroxy-phenylalanine; AADC = aromatic amino acid decarboxylase; DA = dopamine; DBH = dopamine-β-hydroxylase; NE = norepinephrine; PNMT = phenylethanolamine-N-methyltransferase; Epi = epinephrine; AM = adrenal medulla.

Additionally, several authors have demonstrated a connection between NE secretion inside the brain and increased plasma ACTH levels and corticosterone levels in animals. Furthermore, even though the participants were all merely sitting down on a cycle ergometer, some experiments found that pre-exercise catecholamine plasma levels rose linearly from before cognitive testing immediately before exercise to before cognitive testing throughout exercise at 80 percentile MAP. Elevated catecholamine creation and secretion within the brain are probably due to enhanced limbic system activity caused by exercise-induced stress. This is aligned with one of the reference studies that stress is created when a person recognizes the circumstance to be unanticipated and/or over which he or she seems to have no command. Catecholamines have been discovered to be released in the plasma of people and the brain of animals when they are exposed to this sort of mental stress. Thus, elevation in catecholamine levels due to central production in response to stress may lead to improved mental function.

To conclude, the outcomes of this study did not entirely agree with the idea that a physiological/biochemical trigger point causes increased cognitive speed. However, moderate-intensity exercise appears to increase cognition speed, which is probably because of anatomical as well as biochemical alterations in the periphery, as shown in figure 5.3. The inadequacy to correlate the impacts of physical activity on cognitive function, especially central administrative tasks, with the impacts of workouts on focus oriented tasks, which were demonstrated to be influenced differently by exercise at varying strengths, is a key limitation in this study.

5.6.1 Influence of schizophrenia on the brain and peripheral markers

Biological indicators may have characteristics that are unique to a certain disease. These characteristics must meet certain criteria to be called biomarkers. There is currently no biological characteristic in schizophrenia that meets these criteria. The purpose of this study is to provide a critical assessment of existing information on biomarker development in schizophrenia psychosis. Schizophrenia is a disorder characterised by a lack of DA operations in the cortex and overactivity of DA in the subcortex (Callicott *et al* 2003).

The autopsy results showed changes in cortical GABAergic neurons in the brain tissue of individuals with schizophrenia. Neuronal signalling pathways regulate neurons' neural location, creation and development, plasticity, and neuronal integration. Cognitive impairment is believed to be a major characteristic of schizophrenia psychoses, with variable degrees of deficiency in all areas. Here biological (i.e., nonpsychotic twins or other related kins) and clinically dangerous strategies are two study paradigms that have been widely used to evaluate vulnerability to psychopathology (Manoach 2003, Sitskoorn *et al* 2004). By utilising neuropsychological susceptibility markers of transformation in vulnerable patients for psychopathology, it may be possible to pinpoint specific pathogenic mechanisms involved during the early stages of schizophrenia. Micro-array investigations of the expression of genes in tissues from autopsy, particularly the prefrontal cortex, have yielded a plethora of diverse and concordant findings.

The partly independent cell structure is mitochondria with its own genetic material, and a highly preserved oxidative addition of phosphate mechanism is particularly important. The identification of disease-related gene groups will be substantially facilitated by integrating proteomic data (mass spectroscopy and expression scanning) with microarray gene expression. The gene expression, the number of proteins, and the function of these proteins are all tissue and environment-dependent, making it challenging to establish a peripheral biomarker. Proteomics and lipidomics of cerebrospinal fluid (CSF) are critical in the search for possible schizophrenia biomarkers. Metabolic distress, elevated oxidation, and changes in the macromolecular content of the cerebrospinal fluid in schizophrenia patients are biochemical processes that suggest schizophrenia start or development. The proteins and lipids found in CSF are critical to brain health and might serve as biomarkers for schizophrenia. Compositional analyses have discovered a few CSF proteins which alter the of schizophrenia patients. Validation of potential protein biomarkers is still required. The genetic foundation for schizophrenia is still unknown, and specific biomarkers to distinguish people predisposed to the disorder or who are already showing clinical symptoms of the disease are still missing. Immune cytokines, lymphocytes and platelets, endogenous intoxication, and functional genomics are currently available analytical methods. To summarise, schizophrenic psychoses are among the world's most complicated mental illnesses, and it remains to be seen whether valid peripheral biomarkers for them can be found. If schizophrenia is considered a separate entity, the impact size of any biological alteration seen will be quite minimal. This is due to the poorly developed medical science dealing with the classification of diseases and the fact that psychiatric disorders are brain abnormalities, and its pathology might not get expressed in peripheral systems. Such biomarkers would also aid in identifying those at a higher risk of developing this serious mental disease, allowing for earlier diagnosis and management.

5.6.2 TBI-associated dynamicity of biochemical markers

This study deals with assessing chemical indicators about the detriment of brain tissue in patients with severe brain trauma, which usually results from an outside impact on the head or body. Several prevailing neurobehavioral abnormalities are the major outcome of TBI (traumatic brain injury), even if the trauma is relatively small. Also, extended neuropsychological issues have been noted in patients with TBI. Hence, early detection of the potential risk is the key to the patient's recovery and rehabilitation (Ingebrigtsen *et al* 1997). Here discharge of neurobiochemical indicators about cerebral abnormality and their immediate and long term effects is analyzed. To accomplish this task, the blood samples of 69 patients (aged between 16 and 65 years having no past neurological/mental disease or substance abuse) after TBI was taken. To see the short- and long-term implications, the samples were obtained at days one, two and three TBI. And assiduousness of protein Serial NSE and S-100B in blood specimens was estimated. Also, neuroradiological assessment CT, neurological assessment using GCS (Glasgow coma scale) and neuropsychological assessment in which global cognitive and behavioural screening including various assessments of language, memory/learning (NBRS19), mini-mental state examination (MMSE20), frontal lobe score (FLS21), visualperception, executive functions, attention performance, and psychomotor speed were performed. Also, follow up examinations of patients after six months was done. It was observed that patients with neuropsychological disturbance had noticeably high serum concentration and longer period discharge of NSE and S-100B biomarkers (Herrmann *et al* 1999). Also, it was seen that there was a subsequent reduction in serum concentration in the later three days, after the primary increase.

The long-term discharge of biochemical indicators (both neuron and astrocytes) and their elevated levels were related to medium to a higher amount of brain trauma (Ingebrigtsen *et al* 1997). The elevated levels of S-100B concentration in blood in the ancillary unit are also taken as an indicator of blood–brain barrier abnormality and protein S-100B discharge in peripheral blood may point out operational brain abnormalities even in the absence of any pathology in CT scans. Hence protein S-100B can better prognosticate neurobehavioural diseases even after slight TBI than NSE. This elevated deposition of NSE was seen in CSF as well as parametric blood specimen post neuronal distortions. Hence, after a relative investigation of S-100B and NSE bio markers, these have the most pre-estimating capacity for long-term or persisting neuropsychological abnormalities. The results indicate that the serum consolidation about NSE and S-100B contemplates complete seriousness of cerebral impact explained through GCS count and explains the minute abnormalities in neuropsychological aspects. Hence this study is very significant as it deals with the early detection of brain abnormalities with the help of subtle biochemical markers rather than convention radiological techniques such as CT.

Small sample size can be the shortcoming of this study and the patient, including the subclass of relatively cerebral damage, so the generalizability of this study based on recent results is limited. But this study will attribute to the use of different biomarkers in different study designs for early detection of abnormalities rather than relying on conventional techniques. The estimation of neuro-biochemical discharges after brain trauma can hugely help determine the risks of long-term psychological and social impacts in patients having cerebral damage.

5.7 Influence of peripheral sensory stimulus on cognitive brain

In many cases, chronic pain problems, such as low back pain and fibromyalgia, are linked to alterations in the brain's structure and function. Chronic pain has now been linked to decreased grey matter in the brain, and altered cortex functioning in several investigations and the degree of these alterations may be directly related to the longevity and severity of the pain (Seminowicz *et al* 2009). The current study attempted to examine: (1) if parametric nerve damage imposed heavy, prolonged behavioural indications of nerve pain as well as a grey matter reduction inside the prefrontal cortex numerous months after the trauma, as well as modifications in DNA of particular areas methylation inside the brain which can be identified post the primary trauma; and (2) if these modifications are susceptible to the atmospheric alterations. Two groups of male CD1 mice aged eight-to-ten weeks were used. The animals were kept in groups of three to four in the standard habitat, which included a cardboard house and cotton elements. In contrast, the embellished habitat featured three mice per cage, a house cage, a spinning wheel mounted on a plastic house, and pebbles. In the lack of a spinning wheel, pebbles, or other forms of enriching environment, every animal was confined to its isolated cage in the poor environment. All other variables, such as nutrition, bedding, availability to H_2O, and illumination, remained the same. Nerve injury was induced, and behavioural assessment was performed based on mechanical sensitivity, cold sensitivity, motor function, overall activity and anxiety-like behaviour (Seminowicz *et al* 2009). The existence of neuropathic pain was verified three months following damage or sham surgery, and mice were selected arbitrarily to one of four categories: injured with ideal atmosphere, injured with poor atmosphere, pseud with ideal atmosphere, pseud with poor atmosphere. Mice were subsequently re-tested two months later after being subjected to environmental manipulation, and tissue was taken. Their DNA was extracted, and data were evaluated. All information is displayed as an average with a standard error of the average of six standard deviations (SEM). To assess injured and control groups and enriched versus poor groups, a t-test was utilised. ANOVA and Tukey's test was used for several comparisons and interpretations. Whenever the expectation of equality of variances wasn't met, Welch's adjustment was used. Because the data had a Gaussian distribution, the extent of correlated variation within mechanical or cold susceptivity and methylation was determined utilising Pearson's coefficient. Prism was used for statistical analysis (Denk and McMahon 2012).

Chronic, long-term changes in dermal sensitivity to mechanical and chilly stimuli were seen six months following nerve injury. Injured mice had lower mechanical thresholds and higher acetone-evoked behaviours. Animals with nerve injury exhibited significantly poorer motor performance in the rotarod experiment. In the open field experiment six months after injury, varmints with nerve damage displayed anxiety symptoms. Ancillary nerve injury resulted in a decrease in global methylation inside the frontal cortex and amygdala, which was discovered six months later. No significant changes occurred in the thalamus or visual cortex. The second group of mice was removed from usual habitation three months after the peripheral nerve injury and placed in either an upgraded or deficient habitat for two months. A restoration followed it to usual control levels of nerve injury-induced declines in PFC global methylation. The key discovery addressed in this study is the long-term effects of peripheral nerve injury on the mouse methylome. It was also observed that these methylation changes occur distant from the site of the initial damage. The study concluded that inflicting peripheral injury impacted the brain in the form of diminished DNA methylation within the amygdala and prefrontal cortex after the initial lesion. Also mitigating long-term pain in human causes. Furthermore, reducing chronic pain in humans substitutes pain-related alteration in the morphology and operation in PFC (Rodriguez-Raecke *et al* 2009). A few of the study's limitations are that it doesn't establish a causal association between DNA methylation inside the brain and chronic pain or its related diseases, nor does it show a link among these changes in DNA methylation as well as gene statement. Furthermore, the study draws no difference between the effects of nerve injury and chronic pain and its accompanying disorders. Finally, the current study focused on the long-term effects of nerve damage on the brain rather than the development of global methylation changes over time.

5.7.1 Prefrontal cortex and pain processing

The PFC plays the most crucial roles in directorial functions such as analytical functioning, organization and social supervision (Goldman-Rakic *et al* 1996). Also, PFC is essential for pain processing and management. The processing of pain is conditional on the interconnection of PFC to various places in the neocortex area of the brain, such as the thalamus, amygdala, hippocampus, basal ganglia, and periaqueductal grey (PAG) (Apkarian *et al* 2005). If drastic and chronic pain presents, alterations in neurotransmitters, glial cells, gene interpretations and neuro-inflammation are visible. Also, it affects the structure, functioning and links of PFC. The ventrolateral PFC, the medial prefrontal cortex (mPFC), the orbitofrontal cortex, the ventrolateral PFC, the dorsolateral PFC (DLPFC), and the caudal PFC are all parts of the prefrontal cortex.

All the above-mentioned areas play an important part in the processing of pain such as medial PFC (mPFC) conciliates anti-nociceptive (body's reaction to potentially toxic or harmful stimuli, mechanical injury, or adverse temperature) (sensory nervous system) effects. The PFC has an association with other cortical structures due to which it serves as a primary fount of cortical afferents (conveying impulses toward the central nervous system) to the PAG for regulation of pain (Coulombe *et al* 2016). Here one sensorial stimulus after processing is converted to visual input, after which it provides direction to flow the sensory stimulus towards nerve fibre at its entry towards the central nervous system. This also can cause the discomfort to become long term and chronic with the help of its corticostriatal projection. Pain and cognition have a bi-directional relationship as various researches indicate in damage of brain of patients experiencing chronic pain, hence level of cognition can be a predictive measure of reactiveness to the management of pain. The study also provides insight into the interplay between various chemical messengers of the PFC, which seem crucial for the process of antinociception (body's response to potentially toxic stimuli, like harmful chemicals). It was also evident that the connection between chronic discomfort and reduction in neuronal processes can further lead to the inflammation of the nervous tissue. Also, a reduction in medial PFC activities may result in less articulation of discomfort. Also, some studies indicate an alteration in Global Gene Expression due to reduction in the grey matter of the PFC as an outcome of long-term discomfort. Also, abnormal blood oxygenation levels in the mPFC may result from long-term lower back problems and disturb functional congruence towards brain signaling discomfort.

The PFC plays a very important part in managing bio-psychosocial discomfort with the help of utilizing various corrective measures. Also, the PFC plays an important role during placebo analgesia as various scans indicate the association of placebo analgesia with reduced neuronal function into discomfort-reactive cerebral areas (thalamus and insula) and enhancing activity in the PFC. Cognition has a relation with discomfort as well as general anxiety and depression. This study also brings attention towards this. It is evident from the above research that with the help of various measures such as meditation, music, empathy, CBT, TDS, TMS, etc, the pain inflicted damage and loss of grey matter of the PFC is reversible. With the help of multi-disciplinary, bio-psychosocial approaches, reduction in cognitive disability and physical discomfort is possible. Also, crucial executive activities like addressing certain issues, making a proper plan, and smooth social interaction will be possible.

5.7.2 Periodontal tactile input and prefrontal cortex

The cerebral structure location of the PFC is in front of the frontal lobe. It is responsible for various important activities such as cognitive control, influencing attention, executive functions such as planning working memory, prospective memory, flexibility and processing speed (Miller *et al* 2001, Corbetta and Shulman 2002, Pinti *et al* 2015). In this paper, the actuation of PFC while performing some motor activity and impact of peripheral sensory information is studied with the help of functional near-infrared spectroscopy (fNIRS) system (Hoshi *et al* 2003, Veltman *et al* 2003). As fNRIS uses near-infrared light to assess cortical hemodynamic activity for measuring brain activity, CBF was measured. The amount of CBF was elevated around the middle PFC as this area plays an important part in attention and working memory. Also, during the motor task, such as while flexing the toe, shoulder and chewing (Lee *et al* 2013, Yeo *et al* 2013), there were elevated levels of CBF in the PFC (Narita and Otsuka). It can be said that various movement works may have varying levels of influence on CBF in the PFC. Hence tasks involving motion, including removal of sensorial data in peripheral organs, can measure the essential impact of peripheral sensory information on the PFC. To understand this further, an experiment including five young, healthy Japanese subjects having normal dentition was performed, where a 1-hour investigation on PFC activation was estimated in unrestrained conditions with each patient wearing an fNIRS device (WOT-100, HITACHI, Tokyo, Japan). During the experiment, it was defined to facilitate the occlusal force (the force at which the lower jaw mandible and upper jaw maxilla come together) in a controlled environment (soundproof room). The participants were situated on the seat in a complaisant way and told to bite the instrument, which measured the occlusal force (occlusal force transducer) for 30 seconds with a pressure of 27.5 ± 2.5 N. Also for measuring the impact of periodontal tactile sensation upon PFC activity, anaesthesia was given to molar regions of the subjects. And before and after local anaesthesia, the measurements were taken. Also, to guide occlusal force modifications, issues have been provided with instructions involving audio and video information. After synchronizing the results obtained from the transducer and fNIRS, the estimation and comparison of occlusal force and CBF was done having all the four constraints, including pre- and post-anaesthesia. The modification in occlusal force devoid of details and visual and auditory instruction was performed with the help of statistical analysis tools (ANOVA and Bonferroni post hoc tests). The increase in CBF was evident from the various results during the biting. After the post, local sedation values of CBF were lowered with maintaining occlusal force. Hence, the implications of influences on sensory indications of peripheral organs (periodontal ligament) have a minute effect on occlusal force retention still very crucial for stimulation of the PFC. Hence, this study is advancing over several previous works that only compared PFC stimulation in terms of two different movement tasks (such as finger flexing) rather than having any other sensory input during the motor task. Herewith, the use of local sedation the influence of decision making upon the PFC while performing a motion task was eliminated to witness the primary impact of periodontal tactile input; hence this research can be seen as a valuable addition to an understanding of activation in the PFC in terms of external feedback information with proper clarity.

5.8 Influence of peripheral pressure on the interpretation of positive emotions

Emotions tend to affect our cardiovascular activity, such as the blood pressure elevates and heart rate goes up if we are feeling stressed (Diener and Larsen 1993). Negative emotions and feelings of helplessness and hopelessness can lead to chronic stress, which causes hormone imbalance in the body. The body is unprotected from increased cortisol (a stress hormone the adrenal glands release) in the long term, which in turn depletes the brain chemicals required for happiness and negatively impacts the immune system. Chronic stress can decrease our lifespan. The blood clotting patterns can be altered due to its effect. These can become factors causing cardiovascular or brain disease (Williams *et al* 1985, Blascovich and Katkin 1993). It can cause fear and anxiety to induce certain actions such as fight or flight, and these actions require physical energy, which causes high cardiovascular activity that distributes blood to relating peripheral muscles.

Such cardiovascular activity, if often happening for a long period, can put a person at risk for developing coronary heart abnormalities. In this study, it is suggested that positive emotions can help in regulating negative emotions. For example, positive emotions such as contentment and joy affect the brain's dopamine level (Isen 1990). Also, positive sentiments can aid in correcting or regulating the post effect of an adverse feeling or emotion. Further, this study improves on Fredrickson and Levenson (1998), who have primarily examined this hypothesis.

Unlike the initial study, instead of showing a video clip generating fear, participants were asked to prepare a speech to be delivered under constriction of time and this was done to induce stress or anxiety, which is a primary adverse sentiment. In addition, cardiovascular measures such as systolic and diastolic blood pressure have been taken into account. Following this, four video film clips were shown to the participants, which elicited four different emotions, such as 'waves' (showing ocean waves) and 'puppy' (a small playing dog) for positive feelings of contentment and amusement, respectively, and two videos of 'sticks' (coloured sticks piling) and 'cry' (a boy crying) for emotions of neutrality and sadness, respectively. In addition, participants' experiences and their physical markers such as heart rate, pulse amplitudes and transference time in seconds (in peripheral organ such as finger and ear), and diastolic and systolic blood pressure were taken.

The results represent that positive emotions (contentment and amusement) can recover from negative emotions (anxiety, sadness). An additional alternative or substitute description shows the positive sentiments can change the cardiovascular indications generated due to negative sentiments with their peculiar indication or mark. Overall, the study shows the significance of recovery due to positive emotions on the cardiovascular system in the case of cardiovascular reactivity generated due to negative emotions. Hence it is clear that positive emotions help to down-regulate the critical health-damaging cardiovascular reactivity. This effect has proven critically important for those at the most risk of developing coronary heart disease, such as men from African American ethnicity, so these groups have been considered for study due to having a high risk of developing such problems. Hence considering the overall health, the undoing effect of negative emotion is one of the many reasons for pursuing positive emotions.

5.8.1 Blood pressure and emotion crosstalk

In this study effect of blood pressure on an emotional response or emotional recognition has been discussed with the help of hemodynamic measures. It has been seen that an increase in blood pressure reduces or mitigates the emotional reactivity to the effect of any stimulus (Bruehl *et al* 1992, Ghione *et al* 1996, France *et al* 1999, Waldstein *et al* 2005, Jennings and Zanstra 2009).

Total peripheral resistance, resting blood pressure and other cardiovascular measures have been taken in this study. In addition, to study the emotional reaction in the perception affect test (PAT) is done. Here participants from African American ethnicity have been taken. It seems appropriate as they are considered to be at high risk with cardiovascular and hypertensive issues. One hundred and six participants, 55 females and 51 males belonging to the lower socioeconomic background and the population with a pilot study named HANDLES-Pilot (Healthy Aging in Nationally Diverse Longitudinal Samples) were taken. During the experiment, the participants were given tasks with sentences and faces such that they were asked to read 35 sentences and match or engage them with considered underlined object's response with seven responses: happy, anger, surprise, sad, disgust, neutral emotion and fear, for each feeling, five sets of sentences were used. Similarly, during the face task, 35 pictures with faces were shown to the participants with different expositions and participants needed to tell the sentiments indicated (seven emotions mentioned already) by any particular picture, five sets of each emotion were taken. Participants' age, gender and other important factors were recorded before the experiment. To collect the cardiovascular measures a blood pressure measuring instrument was used, and all cardiovascular specifications were estimated throughout every parameter, attained in a relaxed manner. The results showed that increased blood pressure and peripheral resistance have a relationship with decreased perception of stimulus-driven effect. Hence it is evident that an increase in blood pressure may cause neuropsychological issues in persons with established hypertension. Also, recent studies point out that small changes in central nervous system function can come with even a slight increase in blood pressure (2–5).

With the PAT score's help, it can be inferred that blood pressure and TPR (total peripheral resistance) were inversely related to accurate emotional response. This inability to properly acknowledge sentimental indications is persistent along with the interaction of blood pressure and reaction to the sensation of discomfort image along with individually assessed strain; it can cause psychosocial afflictions due to improper emotional synergy with people, such as peers, family, colleagues and seniors and in the long run, can be a cause of chronic stress and also may hamper the quality of all social interaction. Hence this study provides for further development as it is the first to examine evidence of TPR. Also, the obtained PAT results show a typically analogous relationship with TPR. Hence this study elaborates the crucial association of reduced response to both positive and negative life events and blood pressure regulation. This study can help represent the part of the central nervous scheme within autonomous and intravenous operations while in the primary level of development of blood pressure irregularities. Thus, this study provides a strong base for future research in this area.

5.8.2 Positive emotions and symptomatic peripheral artery disease

Peripheral artery disease (PAD) is a common cardiovascular condition in which constricted arteries decrease blood flow to the limbs. Affecting more than 20 crore individuals globally, it severely affects the quality of life and increases the risk of hypertension, and in worst cases, can cause death (Fowkes *et al* 2010). The primary solution to this condition is to improve walking exercises, but it can be quite difficult for patients with PAD to execute them as effectively as they were meant to. Moreover, claudication symptoms can hinder the patient's ability to exercise properly, leading to a poor commitment to an exercise program (Barbosa *et al* 2015). For such reasons, non-painful exercises such as arm cranking, which have been shown to enhance the ambulatory capability and improve the general well-being of the people, have been introduced. The hypothesis of this paper was based on the soothing sensations of happiness during physical activity and severely reduced blood pressure in individuals with symptoms of PAD, which are promoted by arm cranking exercises. Eleven males who met the following criteria were recruited for the experiment: (i) 50–80 years old; (ii) claudication problems restricting the ability to walk in an evaluated treadmill test; (iii) an ankle-brachial index of 0.90 in either one or both legs; (iv) no surgical operations in the previous year; (v) no documented upper limb mobility restriction. All the necessary data were collected from the patients with their permission.

The experimental procedure was such that the patient had to go through two rounds (arm cranking workout and control) in a randomized manner, and the sessions were separated by 48 h. Certain instructions were given to them to follow before the session took place. The pre-intervention required the patients to rest for 10 min in the supine position, and then their blood pressure and pulse rate were recorded in a set of three (Cucato *et al* 2015). The patients performed 15 × 2 min arm cranking sessions, interspaced by 2 min of resting interval time. The exercise intensity was between 80% and 90% of the maximum HR achieved by the leading graded treadmill examination. After the 1st, 5th, 10th, and 15th rounds, assessments of perceived effort (Borg scale) and emotional reactions (positive/negative) were collected.

The individuals sat in the same posture with the arm ergometer but did not perform any workout in the control session. After both procedures, the patients were asked to lie down for an hour in the supine position, and their blood pressure and heart rate were monitored. The Shapiro–Wilk test verified the data's normal distribution, then examined using a two-way ANOVA. The condition-by-time interplay established the net impact of arm crank on BP and HR readings throughout all durations, which was reported as before and after exercise and control. Cardiovascular activity and psychological and biological reactions throughout exercise sessions, the one-way ANOVA and Fisher's post hoc test, were used. Seven patients began the trial with the control session and four with the workout session, and the research revealed that throughout the workout session, the heart rate stayed within the recommended limits, and the subjects felt a medium level of effort, which rose with subsequent sessions. The emotional response of the patients was also found to be positive during all arm crank sessions. Compared to the control session, there was a massive reduction in blood pressure measures; also, an elevation in heart rate was noticed during the post-experimental procedures. The result was such that the arm cranking exercises were considered to be feasible and well-tolerated. Control sessions resulted in a rise in systolic as well as diastolic blood pressure. Some limitations of this experiment included that all the subjects were male and symptomatic; therefore, it should be generalized cautiously. The participants were also consuming various drugs that did not permit interaction amongst workouts and particular categories of drugs. Blood pressure changes were only studied for one hour after arm cranking activity, and additional study is needed to discover if these benefits persist when the individual can walk. Because the 'feeling scale' wasn't used during the cardiopulmonary exercise test, there have been no sentiment assessments among treadmill and arm ergometer workouts. Finally, in people with PAD symptoms, a single session of arm cranking workout led to a reasonable level of perceived exertion without leg pain and positive emotional responses accompanied by a post-exercise reduction in blood pressure for one hour.

References

Abraira V E and Ginty D D 2013 The sensory neurons of touch *Neuron* **79** 618–39

Annweiler C, Beauchet O, Bartha R, Wells J L, Borrie M J, Hachinski V and Montero-Odasso M 2013 Motor cortex and gait in mild cognitive impairment: a magnetic resonance spectroscopy and volumetric imaging study *Brain* **136** 859–71

Apkarian A V, Bushnell M C, Treede R D and Zubieta J K 2005 Human brain mechanisms of pain perception and regulation in health and disease *Eur. J. Pain* **9** 463–84

Attwell D and Laughlin S B 2001 An energy budget for signaling in the grey matter of the brain *J. Cereb. Blood Flow Metab.* **21** 1133–145

Attwell D, Buchan A M, Charpak S, Lauritzen M, MacVicar B A and Newman E A 2010 Glial and neuronal control of brain blood flow *Nature* **468** 232–43

Barbosa J P, Farah B Q, Chehuen M, Cucato G G, Farias Junior J C and Wolosker N *et al* 2015 Barriers to physical activity in patients with intermittent claudication *Int. J. Behav. Med.* **22** 70e6

Basbaum A I, Bautista D M, Scherrer G and Julius D 2009 Cellular and molecular mechanisms of pain *Cell* **139** 267–84

Benson D F, Davis R J and Snyder B D 1988 Posterior cortical atrophy *Arch. Neurol.* **45** 789–93

Blascovich J J and Katkin E S 1993 *Cardiovascular Reactivity to Psychological Stress and Sisease* (Washington DC: American Psychological Association) pp xv–242

Bora E *et al* 2016 Executive dysfunction and cognitive subgroups in a large sample of euthymic patients with bipolar disorder *Eur. Neuropsychopharmacol.* **26** 1338–47

Brandenberger G, Follenius M, Wittersheim G, Salame P, Siméoni M and Reinhardt B 1980 Plasma catecholamines and pituitary adrenal hormones related to mental task demand under quiet and noise conditions *Biol. Psychol.* **10** 239–52

Bruehl S, Carlson C R and McCubbin J A 1992 The relationship between pain sensitivity and blood pressure in normotensives *Pain* **48** 463–7

Brushart T M E 1991 The mechanical and humoral control of specificity in nerve repair *Operative Nerve Repair and Reconstruction* (Philadelphia, PA: JP Lippincott) pp 215–30

Busija D W, Bari F, Domoki F and Louis T 2007 Mechanisms involved in the cerebrovascular dilator effects of N-methyl-d-aspartate in cerebral cortex *Brain Res. Rev.* **56** 89–100

Callicott J H, Mattay V S, Verchinski B A, Marenco S, Egan M F and Weinberger D R 2003 Complexity of prefrontal cortical dysfunction in schizophrenia: more than up or down *Am. J. Psych.* **160** 2209–15

Cappa A, Ciccarelli N, Baldonero E, Martelli M and Silveri M C 2014 Posterior ad-type pathology: cognitive subtypes emerging from a cluster analysis *Behav. Neurol.* **2014** 259358

Cardno A G *et al* 1999 Heritability estimates for psychotic disorders: the Maudsley twin psychosis series *Arch. Gen. Psychiatry* **56** 162–8

Cauli B, Audinat E, Lambolez B, Angulo M C, Ropert N, Tsuzuki K, Hestrin S and Rossier J 1997 Molecular and physiological diversity of cortical nonpyramidal cells *J. Neurosci.* **17** 3894–906

Cavalcante B R, Ritti-Dias R M, Soares A H G, Lima A H, Correia M A, De Matos L D, Gobbi F, Leicht A S, Wolosker N and Cucato G G 2017 A single bout of arm-crank exercise promotes positive emotions and post-exercise hypotension in patients with symptomatic peripheral artery disease *Eur. J. Vasc. Endovasc. Surg.* **53** 223–8

Cerdán S, Rodrigues T B, Sierra A, Benito M, Fonseca L L, Fonseca C P and García-Martín M L 2006 The redox switch/redox coupling hypothesis *Neurochem. Int.* **48** 523–30

Chesney M A and Rosenman R H 1985 *Anger and Hostility in Cardiovascular and Behavioral Disorders* (London: Hemisphere Publishing Corporation)

Collins K J, Exton-Smith A N, James M H and Oliver D J 1980 Functional changes in autonomic nervous responses with ageing *Age Ageing* **9** 17–24

Corbetta M and Shulman G L 2002 Control of goal-directed and stimulus-driven attention in the brain *Nat. Rev. Neurosci.* **3** 201–15

Coulombe M A, Erpelding N, Kucyi A and Davis K D 2016 Intrinsic functional connectivity of periaqueductal gray subregions in humans *Human Brain Mapping* **37** 1514–30

Cucato G G *et al* 2015 Post-walking exercise hypotension in patients with intermittent claudication *Med. Sci. Sports Exerc.* **47** 460e7

Cumming W 1998 Aging in muscle *Injury in the Aging* (Cambridge: Cambridge University Press) p 189

Delfini M C *et al* 2013 TAFA4, a chemokine-like protein, modulates injury-induced mechanical and chemical pain hypersensitivity in mice *Cell Reports* **5** 378–88

Denk F and McMahon S B 2012 Chronic pain: emerging evidence for the involvement of epigenetics *Neuron* **73** 435–44

Diener E and Larsen R J 1993 The experience of emotional well-being *Handbook of Emotions* (New York: Guildford Press) pp 405–15

Drachman D A, Long R R and Swearer J M 1994 Neurological evaluation in the elderly patient *Handb. Clin. Neurol.* **167** 73–88

Eichert N, Robinson E C, Bryant K L, Jbabdi S, Jenkinson M, Li L, Krug K, Watkins K E and Mars R B 2020 Cross-species cortical alignment identifies different types of anatomical reorganization in the primate temporal lobe *Elife* **9** e53232

Eichert N, Watkins K E, Mars R B and Petrides M 2021 Morphological and functional variability in central and subcentral motor cortex of the human brain *Brain Struct. Funct.* **226** 263–79

Einsiedel L J and Luff A R 1992 Alterations in the contractile properties of motor units within the ageing rat medial gastrocnemius *J. Neurol. Sci.* **112** 170–7

Feigin V L *et al* 2014 Global and regional burden of stroke during 1990–2010: findings from the Global Burden of Disease Study 2010 *Lancet* **383** 245–55

Fiorentini A and Berardi N 1981 Learning in grating waveform discrimination: specificity for orientation and spatial frequency *Vis. Res.* **21** 1149–58

Fischl B and Dale A M 2000 Measuring the thickness of the human cerebral cortex from magnetic resonance images *Proc. Natl Acad. Sci.* **97** 11050–5

Fischl B, Liu A and Dale A M 2001 Automated manifold surgery: constructing geometrically accurate and topologically correct models of the human cerebral cortex *IEEE Trans. Med. Imaging* **20** 70–80

Fischl B *et al* 2002 Whole brain segmentation: automated labeling of neuroanatomical structures in the human brain *Neuron* **33** 341–55

Fowkes F G R *et al* 2013 Comparison of global estimates of prevalence and risk factors for peripheral artery disease in 2000 and 2010: a systematic review and analysis *Lancet* **382** 1329–40

France C R 1999 Decreased pain perception and risk for hypertension: considering a common physiological mechanism *Psychophysiol* **36** 683–92

Franzini C 1992 Brain metabolism and blood flow during sleep *J. Sleep Res.* **1** 3–16

Fredrickson B L, Mancuso R A, Branigan C and Tugade M M 2000 The undoing effect of positive emotions *Motiv. Emot.* **24** 237–58

Fredrickson B L and Levenson R W 1998 Positive emotions speed recovery from the cardiovascular sequelae of negative emotions *Cognition Emotion* **12** 191–220

Ghione S 1996 Hypertension-associated hypalgesia: evidence in experimental animals and humans, pathophysiological mechanisms, and potential clinical consequences *Hypertension* **28** 494–504

Goldman-Rakic P S 1996 The prefrontal landscape: implications of functional architecture for understanding human mentation and the central executive *Phil. Trans. R. Soc. London* B **351** 1445–53

Green M J, Girshkin L, Kremerskothen K, Watkeys O and Quidé Y 2020 A systematic review of studies reporting data-driven cognitive subtypes across the psychosis spectrum *Neuropsychol. Rev.* **30** 446–60

Greig C A, Botella J and Young A 1993 The quadriceps strength of healthy elderly people remeasured after eight years *Muscle Nerve* **16** 6–10

Grinsell D and Keating C P 2014 Peripheral nerve reconstruction after injury: a review of clinical and experimental therapies *BioMed Res. Int.* 2014

Gusnard D A and Raichle M E 2001 Searching for a baseline: functional imaging and the resting human brain *Nat. Rev. Neurosci.* **2** 685–94

Hallet M, Pascual-Leone A and Topeka H 1996 *Acquisition of Motor Behavior in Vertebrates* eds J Bloedel, T Ebner and S P Wise (Cambridge, MA: MIT Press) pp 289–301

Herrmann M, Curio N, Jost S, Grubich C, Ebert A D, Fork M L and Synowitz H 2001 Release of biochemical markers of damage to neuronal and glial brain tissue is associated with short and long term neuropsychological outcome after traumatic brain injury *J. Neurol. Neurosurg. Psychiatry* **70** 95–100

Herrmann M, Curio N, Jost S, Wunderlich M T, Synowitz H and Wallesch C W 1999 Protein S-100B and neuron specific enolase as early neurobiochemical markers of the severity of traumatic brain injury *Restor. Neurol. Neurosci.* **14** 109–14

Higaki N, Goto T and Ichikawa T 2016 Periodontal tactile input activates the prefrontal cortex *Sci. Rep.* **6** 1–8

Hoshi Y, Tsou B H, Billock V A, Tanosaki M, Iguchi Y, Shimada M, Shinba T, Yamada Y and Oda I 2003 Spatiotemporal characteristics of hemodynamic changes in the human lateral prefrontal cortex during working memory tasks *Neuroimage* **20** 1493–504

Hughlings J J and Taylor J 1958 On the anatomical and physiological localisation of movements in the brain *Selected Writings of John Hughlings Jackson* vol 52 (New York: Staples)

Ingebrigtsen T, Romner B and Trumpy J H 1997 Management of minor head injury: the value of early computed tomography and serum protein S-100 measurements *J. Clin. Neurosci.* **4** 29–33

Ingebrigtsen T, Romner B, Marup-Jensen S, Dons M, Lundqvist C, Bellner J, Alling C and Børgesen S E 2000 The clinical value of serum S-100 protein measurements in minor head injury: a Scandinavian multicentre study *Brain Injury* **14** 1047–55

Ingebrigtsen T, Waterloo K, Jacobsen E A, Langbakk B and Romner B 1999 Traumatic brain damage in minor head injury: relation of serum S-100 protein measurements to magnetic resonance imaging and neurobehavioral outcome *Neurosurgery* **45** 468–76

Isen A M 1990 The influence of positive and negative affect on cognitive organization: Some implications for development *Psychological and Biological Approaches to Emotion* (Hillsdale, NJ: Lawrence Erlbaum) pp 75–94

Iwamura Y, Tanaka M, Sakamoto M and Hikosaka O 1983 Functional subdivisions representing different finger regions in area 3 of the first somatosensory cortex of the conscious monkey *Exp. Brain Res.* **51** 315–26

Jennings J R and Zanstra Y 2009 Is the brain the essential in hypertension? *Neuroimage* **47** 914–21

Karni A and Sagi D 1993 The time course of learning a visual skill *Nature* **365** 250–2

Karni A, Meyer G, Rey-Hipolito C, Jezzard P, Adams M M, Turner R and Ungerleider L G 1998 The acquisition of skilled motor performance: fast and slow experience-driven changes in primary motor cortex *Proc. Natl Acad. Sci.* **95** 861–8

Katzman R and Terry R 1983 Normal aging of the nervous system *Neurol. Aging* **36** 38

Kaufman A S 1993 King WISC the third assumes the throne *J. Sch. Psychol.* **31** 345–54

Kennedy W R, Navarro X, Sakuta M, Mandell H, Knox C K and Sutherland D E 1989 Physiological and clinical correlates of cardiorespiratory reflexes in diabetes mellitus *Diabetes Care* **12** 399–408

Kouyoumdjian J A 2006 Peripheral nerve injuries: a retrospective survey of 456 cases *Muscle Nerve* **34** 785–8

Kubota Y, Hattori R and Yui Y 1994 Three distinct subpopulations of GABAergic neurons in rat frontal agranular cortex *Brain Res.* **649** 159–73

Lee M Y, Chang P H, Kwon Y H and Jang S H 2013 Differences of the frontal activation patterns by finger and toe movements: a functional MRI study *Neurosci. Lett.* **533** 7–10

Lewin G R, Smith E S J, Reznick J, Debus K, Barker A J and Park T J 2021 The somatosensory world of the African naked mole-rat *The Extraordinary Biology of the Naked Mole-Rat* (Cham: Springer) pp 197–220

Li L, Rutlin M, Abraira V E, Cassidy C, Kus L, Gong S, Jankowski M P, Luo W, Heintz N and Koerber H R *et al* 2011 The functional organization of cutaneous low-threshold mechanosensory neurons *Cell* **147** 1615–27

Li K, Zhang Y, Ning Y, Zhang H, Liu H, Fu C, Ren Y and Zou Y 2015 The effects of acupuncture treatment on the right frontoparietal network in migraine without aura patients *J. Headache Pain* **16** 1–10

Lin A L, Fox P T, Hardies J, Duong T Q and Gao J H 2010 Nonlinear coupling between cerebral blood flow, oxygen consumption, and ATP production in human visual cortex *Proc. Natl Acad. Sci.* **107** 8446–51

Low P A 1997 The effect of aging on the autonomic nervous system *Clinical Autonomic Disorders: Evaluation and Management* (Philadelphia, PA: Lippincott-Raven) pp 161–75

Lundborg G 2000 A 25-year perspective of peripheral nerve surgery: evolving neuroscientific concepts and clinical significance *J. Hand Surg.* **25** 391–414

Ma J I A N Y A, Ayata C E N K, Huang P L, Fishman M C and Moskowitz M A 1996 Regional cerebral blood flow response to vibrissal stimulation in mice lacking type I NOS gene expression *Am. J. Physiol. Heart Circ. Physiol.* **270** H1085–90

Magistretti P J 2006 Neuron–glia metabolic coupling and plasticity *J. Exp. Biol.* **209** 2304–11

Manoach D S 2003 Prefrontal cortex dysfunction during working memory performance in schizophrenia: reconciling discrepant findings *Schizophr. Res.* **60** 285–98

Margolis A, Bansal R, Hao X, Algermissen M, Erickson C, Klahr K W, Naglieri J A and Peterson B S 2013 Using IQ discrepancy scores to examine the neural correlates of specific cognitive abilities *J. Neurosci.* **33** 14135–45

McCormick D A, Connors B W, Lighthall J W and Prince D A 1985 Comparative electrophysiology of pyramidal and sparsely spiny stellate neurons of the neocortex *J. Neurophysiol.* **54** 782–806

McCubbin J A, Merritt M M, Sollers J J III, Evans M K, Zonderman A B, Lane R D and Thayer J F 2011 Cardiovascular emotional dampening: the relationship between blood pressure and recognition of emotion *Psychosom. Med.* **73** 743

McMonagle P, Deering F, Berliner Y and Kertesz A 2006 The cognitive profile of posterior cortical atrophy *Neurology* **66** 331–8

McMorris T and Hale B J 2015 Is there an acute exercise-induced physiological/biochemical threshold which triggers increased speed of cognitive functioning? A meta-analytic investigation *J. Sport Health Sci.* **4** 4–13

McMorris T, Sproule J, Turner A and Hale B J 2011 Acute, intermediate intensity exercise, and speed and accuracy in working memory tasks: a meta-analytical comparison of effects *Physiol. Behav.* **102** 421–8

Mendez M F, Ghajarania M and Perryman K M 2002 Posterior cortical atrophy: clinical characteristics and differences compared to Alzheimer's disease *Dement. Geriatr. Cogn. Disord.* **14** 33–40

Miller E K and Cohen J D 2001 An integrative theory of prefrontal cortex function *Annu. Rev. Neurosci.* **24** 167–202

Nasreddine Z S, Phillips N A, Bédirian V, Charbonneau S, Whitehead V, Collin I, Cummings J L and Chertkow H 2005 The Montreal cognitive assessment, MoCA: a brief screening tool for mild cognitive impairment *J. Am. Geriatr. Soc.* **53** 695–9

Ong W Y, Stohler C S and Herr D R 2019 Role of the prefrontal cortex in pain processing *Mol. Neurobiol.* **56** 1137–66

Öngür D and Price J L 2000 The organization of networks within the orbital and medial prefrontal cortex of rats, monkeys and humans *Cereb. Cortex* **10** 206–19

Penfield W and Rasmussen T 1950 The cerebral cortex of man: a clinical study of localization of function *JAMA* **144** 1412

Peters A and Harriman K M 1988 Enigmatic bipolar cell of rat visual cortex *J. Comp. Neurol.* **267** 409–32

Petrides M 2012 *The Human Cerebral Cortex: An MRI Atlas of the Sulci and Gyri in MNI Stereotaxic Space* (New York: Elsevier)

Petrides M 2018 *Atlas of the Morphology of the Human Cerebral Cortex on the Average MNI Brain* (New York: Academic) *)*

Pinti P, Cardone D and Merla A 2015 Simultaneous fNIRS and thermal infrared imaging during cognitive task reveal autonomic correlates of prefrontal cortex activity *Sci. Rep.* **5** 1–14

Pons T P, Wall J T, Garraghty P E, Cusick C G and Kaas J H 1987 Consistent features of the representation of the hand in area 3b of macaque monkeys *Somatosens. Res.* **4** 309–31

Potvin A R, Syndulko K, Tourtellotte W W, Lemmon J A and Potvin J H 1980 Human neurologic function and the aging process *J. Am. Geriatr. Soc.* **28** 1–9

Raichle M E, MacLeod A M, Snyder A Z, Powers W J, Gusnard D A and Shulman G L 2001 A default mode of brain function *Proc. Natl Acad. Sci.* **98** 676–82

Rodriguez-Raecke R, Niemeier A, Ihle K, Ruether W and May A 2009 Brain gray matter decrease in chronic pain is the consequence and not the cause of pain *J. Neurosci.* **29** 13746–50

Roumazeilles L *et al* 2020 Longitudinal connections and the organization of the temporal cortex in macaques, great apes, and humans *PLoS Biol.* **18** e3000810

Salem D B, Walker P M, Aho S, Tavernier B, Giroud M, Tzourio C, Ricolfi F and Brunotte F 2008 Brain flexibility and balance and gait performances mark morphological and metabolic abnormalities in the elderly *J. Clin. Neurosci.* **15** 1360–5

Sanes J N and Donoghue J P 2000 Plasticity and primary motor cortex *Annu. Rev. Neurosci.* **23** 393–415

Schieber M H 2001 Constraints on somatotopic organization in the primary motor cortex *J. Neurophysiol.* **86** 2125–43

Seal R P, Wang X, Guan Y, Raja S N, Woodbury C J, Basbaum A I and Edwards R H 2009 Injury-induced mechanical hypersensitivity requires C-low threshold mechanoreceptors *Nature* **462** 651–5

Seminowicz D A, Laferriere A L, Millecamps M, Jon S C, Coderre T J and Bushnell M C 2009 MRI structural brain changes associated with sensory and emotional function in a rat model of long-term neuropathic pain *Neuroimage* **47** 1007–14

Siemionow M and Brzezicki G 2009 Current techniques and concepts in peripheral nerve repair *Int. Rev. Neurobiol.* **87** 141–72

Sitskoorn M M, Aleman A, Ebisch S J, Appels M C and Kahn R S 2004 Cognitive deficits in relatives of patients with schizophrenia: a meta-analysis *Schizophr. Res.* **71** 285–95

Smith E S J and Lewin G R 2009 Nociceptors: a phylogenetic view *J. Compar. Physiol.* A **195** 1089–106

Stöber G *et al* 2009 Schizophrenia: from the brain to peripheral markers. A consensus paper of the WFSBP task force on biological markers *World J. Biol. Psychiatry* **10** 127–55

Stuerenburg H J and Kunze K 1999 Concentrations of free carnosine (a putative membrane-protective antioxidant) in human muscle biopsies and rat muscles *Arch. Gerontol. Geriatr.* **29** 107–13

Suzuki A, Stern S A, Bozdagi O, Huntley G W, Walker R H, Magistretti P J and Alberini C M 2011 Astrocyte-neuron lactate transport is required for long-term memory formation *Cell* **144** 810–23

Tajerian M, Alvarado S, Millecamps M, Vachon P, Crosby C, Bushnell M C, Szyf M and Stone L S 2013 Peripheral nerve injury is associated with chronic, reversible changes in global DNA methylation in the mouse prefrontal cortex *PLoS One* **8** e55259

Taki Y, Hashizume H, Sassa Y, Takeuchi H, Wu K, Asano M, Asano K, Fukuda H and Kawashima R 2011 Correlation between gray matter density-adjusted brain perfusion and age using brain MR images of 202 healthy children *Human Brain Mapp.* **32** 1973–85

Todd A J 2010 Neuronal circuitry for pain processing in the dorsal horn *Nat. Rev. Neurosci.* **11** 823–36

Veltman D J, Rombouts S A and Dolan R J 2003 Maintenance versus manipulation in verbal working memory revisited: an fMRI study *Neuroimage* **18** 247–56

Verdú E, Ceballos D, Vilches J J and Navarro X 2000 Influence of aging on peripheral nerve function and regeneration *J. Peripher. Nerv. Syst.* **5** 191–208

Von Elm E, Altman D G, Egger M, Pocock S J, Gøtzsche P C and Vandenbroucke J P 2007 The Strengthening the Reporting of Observational Studies in Epidemiology (STROBE) statement: guidelines for reporting observational studies *Bull. World Health Org.* **85** 867–72

Waldstein S R, Brown J R, Maier K J and Katzel L I 2005 Diagnosis of hypertension and high blood pressure levels negatively affect cognitive function in older adults *Ann. Behav. Med.* **29** 174–80

Williams R B, Barefoot J C and Shekelle R B 1985 The health consequences of hostility *Anger and Hostility in Cardiovascular and Behavioral Disorders* eds M A Chesney and R H Rosenman (Washington, DC: Hemisphere) pp 173–85

Yamamoto Y, Miyashita M, Hughson R L, Tamura S I, Shinohara M and Mutoh Y 1991 The ventilatory threshold gives maximal lactate steady state *Eur. J. Appl. Physiol. Occup. Physiol.* **63** 55–9

Yeo S S, Chang P H and Jang S H 2013 The cortical activation differences between proximal and distal joint movements of the upper extremities: a functional NIRS study *NeuroRehabilitation* **32** 861–6

Yokota S, Takeuchi H, Hashimoto T, Hashizume H, Asano K, Asano M, Sassa Y, Taki Y and Kawashima R 2015 Individual differences in cognitive performance and brain structure in typically developing children *Dev. Cogn. Neurosci.* **14** 1–7

Zhang Y, Li K S, Ning Y Z, Fu C H, Liu H W, Han X, Cui F Y, Ren Y and Zou Y H 2016 Altered structural and functional connectivity between the bilateral primary motor cortex in unilateral subcortical stroke: a multimodal magnetic resonance imaging study *Medicine* **95** e4534

Chapter 6

Yoga and meditation biomarkers for depression

Arindam Bit, Raghavendra Prasad and Shashikanta Tarai

Depressive disorders are catalysts and outcomes of expressive disorder of the brain under abundant non-cooperative cognitive load. Drug administration to address the issue appears to be critical in relevance to the sensitivity of pathophysiological conditions. At the same time, the effect of drug-based therapy is difficult to quantify in this kind of cumbersome symptom. Assessment of the efficacy of the treatment was trivial and purely based on qualitative judgment. The characteristics pattern, behavioural traits, evolution of thoughts, languages and emotional characteristics of human beings are severely inflicted due to depression. Various conclusive studies over cognitive theories speculate that the victims of the depressive disorder always agonise through unembellished suffering with mild cognitive impairments, emotional disorders, inhibitory processing, memory deficit and disorientations, and fast-paced reciprocation towards undesirable life events (McCabe and Healey 2018). The outcome of the cognitive impairments and mood disorders impose a severe strain on activities of the brain, eventually leading to neurodegenerative disorders (Rottenberg *et al* 2005). Frequent mood swings after the disease abates and re-attainment of self-control following a stability in the morbidity at the neuro-physiological level is generally referred to as major depressive disorder (MDD) (Goodwin and Jamison 2007). It is a strenuous task to trace the origin, advancement and recurrence of the depressive disorder, especially considering challenges such as detailed analysis and identification of morbidities and their symptoms, which will also diminish the chance of diagnosis at the proper time and may not be able to prevent it in the near future.

In our traditional ancient Vedic medicine and practices, yoga and meditation were considered the most holistic therapeutic techniques for addressing MDD. Yoga is accepted as a therapy for physical, social and psycho-cognitive treatments for stress reduction, emotional regulation and spiritual development. It has been proposed that Yoga practice-prana (breathing), dhyana (mediation) and asana

doi:10.1088/978-0-7503-3383-2ch6

(movement) enhance the scope of attention, cognitive control and executive functions, positive emotion and adaptive efficiency of patients suffering from depression (figure 6.1).

6.1 Depressive disorders

The depressive issue happens at any age; however, it usually begins at around the 20s, or 30s. In essential consideration settings, upwards of 30% of patients report depressive side effects, yet <10% have significant stress. The term despondency is frequently used to portray the low or disheartened temperament that comes from disillusionment (e.g., money related cataclysm, catastrophic event, genuine sickness) or misfortunes (e.g., the demise of a friend or family member). In any case, better terms for such states of mind are debilitation and sorrow. Researchers proposed a biological plausibility and a multilevel theory that described neural, physiological, molecular, and genomic mechanisms that connect social-environmental stress knowledge with internal biological processes that are strongly responsible for depression pathogenesis (Slavich and Irwin 2014). Critical management of the major depressive disorder in children and youngsters determined that utilisation of antidepressant drugs in the essential handling of significant depressive symptoms does not appear to offer a substantial benefit for them (Cipriani *et al* 2016). An investigative study that analysed the consequence of mindfulness-based cognitive therapy (MBCT) in combating depressive disorders suggested a need for additional rigorous approaches that can evaluate superior heights of underlying specificity (van der Velden *et al* 2015). It was discovered that the patterns and associates of comorbid DSM-IV anxiety ailments among individuals with DSM-IV MDD are parallel across World Mental Health (WMH) reviews across the globe. The findings also elevated enquiries about the comparative status of tempǒrally prime apprehension disorders as risk markers (Kessler *et al* 2015). So many studies still suggest that adequate measures and guidelines are to be drawn to combat depressive

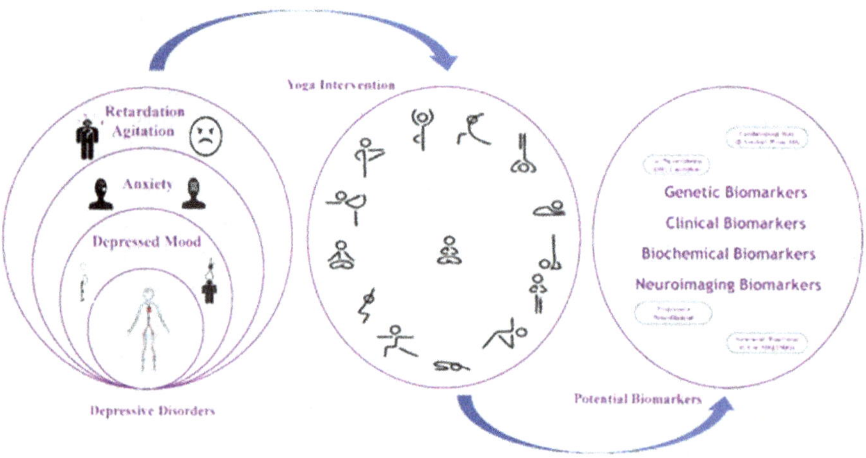

Figure 6.1. Developing biomarkers through yoga for depressive disorder.

disorders. The general types of depressive disorders, along with available therapeutic solutions/methods, are stated below.

Furthermore, depressive disorders can be deeply researched in the prospect of the following manners to have a better understanding of the disorders:

1. Neurocognitive aspects.
2. Neurobiological/neurological aspects.
3. Neurocomputational aspects.

The various types of depressive disorders are given below in table 6.1.

A comparative tabulation is given in table 6.2 with some of the discovered symptoms in terms of neurocognitive, neurobiological, and neurocomputational perspectives. A graphic representation of the identification of appropriate biomarkers is presented in the form of a diagram in figure 6.1

6.2 Understanding yoga through philosophy

Old fundamental content on Yoga was composed by Sage Patanjali 400 years B.C. This content was exchanged through the ages by oral portrayals (Shruti). That is the reason the entire learning of Yoga is compactly encompassed in 196 lines of Sanskrit Sutras by Patanjali altogether, with the goal that understudies can undoubtedly recall these sutras. The Yoga Sutras concentrated basically on expelling all abundance of thought from the psyche and focusing on a solitary thing, yet they were later consolidated more intensely than some other antiquated yoga compositions in the present day, 'corporate' Yoga.

Yoga progression is pronounced in eight phases (ashtanga-yoga, 'eight-membered Yoga'). The following moral, physical and psychological provisions depict the primary states of mind and morals required towards endeavouring the physical and mental preparation of Yoga securely.

6.2.1 Classification of ashtanga-yoga

Moral provisions

Yama—'principles' indicate Ahimsa (nonviolence), Satya (truth), Asteya (non-stealing), etc.

Niyama—'discipline' indicates purity, serenity, strictness, and devotion to God.

Physical provisions

Asana—'postures' indicates physical stances for making the body agile and strong.

Pranayama—'breath control' indicates the tempo of breathing.

Pratyahara—'withdrawal of the senses' involves control of the mind.

Psychological or inner aids

Dharana—'holding on' indicates the ability to confine consciousness of externals to one entity for a prolonged time frame.

Dhyana—'concentrated meditation.'

Samadhi—'salvation' indicates the exit from the cycle of rebirth.

Table 6.1. Classification of depressive disorders.

Types of depressive disorder	Symptoms	Therapy
Major depression	1. Loss of concentration. 2. Restless and disturbed. 3. Weight loss/gain.	1. Medication with antidepressants. 2. Talk therapy. 3. Electroconvulsive therapy (ECT). 4. Repetitive transcranial magnetic stimulation (rTMS).
Persistent depressive disorder	1. Change in appetite. 2. Trouble in decision making. 3. Lack of morale.	1. Psychotherapy. 2. Medication.
Bipolar disorder	1. Mood swing.	1. Medication with antidepressants drugs such as Seroquel, Latuda, etc.
Seasonal affective disorder (SAD)	1. Feeling lack of warmth.	1. Antidepressants. 2. Light therapy.
Psychotic depression	1. Hallucinations. 2. Misapprehensions. 3. Distrust.	1. Antipsychotic drugs. 2. ECT.
Atypical depression	1. Sleeping more than usual. 2. Oversensitive to criticism.	1. Antidepressant: SSRI (selective serotonin reuptake inhibitor). 2. Antidepressant: MAOI (monoamine oxidase inhibitor).

Table 6.2. Neurocognitive, neurobiological and neurocomputational perspectives.

Aspects	Type of disorders	Symptoms/methods	Results and findings
Neurocognitive	Major depressive disorders (MDD)	Cognitive dysfunction	The swiftness of dispensation, decision-making parameter, working memory, and erudition/temporary memory appear to be more strongly affected (Mohn and Rund 2016).
	Post-stroke depression	Somatic	Psychological, neurocognitive and somatic symptoms of depression vary with each other in terms of diagnostic sensitivity (Coster *et al* 2005).
	MDD	The severity of the depression	The association exists between depression severity and neurocognitive function (McClintock *et al* 2010).
Neurobiological	MDD	'Downstream'—neurochemical mechanisms, lack of adherence	Therapeutic differences and their responses contribute to inadequate treatment impact with various clinical and neurobiological factors, including noncompliance, underdosing, etc (Trivedi *et al* 2008).
	Depression	Down-regulation of the hypothalamic-pituitary-adrenal axis and hippocampus	Genes that are responsible for getting affected or develop resistance against the syndrome can be identified to tackle depression with the help of neurobiological studies (Nestler *et al* 2002).
	Maladaptive stress	Guilt and suicidality (pathophysiology perspective)	Combination of behavioural, molecular and electrophysiological techniques proves that there is a change in neuroplasticity in specific neural circuits due to maladaptive stress (Krishnan and Nestler 2008).
	MDD	Pathological alterations are exhibited due to the active part of glucocorticoids, inflammatory cytokines and brain-derived development features. Structural and functional changes in the hippocampus.	Structural, functional and molecular modifications in numerous brain zones can be addressed by antidepressant pharmacotherapy (Maletic *et al* 2007).

(Continued)

Table 6.2. (*Continued*)

Aspects	Type of disorders	Symptoms/methods	Results and findings
Neurocomputational	Anhedonia	DSM-IV criteria for MDD	Victims of MDD exhibited a significant reduction in reward responsiveness. Orientation of hedonic processing found to be down-functional in depression (Pizzagalli *et al* 2008).
	Depression and schizophrenia	Irregularities were exhibited due to the value and prediction errors.	Dopamine irregularities in depression and schizophrenia are suggested by dopamine encoding prediction errors (Gradin *et al* 2011).
	Major depression concerning anhedonia	Learning to predict both positive and negative reinforcement	Negative bias or dampening found in a group of stress exhibited patients is entirely dependent on the neuropsychological task (Chase *et al* 2010).

The art of Yoga thinks about each part of human life. Therefore, Yoga plans to instruct sadhana to a typical individual and leads them to samadhi. Accepting this as a premise, the eight phases of advancement are characterised in the art of Yoga.

6.2.2 Hatha yoga and its framework

The term Hatha Yoga has been frequently used to represent the act of asana (stances). The term 'ha' implies the prana (indispensable) force overseeing the physical body, and 'tha' indicates the conscious (mental) constraint that gives Hatha Yoga an impetus to enliven the two energies that administer our lives. More accurately, the strategies portrayed in Hatha Yoga blend and sanitise the body frameworks and centre the psyche in anticipation of further developed chakra and kundalini rehearse.

The Hatha Yoga framework incorporates asana alongside the six shatkarmas (physical and mental detox methods), mudras and bandhas (psycho-physiological vitality discharge strategies) and pranayama (pranic arousing refinements). Calibrating the human identity at progressively unobtrusive levels prompts higher conditions of mindfulness and reflection.

1. *Yogasana—Yoga postures.*
2. *Six shatkarmas—corporeal and psychological detox techniques.*
3. *Mudras—psychophysiological energy proclamation practices.*
4. *Pranayama—breathing exercises.*

6.2.3 Prana (breathing), dhyana (meditation) and asana (movement)

Prana (breathing)

Prana is a vitality, essence, control. Prana is the establishment and quintessence of all life, the vitality and essence which pervades the whole planet. Prana streams through every being that prevails. Prana is divided into the following five main functions: *Prana, Apana, Udana, Vyana and Samana.*

Prana

Prana is an exceptional capacity of the Galactic Prana, which provides the humanoid body with necessary oxygen. Its vitality streams from the anterior naris to the level of the heart. Pure air is crucial for wellbeing; be that as it may, atmosphere alone is not the conclusive factor for health. A few people are inclined to disease, despite being out in the natural air as often as possible. Then again, individuals who live in the enclosed periphery or rural areas with generally deprived air quality stay sound. The well-being is not affected by outer factors, as it were. Our inward condition likewise represents well-being by the intensity of opposition and the internal will—Atmabala—the internal imperative.

Apana

Apana impacts some of the lower portions of the body, starting from the umbilicus to the ends of the feet. Prana controls the disposal procedure. Infections that influence the subordinate guts, digestive organs, kidneys, renal systems, limbs, etc, are the consequence of irritated ApanaPrana. The methods such as Nauli (purification method), AgnisaraKriya (cleansing technique), Ashvini Mudra and Mula Bandha reinforce and cleanse ApanaPrana.

Vyana

Vyana sequences through the nerve canals of the human body. It has an impact upon the entire physique and especially on the Nadis. Deprived flow, debilitated nerve incitement and mental meltdowns start from an inadequacy in VyanaPrana. VyanaPrana is initiated and reinforced in the act of Kumbhaka (breath maintenance). There is a programmed delay among inward breath and exhalation with every characteristic, loosened up breath that we take. While performing pranayama, this interruption is deliberately extended. When we hold our breath, we withhold vitality in the body with a resultant development in weight. This weight will have the impact of discharging vitality obstructions. Kumbhaka invigorates the sensory system.

Any individual who has consolidated Kumbhaka and Maha Bandha's strategies knows the consequent, excellent impression of peace that moves over the body. This is the purpose behind having the capacity to contemplate in a better sense after this training. The expanded stream of VyanaPrana creates the inclination all through the entire body.

Udana

UdanaPrana is the rising vitality that streams from the heart to the head and mind. UdanaPrana goes with the enlivening of the Kundalini force. It is with the help of UdanaPrana that the celestial body isolates itself from the physical body. A solid UdanaPrana facilitates the period of death. UdanaPrana takes control, and the body turns out to be light, and one may pick up the capacity to suspend. When UdanaPrana is in our possession, outer hindrances, for example, water, earth or stones, never again deter us. Serious routine regarding the Yoga breath practices also gives the feeling of floating on water, or notwithstanding drifting noticeable all around.

Samana

Samana is an essential Prana that interfaces two primary Chakras (focal energy points in the spinning disk as inferred in ancient meditation practices): Anahata energy point and Manipura energy point. The human body receives the vitality of the nourishment circulated by SamanaPrana. We know that sustenance impacts our physical body, as well as influences our mind and cognisance. The nature of our prana (a wide range of prana) is straightforwardly connected with the heart of our sustenance. Unadulterated, sattvic (pure, genuine, ethical, energetic), vegetarian sustenance and the performance of pranayama shall give a sound and adjusted body forever.

Manipura Chakra, or the energy point, is impacted through Samana Prana, whose relating component is naturally fire. When Yogis have their mastery over Samana Prana, it is purely nothing but an unadulterated fire inside them. Those in whom Samana Prana is unadulterated are encompassed by a brilliant air, or, in other words, by individuals who do not perceive emanations.

This prana is reinforced by the act of Agnisara Kriya and Nauli. The performance of the two Kriyas above forestalls stomach related issues and Diabetes. It likewise enhances one's protection from irresistible illness and disease because of the stomach-related fire that is stirred in the entire body and filters and cleans in return. The best system for arousing Samana Prana is Kriya Yoga. The act of Kriya Yoga creates comfort in the whole body due to the ascendence of Samana Prana. An extremely mindful individual can watch the air of a Kriya professional becoming more splendid and more grounded with each round of training.

Dhyana (meditation)

Dhyana is the seventh appendage of Yoga, expanding upon asana (corporal stance), pranayama (the art of breath regulation), pratyahara (regulator of the faculties, moving the meditation to within), and Dharana (fixation). The word 'Dhyana' originates from the Sanskrit word '*dhyana*', which signifies 'to consider.' Thus, Dhyana includes fixation and reflection on the point of centre to know the reality about it.

This more profound centralisation of the brain is simply the instrument information where one can isolate figment from the real world, and in the end, achieve a definitive objective of Yoga: samadhi (euphoria, or association with the source).

Jnana yoga

Jnana Yoga is depicted by convention to get the most noteworthy reflective state and inward information. This is because Jnana signifies 'information'; however, with regards to Yoga, it implies thoughtful mindfulness, which prompts illuminative knowledge.

It is anything but a technique by which we endeavour to discover normal responses to everlasting inquiries; instead, it is a piece of contemplation prompting self-enquiry and self-acknowledgement.

Asana (movement)

According to a textbook of Hatha Yoga called 'Gherand Sanhita', there are all **8.4 million asanas.** But the book pronounces 32 asanas, **Pradipika** pronounces 15 asanas, **Hatha Ratnavali** indicates 34 asanas, **Goraksha Samhita** talks about 84 asanas, etc. So, although learning the asanas is a theme of exploration, this is just a primer to the views on asanas to encourage additional efforts in this field. Some of the yogasanas are depicted in the figure and tabulated below in table 6.3, along with their details.

6.3 Yoga—neuroscience intersection

According to Ham-D (Hamilton Depression Rating Scale), factors like unhappy mood, guilt, self-harm, sleeplessness (beginning stage, in-between and deferred stages), work and benefits, obstruction, anxiety, nervousness in cognitive and somatic perspectives, somatic indications such as gastrointestinal, general problems, venereal symptoms, hypochondriasis, weight reduction, distrustfulness are a few of those considered as an inclusive component to address and gauge depression.

Outside of its spiritual and religious goals, there is little doubt that Yoga has various therapeutic influences over the collective health and other elements,

Table 6.3. Various asanas.

Asana	Posture/gesture indicators	Asana	Posture/gesture indicators
Datta Mudra	Neck	Eka Pada Sahajahasta Bhujangasana	Cobra with sole of foot touching thigh
Shavasana	Corpse	Adhvasana	Downward facing pose
Swastikasana	Auspicious	Eka Pada Sulabha Pawanmuktasana	Easy gas release pose one leg
Tadagasana	Pond	Sarwangasana	Stance with shoulder
Vajrasana	Thunderbolt	Vakrasana	Twisted pose
Uttanpadasan	Legs	Ashwini Mudra	Horse gesture in shoulder stance
Makarasana	Crocodile	Matsyasana	Fish pose
Parvatasana	Mountain	Halasana	Plough pose
Vrikshasana	Tree	Naukasana	Boat pose
Hasta Sanchalan	Arms	Pawanmuktasan	Bent neck
Pada Sanchalan	Drive of legs	Dhanurasana	Bow pose
Janu Sanchalan	Drive of knees	Padmasana	Lotus pose
Skandha Sanchalan	Drive of shoulders	Shalabhasana	Locust pose
Sukha Pranayam	Deep breathing	Paschimottanasana	Half forward bend
Janu Hastasana	Hand to knee	Ardha Matsyendrasana	Half spinal twist
Hasta Shirasana	Hand to chin	Trikonasana	Triangle pose
Patangasana	Kite pose	Utkatasana	Toe balance pose
Chakrasana	Wheel pose	Padangushtasana	Single toe balance pose

including those parameters from Ham-D for gauging depression of the human being. According to Johns Hopkins University, Yoga can be used as an instrumental tool to improve strength, poise, flexibility, heart health, positive attitude, etc. In one of the primary studies conducted by Dr Streeter and his team in 2007, it was revealed that Yoga significantly contributes to the improvisation of mood by regulating the movement of the Gamma-aminobutyric acid (GABA) system positively. The team also demonstrated the upsurge of thalamic GABA levels post-practice of Iyengar yoga compared with metabolically-coordinated walking amongst healthy people (Streeter *et al* 2007). Furthermore, it has been proven that Yoga intervention has lowered the cortisol levels by downwards regulation of the hypothalamic-pituitary-adrenal (HPA) axis. It was also displayed that psychiatric ailments like autism and schizophrenia are closely associated with low oxytocin levels, which emerges as an outcome of reducing social bondings (Bhargav *et al* 2021). In a recent systematic review, scientists illustrated positive impacts of Yoga over the structure and function of the brain locales such as the default mode network (DMN) region, hippocampus region, amygdala region, prefrontal cortex region, cingulate cortex and also the prevalent brain networks (Gothe *et al* 2019).

Foreseeing further concrete scientific evidence, it can be conclusively stated that Yoga and meditation can be an actual noninvasive tool to combat all depressive disorders when practised with utmost guidance.

6.4 Behavioral and psycho-physiological effects of yoga interventions

A recent study points out that the yoga intervention created a constructive impact in decreasing alcohol consumption and enhanced the social behaviour of the students without any disruption in attention, even during stressful tasks. The study outlined that Yoga effectively tackled and decreased the problems, and it also boosted the positive results among the students. Furthermore, yoga intervention decreased the adverse outcomes and tremendously contributed to the development of prosocial behaviours, such as praising others, offering reassurance to others, offering assistance, and exploring and identifying the best in individuals (Fishbein *et al* 2016).

Conclusive evidence evolved from research in 2012 stating that Yoga intervention addresses a pool of psychological, emotional, and corporal sides of the individual. During their comparative analysis with physical education, a study of covariance test (ANCOVA) published by them exhaustively deliberated positive contribution of Yoga intervention concerning parameters like the mood states, schedule for children (positive and negative affects), professed anxiety scale, list of positive psychological attitudes, flexibility scale, state-trait anger expression inventory, etc. It was further exhibited that self-regulatory skills were obtained by individuals who practice Yoga which eventually led to improvised mental health by downregulating stress (Noggle *et al* 2012).

Numerous scientific studies and their outcome indicates the active role of Yoga in combatting depressive disorders. Therefore, cumulative analysis of the impact of Yoga in terms of behavioural and psycho-physiological traits is given in table 6.4.

6.4.1 A harmonical 432 MHz: OM

Further, meditation, along with the mantra 'OM' as the highest sacred tone, might change brain structure. One study found brain differences in meditators associated with non-meditators in the frontopolar and orbitofrontal cortex, insula, amygdala

Table 6.4. Impact of yoga on behavioral and psycho-physiological traits.

Post yoga intervention	
Reduced parameters	Increased parameters
Discomposed nature	Positive affect
Tension/agitation/pressure	Positive psychological traits
Despair	Life purpose and satisfaction
Annoyance/wrath	Self-confidence
Negative affect	Anger management
Stress	Resilience

regions, medial portions of cerebral hemispheres (cingulate cortex), superior longitudinal fasciculus and callosal commissure regions. These regions influence interoceptive and exteroceptive awareness, memory, emotive regulation, intra- and interhemispheric communiqué amid brain regions (Fox *et al* 2014). Studies have also mentioned that changes in temporal dynamics of oscillation are exhibited after meditation through the OM mantra (Kumar *et al* 2010). The meditation performed through OM enables mental and physiological relaxation concerning the galvanic skin response (Telles *et al* 1995). Functional magnetic resonance imaging (fMRI) study (Kalyani *et al* 2011) has exposed noteworthy inactivation of hippocampus regions during meditation through OM. When heard over some time, the OM sound positively affects the neural cortex regions (Kumar *et al* 2015). The time and frequency domain analysis on the 'OM' chant signal has found evidence that stress is found to be reduced in human beings when 'OM' chanting is done, and it also gives tranquillity and harmony to a strained mind (Gurjar and Ladhake 2008).

In terms of time-domain analysis, constructive and adverse early sensory modules such as P100, N170, N200, and P200 (within 100–200 ms) characterise improved amplitude when affected people with depression process emotive faces, voices and words. These sensory modules portray the early acknowledgement of sad stimuli with higher amplitudes than the happy stimuli. For understanding the pathogenesis and clinical bias towards repudiation in depressed patients, the performance of sensory modules is essential. Somehow, the study conducted by Burkhart and Thomas in the year 1993 stays exceptional when compared to most of the current studies, which reveals the enhancement of the amplitude of these early components. However, some studies account that dejected patients have reduced the amplitude of potentials in the N2 latency in frontal, central and parietal regions. Here the decrease in N2 characterises the allowance of adverse facial expressions, enabling a higher possibility of suicidal ideation.

6.5 Biomarkers

A biomarker characterises a tool perhaps serving doctors in foreseeing commencement, analysis, and evolution of an ailment and assessing the responses to the treatments that modify the disease. The Biomarkers Definitions Working Group has defined a biomarker as 'a characteristic that is objectively measured and evaluated as an indicator of normal biological processes, pathogenic processes or pharmacological responses to a therapeutic intervention'. It will be a complicated process for a standalone biomarker to adjudge the complexity of the disorder. Biomarkers can be effectively used for prognosis and diagnosis of any ailments. Combinations of biomarkers are suggested to decode the complexity and the progression of a disorder. A progression biomarker (a neutrally quantifiable trait) that fluctuates over time in a way that can be associated with the progression of ailment. This kind of marker is usually used in clinical trials and potential disease-modifying treatments. A diagnostic biomarker (or risk marker) is a quantifiable physical trait related to the ailment's occurrence. A detailed analysis of the biomarkers is done in table 6.5, and their potentials are analysed for their usability.

Table 6.5. Biomarkers analysis.

Biomarkers	Categories	Plausible potentials
Genetic	a-syn (SNCA) Leucine-rich repeat kinase 2 (LRRK2)	Monitoring genetical changes.
Clinical	Depression Constipation Hyposmia REM sleep behavioural disorder Olfactory dysfunction	Recognising individuals who are at risk of more significant progression (e.g., with growth of cognitive impairment).
Biochemical	Metabolic factors Insulin-like growth factor 1 (IGF-1) Oxidative stress Neuroinflammation	Axial motor impairment and cognitive dysfunction.
Neuroimaging	Positron emission tomography (PET) Single photon emission computed tomography (SPECT) Transcranial sonography (TCS) Functional MRI (fMRI)	Changes in the brain's functional connectivity are spotted. Cognitive declination is observed.

The biomarkers can be broadly classified as follows:

1. Genetic biomarkers;
2. Clinical biomarkers;
3. Biochemical biomarkers;
4. Neuroimaging biomarkers.

6.5.1 Neurological disorders and biomarkers

Most neurological ailments like Alzheimer's, Parkinson's, Multiple Sclerosis are based on motor components, and sensory details rely upon treatment methods to prognose the disease in their nascent stages. The diagrammatic representation of a classification of neurological disorders is represented in the form of a diagram in figure 6.2.

Essential traits of an ideal biomarker

1. It should be able to track the neurodegeneration by changing itself.
2. It must exhibit an established connection with the disease.
3. It must have a flexible longitudinal association with disease progression data.
4. It must be sensitive, reflecting small changes in disease progression.
5. It should be safe to try and measure.
6. It must be ideally linear for measurement purposes irrespective of circumstances.
7. It should be feasible to use across different ages, sex, ethnicity groups.

Need for biomarkers

Biomarkers will pave the way for a breakthrough in predicting and diagnosing diseases much earlier. Customisation of biomarkers will lead to assessing the effects

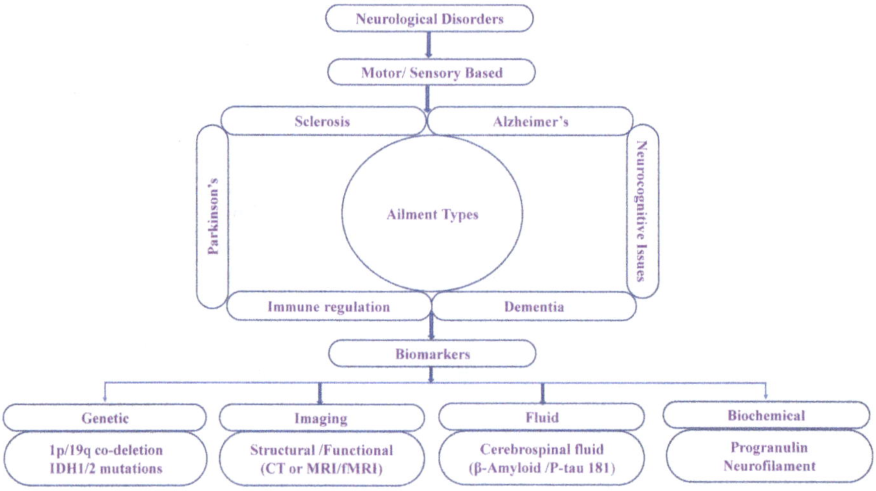

Figure 6.2. Schematic diagram—neurological disorders and biomarkers.

of certain drugs handled during clinical trials. Simply, biomarkers will help in conducting faster, cheaper and safer trails. Various studies across domains suggest an urgent requirement of discovering disease-specific biomarkers that will support the prognosis and analysis of disease.

A chronic neuropathy disease like chronic inflammatory demyelinating polyneuropathy (CIDP) do not have any targeted biomarker to help in the ailment of the condition, which is identified by symptoms like symmetrical proximal and distal muscular dystrophy (DD), loss of sensory perception, and weakened balance (Brannagan 2011). Therefore, there is a stringent requirement for developing new biomarkers to minimise the gap between the observational steps to be taken to tackle the disease. Therefore, a relationship between the disease's pathology to be established along with a neat characterisation of biomarkers in terms of their sensitivity, specificity, and viability in adaptation is needed (Ward *et al* 1996).

There are a few concerning factors that immunotherapies are often associated with immune-corelated toxicity and contribute to high expenses such as classifying biomarkers to govern the type of patients expected to yield clinical benefit from immunotherapy and be vulnerable to adverse side effects is a captivating clinical and communal need (Masucci *et al* 2017). Mild cognitive impairment (MCI) and Alzheimer's disease (AD) are found to remain stubborn against general therapeutic intervention. The pathway of developing biomarkers to address the preclinical condition of MCI/AD is a boon to address this ailment (Fiandaca *et al* 2014).

Drug-induced liver injury (DILI) can be curtailed through metabolomics, where biofluids are collected to determine the initial biomarkers of noxiousness, which might contribute with precise pointers of liver damage helping in the ailment (Iruzubieta *et al* 2015). Even though studies indicate that biomarkers are not required systematically to guide every decision, in certain specific approaches, these may help us with some finite details regarding the ailment (Dianti and Luna 2018). The current scientific community is eagerly shifting its focus towards biomarkers to address diseases like amyotrophic lateral sclerosis (ALS), where the potential biomarkers can effectively help in the drug development and the cure of such diseases (Wagner 2009).

6.5.2 Quest for biomarkers in the intersection of neuroscience with yoga and meditation

Understanding the role of biomarkers in tackling neurological disorders has become the need of the hour to validate an authenticated biomarker. By the philosophical and scientific evidence favouring Yoga interventions, it's time to look in this direction.

A scientific observation reported that after the intervention of Yoga, there was a noteworthy upsurge in αHF. The sensitivity of the baroreflex was enumerated by the α-index, at high frequency (HF; 0.15–0.35 Hz, reflecting parasympathetic nervous system activity) and mid-frequency (MF; 0.05–0.15 Hz, reflecting sympathetic nervous system activity), consequent from the spectral and cross-spectral investigation of impulsive variations in heart rate and blood pressure. It was seen that there was an increase in VO_2 after Yoga; heart rate diminished taking after Yoga, though there was no alteration of systolic blood pressure post-yoga. Furthermore, there was a noteworthy increment within the crest control values of heart rate changeability (HRV) within the MF but not HF (Bowman *et al* 1997).

Self-Assessment Manikin (SAM), an assessment technique, was developed to quantify and rate pleasure, arousal and dominance and compared with an environmental psychology approach called the semantic differential scale devised by Mehrabian and Russell in 1974. The differences in the dominance dimension from the comparison suggested that SAM may be the better of the two in terms of the personal response to an affective stimulus (Bradley and Lang 1994). The study of mindfulness conducted by Dr Brown and his team concluded that there were credible positive impacts as an outcome of the mindfulness program among individuals. They also admitted that a comprehensive research study might be required to address the development of 'mindfulness' consciousness that develops naturally and the role of psychological and social environments supporting or hindering its growth. This consideration program aimed to illustrate the part of mindfulness, measured in both inter- and intraindividual terms, in mental well-being (Brown and Ryan 2003).

Another fascinating investigation on the influence of mindfulness meditation on brain and immune functionality was studied, and it was initially predicted that there would be substantial fluctuations in prefrontal and central electrode positions. However, later the findings consistently led to the central leads (C3/C4). Affect related asymmetries were generally observed in the regions of C3/C4. It was concluded that a short duration drill program in mindfulness meditation (MBSR) has palpable effects on the brain and immune function, which emphasises the requirement for supplementary research on the life penalties of this intervention (Davidson *et al* 2003).

6.6 Discussions

An alternative safeguards traditional therapeutic solution to address the above-stated problem was proposed to be effective yogic postures and meditation. At the same time, the outcomes of such practices were measured qualitatively solely. And thus, they are not in practice commercially frequently in India. A quantitative measurement tool for selective types of Yoga and meditation, along with reciting 'OM', may be accommodated to address the issues. EEG and fNIRS signals obtained directly from the affected brain (noninvasive method) under therapeutic conditions will be extrapolated for features classification. These classifiers will be used as biomarkers for the quantitative judgment of effective treatment. This will also begin a cross-talk amongst neurogenetic pleomorphisms and neurocognitive aspects of depression, thereby supplementing our exertions to avert and treat cognitive deterioration and enhancing enduring consequences for those suffering from depressive ailments.

The proposed solution will be focusing on the outcome of the Yoga and mindful meditation act of 'OM' recitation over the group of depressed and control subjects, and ERP components along with PSD spectrum of alpha, delta, and theta frequencies will be evaluated to obtain a temporal biomarker. Simultaneously, functional near-infrared spectroscopy (fNIRS) will be employed to record BOLD of brain hemodynamics during these experiments to get spatial biomarkers in co-relation with temporal markers. These signal-based biomarkers will be further classified by using different machine-learning algorithms.

Preceding studies have concentrated on the outcomes of depression-based mindfulness and Yoga programs in the urban area that were applied to the classroom context (Greenberg and Harris 2012, Weare 2013). It has been observed that children have developed more considerable cognitive resources, including emotional directive assistances, de-escalating undesirable emotions, endorsing calmness, assistance for reducing depression; dynamic regulations; enhanced mental and corporeal health; and enhanced social-emotional, cognitive, and behavioural outcomes (Zoogman *et al* 2014). Mindfulness and Yoga programs are assumed to have possible assistances for youth living in stressed atmospheres by extenuating the detrimental effects of chronic stress exposure through promoting self-supervisory capacities (Brown *et al* 2003, Mendelson *et al* 2010, Zenner *et al* 2014). Furthermore, it might advance the behavioural outcomes among the younger generations by positively influencing youths' emotional and cognitive parameters (Mendelson *et al* 2010, Gould *et al* 2014). A mindful Yoga intercession had a valuable impression on substance use and its psychological and anatomical correlations in speculative youngsters compared to control clusters (Fishbein *et al* 2016). Yet, despite this mounting knowledge base, maximum studies are steered with random trials following a qualitative behavioural approach. Though research has begun to appraise the effects of meditation and Yoga training programs on quantifiable and qualitative youth outcomes exposed to depression (Diamond and Lee 2011, Noggle *et al* 2012, Khalsa *et al* 2012, Serwacki and Cook-Cottone 2012, Lagor *et al* 2013, Zenner *et al* 2014), few investigators have discovered the neurocognitive viewpoints of patients that bring a change in their neuro-cognitive outcomes.

Numerous studies have recorded the effectiveness of Yoga and meditation since it has reduced depression and anxiety and improved attention and concentration

(Matchim and Armer 2007, Teixeira 2008, Uebelacker *et al* 2010). Development of the prefrontal neural circuit serves the progressive amalgamation, endorsing the ability to exert effortful control over cognitive resources in emotional circumstances. Furthermore, neuro-developmental processes in prefrontal regions facilitate psycho-social adaptations during adolescence (Steinberg 2005). Neuroimaging and EEG studies advise that the emphasised mindfulness endorsed by Yoga affects the fundamental neuro-biologic mechanisms that target regulatory and affective processes (Davidson *et al* 2003, Pagnoni *et al* 2008, Davidson and McEwen 2012). A review made by Davidson *et al* (2012) offers an indication for the effects of mindfulness-based practices on brain plasticity, concluding that there is a possibility of reducing stress reactivity through amendments in brain regions that regulate emotive responses. Whether prefrontal or mid frontal regions enhance neural plasticity and modulate the attentional and emotional control mechanisms or some other areas are involved in controlling the conflict situations between action-emotion and attention will be experimented with among stress-induced participants with depression who have practised Yoga for more than six months. Obtained experimental results will be compared with the results of a control group of students.

The scientific attention in Yoga has amplified significantly in recent years and several biological effects of Yoga, including physical stances (Bowman *et al* 1997, Miyamura *et al* 2002, Joshi and Telles 2009, Pomidori *et al* 2009, Yadav and Mutha 2016) and meditation (Sarang and Telles 2006), have been explored. Yoga is accepted as a therapy for physical, social and psycho-cognitive treatments for stress reduction, emotional regulation and spiritual development. Most of these previous studies have emphasised the qualitative data in questionnaires following and before the mindful Yoga practice. So far, little if any research has endeavoured to understand behavioural and neurocognitive mechanisms behind the benefits of mindful Yoga practice among stress-induced participants with depression severity when encountering various conflicting and competing situations in their professional careers.

6.7 Conclusion

Designing EEG experiments based on competing trails and conflicting stimuli of emotion and attention, the proposed research aims to investigate how Yoga practice-prana (breathing), dhyana (mediation) and asana (movement) enhances the scope of neuro-cognitive control and executive functions of the clinical participants of our study group. Behavioural response time and accuracy and neural amplitudes of various brain regions will be collected from the Yogic and Control group of Chhattisgarh. We predict that Yoga will improve psycho-physiological stress responses in at-risk youngsters and disrupt substance use behaviour, plummeting the usage of alcohol, cannabis and illegal drugs. Further, we hypothesise that the Yoga intervention would change the neural plasticity that brings a change in patient's behaviour, and behavioural modifications would get positive outcomes.

References

Bhargav H, George S, Varambally S and Gangadhar B N 2021 Yoga and psychiatric disorders: a review of biomarker evidence *Int. Rev. Psych.* **33** 162–9

Bowman A J, Clayton R H, Murray A, Reed J W, Subhan M M and Ford G A 1997 Effects of aerobic exercise training and Yoga on the baroreflex in healthy elderly persons *Eur. J. Clin. Invest.* **27** 443–9

Bradley M M and Lang P J 1994 Measuring emotion: the self-assessment manikin and the semantic differential *J. Behav. Ther. Exp. Psych.* **25** 49–59

Brannagan T H 2011 Current diagnosis of CIDP: the need for biomarkers *J. Peripher. Nerv. Syst.* **16** 3–13

Brown K W and Ryan R M 2003 The benefits of being present: mindfulness and its role in psychological well-being *J. Pers. Soc. Psychol.* **84** 822–48

Chase H W, Frank M J, Michael A, Bullmore E T, Sahakian B J and Robbins T W 2010 Approach and avoidance learning in patients with major depression and healthy controls: relation to anhedonia *Psychol. Med.* **40** 433

Cipriani A *et al* 2016 Comparative efficacy and tolerability of antidepressants for major depressive disorder in children and adolescents: a network meta-analysis *Lancet* **388** 881–90

Coster L, de, Leentjens A F G, Lodder J and Verhey F R J 2005 The sensitivity of somatic symptoms in post-stroke depression: a discriminant analytic approach *Int. J. Geriatr. Psych.* **20** 358–62

Davidson R J, Kabat-Zinn J, Schumacher J, Rosenkranz M, Muller D, Santorelli S F, Urbanowski F, Harrington A, Bonus K and Sheridan J F 2003 Alterations in brain and immune function produced by mindfulness meditation *Psychosomat. Med.* **65** 564–70

Davidson R J and McEwen B S 2012 Social influences on neuroplasticity: stress and interventions to promote well-being *Nat. Neurosci.* **15** 689

Diamond A and Lee K 2011 Interventions shown to aid executive function development in children 4–12 years old *Science* **333** 959

Dianti M and Luna C M 2018 Do we need biomarkers for the follow-up and shortening of antibiotic treatment duration? *Curr. Opin. Critical Care* **24** 361–9

Fiandaca M S, Mapstone M E, Cheema A K and Federoff H J 2014 The critical need for defining preclinical biomarkers in Alzheimer's disease *Alzheimer's Demen.* **10** S196–S212

Fishbein D, Miller S, Herman-Stahl M, Williams J, Lavery B, Markovitz L, Kluckman M, Mosoriak G and Johnson M 2016 Behavioral and psycho-physiological effects of a yoga intervention on high-risk adolescents: a randomised control trial *J. Child Family Stud.* **25** 518–29

Fox K C R, Nijeboer S, Dixon M L, Floman J L, Ellamil M, Rumak S P, Sedlmeier P and Christoff K 2014 Is meditation associated with altered brain structure? A systematic review and meta-analysis of morphometric neuroimaging in meditation practitioners *Neurosci. Biobehav. Rev.* **43** 48–73

Goodwin F K and Jamison K R 2007 *Manic-depressive Illness: Bipolar Disorders and Recurrent Depression* (New York: Oxford University Press) pp 3–9

Gothe N P, Khan I, Hayes J, Erlenbach E and Damoiseaux J S 2019 Yoga effects on brain health: a systematic review of the current literature *Brain Plastic.* **5** 105–22

Gould L F E, Mendelson T, Dariotis J K, Ancona M, Smith A S R, Gonzalez A A, Smith A A and Greenberg M T 2014 Assessing fidelity of core components in a mindfulness and yoga intervention for urban youth: applying the CORE Process *New Direct. Youth Dev.* **142** 59–81

Gradin V B, Kumar P, Waiter G, Ahearn T, Stickle C, Milders M, Reid I, Hall J and Steele J D 2011 Expected value and prediction error abnormalities in depression and schizophrenia *Brain* **134** 1751–64

Greenberg M T and Harris A R 2012 Nurturing mindfulness in children and youth: current state of research *Child Dev. Persp.* **6** 161–6

Gurjar A A and Ladhake S A 2008 Time-frequency analysis of chanting sanskrit divine sound 'OM' mantra *IJCSNS Int. J. Comp. Sci. Network Sec.* **8** 170–5

Iruzubieta P, Arias-Loste M T, Barbier-Torres L, Martinez-Chantar M L and Crespo J 2015 The need for biomarkers in diagnosis and prognosis of drug-induced liver disease: does metabolomics have any role? *BioMed Res. Int.* **2015** 1–8

Joshi M and Telles S 2009 A nonrandomised non-naive comparative study of the effects of kapalabhati and breath awareness on event-related potentials in trained yoga practitioners *J. Altern. Complemen. Med.* **15** 281–5

Kalyani B G, Venkatasubramanian G, Arasappa R, Rao N P, Kalmady S V, Behere R V, Rao H, Vasudev M K and Gangadhar B N 2011 Neurohemodynamic correlates of 'OM' chanting: a pilot functional magnetic resonance imaging study *Int. J. Yoga* **4** 3

Kessler R C *et al* 2015 Anxious and non-anxious major depressive disorder in the World Health Organization World Mental Health Surveys *Epidemiol. Psych. Sci.* **24** 210–26

Khalsa S B S, Hickey-Schultz L, Cohen D, Steiner N and Cope S 2012 Evaluation of the mental health benefits of yoga in a secondary school: a preliminary randomised controlled trial *J. Behav. Health Ser. Res.* **39** 80–90

Krishnan V and Nestler E J 2008 The molecular neurobiology of depression *Nature* **455** 894–902

Kumar S, Nagendra H R, Manjunath N K, Naveen K V and Telles S 2010 Meditation on OM: relevance from ancient texts and contemporary science *Int. J. Yoga* **3** 2

Kumar U, Guleria A and Khetrapal C L 2015 Neuro-cognitive aspects of 'OM' sound/syllable perception: a functional neuroimaging study *Cognit. Emot.* **29** 432–41

Lagor A F, Williams D J, Lerner J B and McClure K S 2013 Lessons learned from a mindfulness-based intervention with chronically ill youth *Clin. Pract. Pediatr. Psychol.* **1** 146–58

Maletic V, Robinson M, Oakes T, Iyengar S, Ball S G and Russell J 2007 Neurobiology of depression: an integrated view of key findings *Int. J. Clin. Pract.* **61** 2030–40

Masucci G V *et al* 2017 The need for a network to establish and validate predictive biomarkers in cancer immunotherapy *J. Transl. Med.* **15** 223

Matchim Y and Armer J M 2007 Measuring the psychological impact of mindfulness meditation on health among patients with cancer: a literature review *Oncol. Nurs. Forum* **34** 1059–66

McCabe R and Healey P G T 2018 Miscommunication in doctor–patient communication *Top. Cogn. Sci.* **10** 409–24

McClintock S M, Husain M M, Greer T L and Cullum C M 2010 Association between depression severity and neurocognitive function in major depressive disorder: a review and synthesis *Neuropsychology* **24** 9–34

Mendelson T, Greenberg M T, Dariotis J K, Gould L F, Rhoades B L and Leaf P J 2010 Feasibility and preliminary outcomes of a school-based mindfulness intervention for urban youth *J. Abnorm. Child Psychol.* **38** 985–94

Miyamura M, Nishimura K, Ishida K, Katayama K, Shimaoka M and Hiruta S 2002 Is man able to breathe once a minute for an hour? The effect of yoga respiration on blood gases *Jpn. J. Physiol.* **52** 313–16

Mohn C and Rund B R 2016 Neurocognitive profile in major depressive disorders: relationship to symptom level and subjective memory complaints *BMC Psych.* **16** 108

Nestler E J, Barrot M, DiLeone R J, Eisch A J, Gold S J and Monteggia L M 2002 Neurobiology of depression *Neuron* **34** 13–25

Noggle J J, Steiner N J, Minami T and Khalsa S B S 2012 Benefits of yoga for psycho-social well-being in a US high school curriculum: a preliminary randomised controlled trial *J. Develop. Behav. Pediatr.* **33** 193–201

Pagnoni G, Cekic M and Guo Y 2008 'Thinking about not-thinking': neural correlates of conceptual processing during zen meditation *PLoS One* **3** e3083

Pizzagalli D A, Iosifescu D, Hallett L A, Ratner K G and Fava M 2008 Reduced hedonic capacity in major depressive disorder: evidence from a probabilistic reward task *J. Psychiatric Res.* **43** 76–87

Pomidori L, Campigotto F, Amatya T M, Bernardi L and Cogo A 2009 Efficacy and tolerability of yoga breathing in patients with chronic obstructive pulmonary disease: a pilot study *J. Cardiopulm. Rehabil. Prev.* **29** 133–7

Rottenberg J, Gross J J and Gotlib I H 2005 Emotion context insensitivity in major depressive disorder *J. Abnorm. Psychol.* **114** 627–39

Sarang P S and Telles S 2006 Oxygen consumption and respiration during and after two yoga relaxation techniques *Appl. Psychophysiol. Biofeedback* **31** 143–53

Serwacki M L and Cook-Cottone C 2012 Yoga in the schools: a systematic review of the literature *Int. J. Yoga Ther.* **22** 101–9

Slavich G M and Irwin M R 2014 From stress to inflammation and major depressive disorder: a social signal transduction theory of depression *Psychol. Bull.* **140** 774–815

Steinberg L 2005 Cognitive and affective development in adolescence *Trends Cogn. Sci.* **9** 69–74

Streeter C C, Jensen J E, Perlmutter R M, Cabral H J, Tian H, Terhune D B, Ciraulo D A and Renshaw P F 2007 Yoga asana sessions increase brain GABA levels: a pilot study *J. Altern. Complement. Med.* **13** 419–26

Teixeira M E 2008 Meditation as an intervention for chronic pain: an integrative review *Holistic Nurs. Pract.* **22** 225–34

Telles S, Nagarathna R and Nagendra H R 1995 Autonomic changes during 'OM' mediation *Indian J. Physiol. Pharmacol.* **39** 418–20

Trivedi M H, Hollander E, Nutt D and Blier P 2008 Clinical evidence and potential neurobiological underpinnings of unresolved symptoms of depression *J. Clin. Psych.* **69** 246–58

Uebelacker L A, Epstein-Lubow G, Gaudiano B A, Tremont G, Battle C L and Miller I W 2010 Hatha yoga for depression: critical review of the evidence for efficacy, plausible mechanisms of action, and directions for future research *J. Psych. Pract.* **16** 22–33

van der Velden A M, Kuyken W, Wattar U, Crane C, Pallesen K J, Dahlgaard J, Fjorback L O and Piet J 2015 A systematic review of mechanisms of change in mindfulness-based cognitive therapy in the treatment of recurrent major depressive disorder *Clin. Psychol. Rev.* **37** 26–39

Wagner K R 2009 The need for biomarkers in amyotrophic lateral sclerosis drug development *Neurology* **72** 11–12

Ward J B, Henderson R E and Henderson R E 1996 Identification of needs in biomarker research *Environ. Health Perspect.* **104** 895–900

Weare K 2013 Developing mindfulness with children and young people: a review of the evidence and policy context *J. Child. Ser.* **8** 141–53

Yadav G and Mutha P K 2016 Deep breathing practice facilitates retention of newly learned motor skills *Sci. Rep.* **6** 1–8

Zenner C, Herrnleben-Kurz S and Walach H 2014 Mindfulness-based interventions in schools- a systematic review and meta-analysis *Front. Psychol.* **5** 603

Zoogman S, Goldberg S B, Hoyt W T and Miller L 2014 Mindfulness interventions with youth: a meta-analysis *Mindfulness* **6** 290–302

Chapter 7

Blood derived neurotrophic factors and their influence on neurocognitive mechanisms

Arindam Bit, Sayantani Biswas and Shashikanta Tarai

It is known that the network structure of the brain is very complex. Brain structures have different nodes. A brain network is formulated by joining nodes present in separate layers. This structure is updated periodically by suitable training. The advantages of training are improving synaptogenesis (figure 7.1), transforming a brain network into a greater small-worldness, and improving learning, storage capacity, and working. With the help of brain-derived neurotrophic factor (BDNF), we can establish the relationship between exercise and the function of the brain. The allele variant and rs7294919 have a connection with the hippocampal volume. Evidence of converging line shows that the area of the brain is not limited to intelligence. Two factors called integrity and a high degree of organisational efficiency of white matter structure are necessary for intelligence. Rich-club networks and resting-state networks (RSNs) play an essential role in cognitive neuroscience. Instruments have been used to convert diffusion tensor imaging (DTI) data to model rich-club structure. These conversions examine the dysfunction of a patient with schizophrenia diseases. Distance between nodes can be decreased with the help of a power complete small-world model configuration with more advantages like level of clustering and global efficiency, most minor routing path, maximum interconnected nodes. The small-world model was a replica of brain networks along with their functionality. More failure damages the flexibility of small worldness in the ageing process. With these phenomena, the high degree of nodes has been influenced. In other words, we can say that the recovering process of failed nodes is inversely proportional to age.

The result of positron emission scanning shows the activation of the dorsal lateral prefrontal cortex (DLPFC), superolateral sensorimotor cortex (SLSMC), lateral sensorimotor cortex (LSMC), and supplementary motor area (SMA) has been done

doi:10.1088/978-0-7503-3383-2ch7

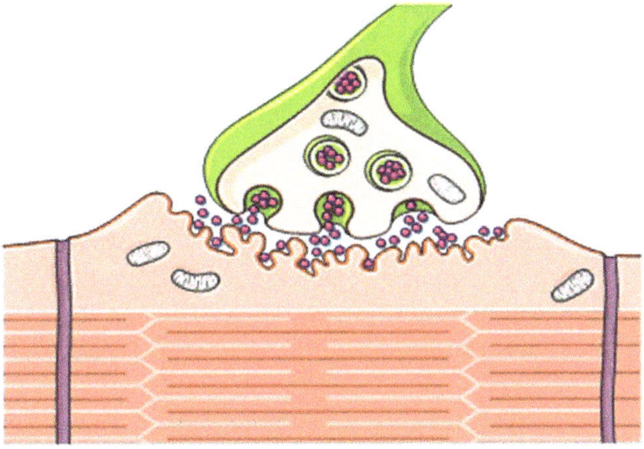

Figure 7.1. Role of training for improvement of synapses.

by imaginary exercise. Note that imaginary exercise was the only method for activation of DLPFC. DLPFC is a significant thing for function and working memory. The periaqueductal grey is a considerable part of the brain structure used to govern the central command. The energy cost of the node is affected by many factors such as no variables, length of the system, hubs. The hubs and interconnection of nodes depend upon the neurons to support synaptogenesis. In the brain structure, higher nodes are mostly spoiled, due to which the structure's length increases and efficiency decreases. The flexibility property of connectivity is poor in a preferred pointed node in a small world due to the interconnection of the sharp node being very high.

The brain network consists of the functioning of neuron activity. The weights of layers are highly dependent upon the myelination degree. DTI is used to check out the myelination degree. DTI is also used to describe the connection of nodes and hubs in the brain network. These characterisations have been done by streamline tractography, including separate parcellation map and functional magnetic resonance imaging. The presence of a rich hub in the brain network is essential. It was found that the connection between structural and functional connectivity was increased in those patients having schizophrenia.

7.1 K-link models

The power-law model governs K-links. A differential equation is used to describe the variation of K-links over time. The mathematical modelling of rich-hub has been done by using the analysis of DTI data. These data have been obtained from patients with schizophrenia. The data enlisting more robustly is known as the weighted rich-club effect. Some nodes are rising to a high degree in the brain network structure, which indicates that the nodes have higher information within the network transition. Synapse scaling in massive amounts produces a disorder in a small-world network. Degradation of spatial memory indicates mental damage, and it is

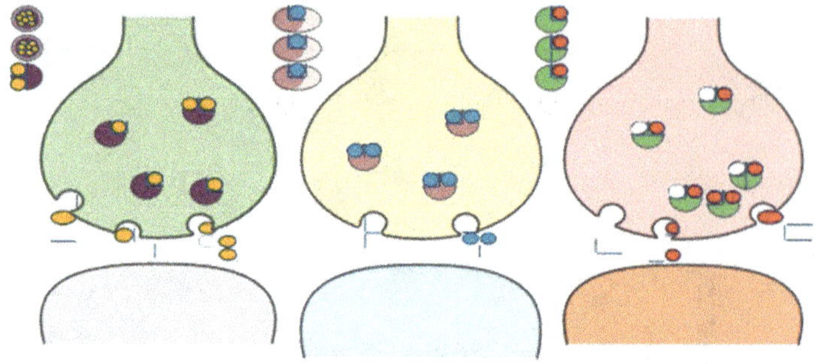

Figure 7.2. Schematic diagram of synaptic plasticity.

connected to Alzheimer's disease (AD). Persons/children who do regular exercise have a better mental capability to handle what they are faced with. Exercise allows us to protect ourselves from mental disorders as well as inevitable stress. Aerobic exercise increases the BDNF levels and amount of the anterior hippocampus, including the dentate gyrus (DG). The communication between brain and muscle has been improved by concurrent reviving of brain and muscle (Voss *et al* 2013). These conveying processes improve the mental benefits. The result of straightforward reviving of brain and muscle are detaching by reducing the movement of message in between them. These phenomena provide intuition into the importance of the conveying process. During the younger and aged brain, BDNF levels were increased by exercise in the hippocampus.

The impact of exercise was observed in highly plastic or transformable areas, responsive to environmental stimuli on BDNF (Neeper *et al* 1995). Tropomyosin receptor kinase B (TrkB) is used as a sense organ component for brain-derived neurotrophic factors. A fully-fledged structure of BDNF known as mBDNF was prepared from the proteolytic cleavage of a precursor protein, proBDNF. BDNF regulates dopaminergic, cholinergic, and GABAergic (gamma-aminobutyric acid) systems (Ding *et al* 2011). mBDNF has different responsibilities such as synaptogenesis inductor, participation in synaptic transmission, and acting on intracellular movement for small structures. In addition, it is found that skeletal muscle exercise regulates other genes of BDNF.

The above study provides information about how training factors are essential and the advantages of training in brain network configuration (Gard *et al* 2014). However, the impact of cognitive exercise and substantial action on neuronal plasticity is still an untouched area.

7.2 BDNF and hippocampal synaptic plasticity

The neurotrophic factor generated by the brain is called the brain-derived neurotrophic factor (BDNF). These factors help for the durability of nerve cells, production as well as proliferation. BDNF is involved in other ways of hippocampus based intellect. Hippocampal synaptic plasticity (figure 7.2) has played a different role in our outside bodies. Most of the time, synaptic plasticity was learned on BDNF. Synaptic plasticity is available in two ways inside a hippocampus, named as a long-term potentiation (LTP) and long-term depression (LTD). These two things were essential factors for long-lasting spatial memory. This study shows the presence of LTP and LTD in BDNF of fluently acting mice. Inside the body, synaptic plasticity was another form of BDNF, and the survival rate of synaptic plasticity was below 4 h. An item placed memory was damaged by $BDNF^{+/-}$ in a mouse, and provoked LTD with the help of item placed training and memory associated with the LTP was also missing. This chapter highlights the importance of the involvement of BDNF for spatial training via LTD and LTP.

$BDNF^{+/-}$ mice were considered for the study. After three weeks of being born, mice were isolated from their origin (Korte *et al* 1995). In our experiment, male mice were used alone. First, the mice were anaesthetised. After this process, an appropriate probe was placed inside the hippocampus, which is located inside the right hemisphere. After these arrangements, the electric signal generated by mice were recorded. During the recording, the mice are wandering freely inside the room. Note that the mice were placed inside the room one day before starting the experiments for acquiring the accurate signal.

In a CA1 region, we measured an excitatory synaptic movement for the same field excitatory postsynaptic potential (fEPSP). This obtained signal was amplified with the help of a differential amplifier. After amplification, it was converted into a digital signal via a data acquisition assembly. At each point, we measured five successive signals. These signals were measured at a 40 s time interval and taking the average of these measured signals. At the sixth point, observable work was applied, and synaptic movement was observed for 14 400 s. All the animals were observed at a baseline to check the reliability of the signal. Note that the deviation of the generated signal was not more than 10% of the baseline value.

To observe the spatial perception memory, we performed item placed perception phenomena. The research found that a direct connection is available between item placed work training and hippocampal LTD. In these types of exercise, two different and unique items were placed in front of the mouse in the recording room. After 10 min, both items were removed from the recording room. At this time, a potential was generated in the CA1 area of the mouse. This induced potential was observed. This process was repeated up to three times after a one-day interval. Item examination time was expressed in terms of total examination time (Clarke *et al* 2010). The collected data rested by t-test with a mean of 50%, and the significance level was settled to $P < 0.05$.

Hippocampal LTP was used to trigger the spatial reference memory. The cookie finding method was used to test the spatial reference memory test. Each animal was trained to find cookies hidden under the animal's bedding in this testing. Seven successive trials were used to prepare the animal. Two trials were performed in one day. One was performed in the evening, and another was conducted in the morning (Novkovic *et al* 2015). Time to find a goal was defined when the mouse found the cookies. The entire thing was recorded in a camera located in the room. The distance cover defines the spatial memory of mice by the mouse to the location of food. The recorded electrical signal was analysed by factorial analysis of variance called (ANOVA).

The result data shows that the holding of synaptic melancholy on BDNF is related to another configuration of plastic that needs to require a complex encryption structure. The result also indicates that the training ease LTD damaged in $BDNF^{+/-}$ was very poor in mice, closely joining a shortage in spatial recognition memory. Similarly, $BDNF^{+/-}$ mouse is damaged in spatial reference memory. The average velocity of WT mice and $BDNF^{+/-}$ was almost the same (Buchler *et al* 2011). The result indicates that the BDNF is necessary for the LTD activated by object place training and different pattern of stimulation. BDNF found in hippocampal synaptic plasticity was dependent on the frequency. It is unnecessary for all synaptic forms depending upon the BDNF, but BDNF was required for LTP. Theta burst simulation (TBS) and LTD generate LTP. Non-identical kinds of LTP and LTD are somehow joined to every hippocampus-based training category (Sakata *et al* 2013). With the help of LTP and LTD interplay, we can alter the synaptic information storage. It was needed to regulate the synaptic structure, and very little amount of BDNF was required.

7.3 Pillars of AD

There is no structure and dimension of the issue associated with memory. Memory loss problems are directly proportional to age. This problem is called Alzheimer's disease (AD). As we age, our thinking power goes down our memory steadily declines. In the US, AD secures the sixth position in the entire category of diseases. But according to the National Institute on Ageing it is in third position. Preservation of AD by pharmaceutical effort is undependable. Minimisation of AD by acceptable science and sense is a better way. Research has found that organised lifestyle and psychological well-being play a significant part in reducing AD. The concept behind reducing AD is to bring balance and a bond between brain cells, different people, and one's well-being. The current chapter provides a four-way strategy to reduce or reverse the effect of AD.

7.3.1 Pillar 1: diet and supplements

Preservation of AD strongly depends upon the diet. Because if you have a balanced diet, it changes your lifestyle, which is responsible for reducing AD. Many types of research prove that people who avoid processed meals and adopt natural food have minimal mental disorder. Performance rating of intellective phenomena was increased by affecting the different factors by use of substances present in a healthy diet. These factors defined synaptic plasticity, synaptic membrane fluidity, glucose utilisation, mitochondrial function, or reducing oxidative stress. There are lots of diet plans given by the different associations named as Alzheimer's Research and Prevention Foundation (ARPF) diet, Americanized versions of the Mediterranean diet, MIND (Mediterranean-DASH Intervention for Neurodegenerative Delay) and DASH (Dietary Approaches to Stop Hypertension) diets. Notice that all the diet plans given by the different associations have some typical food, which is as follows (Morris *et al* 2014):

1. **Vegetarian food:** Sometimes also called vegetable diet. These diet plans contain plant protein. Sources of these types of protein are fruits and vegetables, nuts and seeds, grains, etc.

2. **Juicing:** The primary sources of vitamins and minerals are juice. It improves brain functionality. It gives relief to the brain from stress by antioxidants present in it. In addition, the substance present in it controls the signal transmission between brain cells.
3. **Supplements:** Different associations advised that we can take multi-vitamins and multi-mineral based nutrients. Generally, we prefer to take omega-three oils-based supplements, which improve brain cell strength and performance.

7.3.2 Pillar 2: physical and mental exercise

The second way which plays an essential role in reducing the effect of Alzheimer's disease is physical and mental activity. Exercise enhances the circulation of blood from the heart to the brain. These factors increase the amount of BDNF. BDNF is responsible for the proliferation and differentiation of cells related to the brain (Kottke 1965). The dentate gyrus holds memory and thinking functionality, which is a significant part of the brain. Previous literature shows that if an elderly person performs running on a tread mill for 30 min three to four times per week, this increases the number of cells in the dentate gyrus part of the brain, improving brain functionality.

Similarly, brain functionality can improve by 9000 s of cardio exercise along with some strength exercise. Similarly to physical exercise, mental exercise improves the resistance power for preservation from AD. Mental exercise can be done via reading a book, listening to music, art drawing, playing Sudoku, doing crosswords, etc. All these things act as a stimulation source for brain cells.

7.3.3 Pillar 3: psychological well-being (PWB)

There is an indirect relationship establish between meditation and PWB (Boyle *et al* 2010). If we do meditation, it enhances several properties like the adaptability of self and others, increase of self-possession, reduction of negative thoughts, personal growth, and the primary important factor of providing a base for self-standing survivability. All these properties improve the PWB. Mental failure, cholesterol is reducing by this factor (Sheardova *et al* 2017). Previous research indicates that a well-known relationship is established between spirituality, cognitive health and ageing. The impact of AD can be reduced by a sharp mind as well as happy living life.

7.3.4 Pillar 4: yoga and meditation

The most significant factor for AD is heavy pressure on the mind; this phenomenon is called chronic stress. Chronic stress has a harmful effect on the genes, and people live an unhealthy life which is the starting point of AD. Chronic stress can be minimised by doing 720 s of yoga or meditation. This meditation was known as a kirtankriya (KK) (Newberg *et al* 2010). KK has a significant impact on improvement of mind. If we do KK daily, it boosts the blood flow to the anterior cingulate gyrus (ACG). This ACG is an essential part of the brain, which is responsible for the regulation of stress as well as emotions. The prefrontal cortex (PEC) was a necessary part of the brain. The PEC is the first part of the body affected by AD. Research shows that the dimension of PEC and ACG was increased after doing KK for 720 s a day for eight weeks (figure 7.3) (Hne 2014). The following advantages of KK are listed in table 7.1, and practical benefits are listed in table 7.2 (Yang *et al* 2016).

7.4 Different onsets of AD

The most common disease of the brain is memory loss, called Alzheimer disease (AD). AD affects the different parts of the brain, which is shown in figure 7.4. Generally, early-onset Alzheimer disease (EOAD) is identified by various general symptoms. EOAD can damage the properties of the eye and the functionality of memory. The area of AD is very complex and boundless in neurology. This chapter highlights the homogeneity and non-homogeneity between EOAD and late-onset AD (LOAD) based on medical parameters such as neuropsychology, neuropathology, genetics and neuroimaging. AD can considerably contribute to memory loss (Kaiser *et al* 2012). In some situations, AD can affect the different parts of the body and save the remembering capacity of memory. Detection of problems related to the temporal lobe and posterior hemisphere is the right choice for solving AD's problem. It is found that there is a difference between the psychological report of the brain of an average person and an AD-associated person. Comparing the saving of memory of EOAD and LOAD shows that memory saving is high in EOAD compared to LOAD. The research indicates that LOAD damages the memory more than EOAD, whether the event is recent or later, but LOAD dominates the memory most of the time. If we perform recognition of display naming test on EOAD and LOAD, we find that EOAD has more effect on naming tests as compared to LOAD.

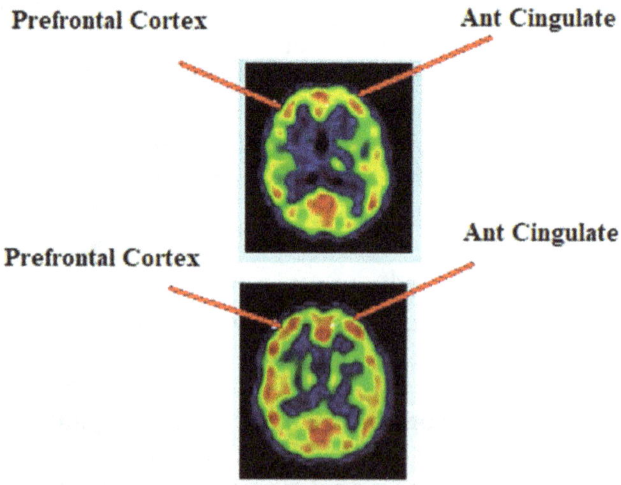

Figure 7.3. Impact of yoga/meditation on size of prefrontal cortex and ant cingulate.

Table 7.1. Property of kirtankriya.

Minimisation of stress	Increases sleeping capacity	Decreases memory failing
Boosts energy amount	Reduces depression	Increases PWB
Increases gene	Increasese blood flow in the targeted area	Minimises fear factor for AD

Table 7.2. Physical property of kirtankriya.

Require only 720 s	Equipment-less
Complex and costly learning	Fully safe

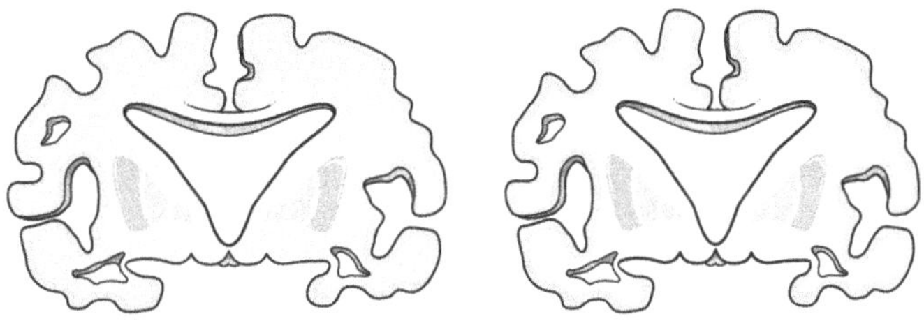

Figure 7.4. Alzheimer's diseases brain comparison. (a) Normal brain; (b) diseases brain.

EOAD has weak power to hold information in the mind for a short time compared to LOAD (Kalpouzos *et al* 2005). Maximum faults have been displayed in EOAD. EOAD provides good results for visuospatial functionality as compared to LOAD. Better results are shown by the EOAD patient for motor behaviours. If we compare the development of EOAD and LOAD for written language, executive function, attention, visuospatial abilities and motor skills, EOAD shows poor performance and LOAD shows good performance (van der Flier *et al* 2011).

From the sources of different studies, it was observed that EOAD outside of the temporal lobe was more significant than LOAD. Similarly, we find a non-typical value for other proteins such as amyoid beta, total tau protein, and phosphorylated tau protein (Ossenkoppele *et al* 2015). We get the same non-typical value for the above parameters. Different genes like CLU, CR1, PICALM, SORL1, BIN1, CTNNA3, GAB2, DNMBP, ABCA7, TREM2, and TOMM40 have been studied for LOAD. The Genome-Wide Association has done these studies. Memory damage and brain functionality can be measured by the advanced techniques known as computer tomography (CT) and magnetic resonance (MR). MR has a high-performance rating compared to CT for observation and evaluation of the cerebral part of the brain. Different studies have been done for the value of grey matter for EOAD and LOAD (Pievani *et al* 2013).

The pattern obtained for EOAD is in the field of awareness, controlling signal and speech. The comprehensive impairment study for the cerebral part has been

Table 7.3. Characteristics of EOAD and LOAD.

Parameter	LOAD	EOAD
Age of onset	Above 65	Below 65
From of onset	Memory loss	No memory loss
Progression	Slower	Faster
Neuropsychology	Poorer memory	Poorer executive function as well as motor skill
Structural MRI	Pattern obtained for hippocampal	Pattern obtain for frontal/temporal
PET-FDG	Lower metabolism in the medical temporal lobe	Lower metabolism in the temporoparietal cortex
PET C-PiB	Maximum	Maximum

performed on the same class of patients. EOAD shows more patterns for the dorsal striatum as compared to LOAD for the ventral striatum. Frontal functionality has been lower as compared to damage of memory in EOAD. More pattern has been observed in EOAD for grey and white matter. It was unable to find a pattern for LOAD in the hippocampal region. EOAD has more impact on the neocortical part of the brain. For subcortical as well as ptamen, EOAD shows more progression.

Neuroimaging techniques permit the doctor to examine the working of the brain. These techniques are positron emission tomography (PET) and F-fluorodeoxyglucose (FDG). These techniques allow measurement of glucose intake rate. Single positron emission tomography (SPET) is used to measure the image of blood flow to the brain. MRI is used to measure the source of impulses inside the brain. The pattern performance of LOAD for the temporal lobe is limited (Riverol and López 2011). More damage occurs for the neocortex in EOAD. EOAD group patients show more pattern for connectivity of the dorsolateral network. This response is the reverse for LOAD for the same situation (Gour *et al* 2014). From the above observation, we find that EOAD has some similarities and dissimilarities shown in table 7.3 (van der Flier *et al* 2011).

An EOAD patient is profoundly affected in memory function, visuospatial function and motor skills and minimum power loss. Density and amuloid plaques phenomena show more in EOAD as compared to LOAD. In addition, EOAD shows more progression, diffusion pattern and extension atrophy. PET and SPET for functional imaging were more dominant for EOAD.

7.5 Music and its influence on BDNF generation

Music can alter the biological system; sometimes, it is used to control the mood. Music can improve the status of psychological health. If we provide musical training to the brain from childhood, then it produces neuroplasticity. People who listen to Mozart Sonata K.448 have significant growth in a spatial-temporal part of the brain compared to other music (figure 7.5). Grey matter design has been linked by musical training in the ventral premotor cortex. It has been observed that music affects the spatial performance of an animal. The above finding represents that music has played a significant role in growing neuroplasticity in early growing stages. In synaptic plasticity, brain derived neurotropic factor (BDNF) and its receptor TrKB were responsible for the enlargement of memory in adult mammalian (Heldt *et al* 2007). BDNF factor was increased in hippocampal based work by the correlation. It can be observed that the signalling of BDNF/TrKB can be changed with the help of Mozart music during pregnancy in adult mice hippocampus (Chikahisa *et al* 2006). With the help of Morris water maze (MWM) work, we can measure the hippocampal training, which is crucial. This article observed the improvement of spatial memory by exposure to music. This work also focused on establishing a relationship between BDNF/TrKB of hippocampal sub-region and spatial memory.

An equal number of two classes has been created from the 30 randomly selected young rats. One lesson is subjected to music called Mozart Group (MG), and the second class is without music called control Group (CG). These young rats are moved to the cage, with proper humidity and temperature and twelve hours of light/dark cycle. The condition for placing rats is five rats per cage.

Music group rats were exposed to music for 12 h. Time for exposure of harmony is maintained between 8 AM and 8 PM. The music and ambient noise intensity were measured at 65–75 dB and 65 dB, respectively. Circular MWM pools were created by PVC plastic with the following dimensions: Walls height 50 cm and radius 65 cm. 26 °C water is placed inside the MWM up to 25 cm. four quadrants have been created in the pool nameda target, left, right and opposite quadrant. The collection is located in a sound separate testing room. Now the next task was that rats were placed inside the pool for 2 min and after that permitted to rest for 20 s. The rats were placed in his initial position in each trial and allowed to swim until the next platform was reached or 60-s swimming. The camera and WMT-200 software recorded the performance of rats in the pools. Latency time is defined as an interval of time between lowering the rats into the pool and moving to the next platform. Latency time was used to measure the spatial reference memory. SPSS software was used to measure the statistical analysis. General linear models have been used by

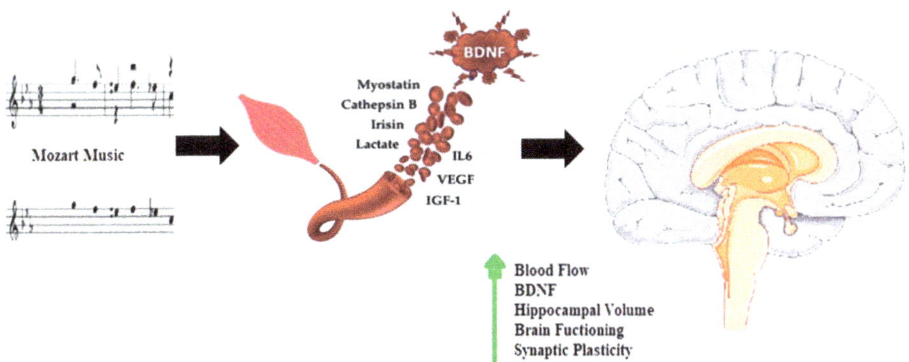

Figure 7.5. Effect of Mozart music on the functioning of brain.

variance (ANOVA) to measure latency time. Image pro-plus software was used to analyse the targeted part of immunohistochemistry (IHC). For calculating the amount of protein and positive cells in BDNF/TrKB, we use a one way ANOVA. To find out the significant changes in each group, we use the post hoc method and LSD method with a level of statical significance $P < 0.05$.

The result for latency (spatial memory performance) was decreased for MG and CG groups. There were severe changes obtained for both groups ($P < 0.01$). The performance of MG was better than CG. The relative optical density was directly proportional to the BDNF/TrKB (Angelucci *et al* 2007) expression level. BDNF protein in the dCA3 and dDG portions was higher for MG than for the CG group. The above result is the same for the dCA1 area.

Similarly, the amount of TrKB is higher for dCA3 and dDG portion for MG than CG. There is no significant change for TrKB in the dCA1 area for MG and CG. The value of BDNF/TrKB positive cells in MG is higher than CG for dCA3 and dDG regions.

The spatial learning and memory value was measured in the dorsal hippocampus (DH) by MWM and protein expression level. The result indicates that music significantly impacts spatial learning and BDNF/TrKB for the MG group compared to CG for dCA3 and dDG region, and no variation was found for the DCA1 region. A better result has been obtained for brain structure if we give training on higher learning sensitive period. Mozart K.448 and Schubert music significantly impact work associated with spatial-temporal (Nantais and Schellenberg 1999). The spatial score value in the presence of these two pieces of music has a higher magnitude than silence. The result also shows that music improves memory size. Recent studies indicate that the level of cell death can be reduced, and neurotrophic factors, neurogenesis, synaptogenesis, dendritic spine number, dendritic arborisation was boosted by the music. CA3 area of the brain was important for object-trace-odour work for measurement of spatial part. The above happened because common cells are present in between CA3 and CA1. The experimental result gives Mozart music importance for the regulation of neuronal plasticity, which boosts the spatial memory capability (Agster and Burwell 2013). Ventral hippocampal and other cortical areas of memory affected by the music are still an untouched area. Apart from these two kinds of music, other music forms can produce the same effect in humans, and other animals require more research.

7.5.1 Anxiolytic impact of music openness on BDNF

Brain-derived neurotrophic factor (BDNF) has a place with the neurotrophin family that plays a significant role in neuronic separation, endurance, and colligation versatility. BDNF ties to the tropomyosin receptor kinase B (TrkB), communicated in high focus inside the focal sensory system. It is accounted for that BDNF is concerned with the pathophysiology of temperament issues (Biffo *et al* 1995). In ongoing investigations, it has been found that BDNF might be a crucial part that aids in the balance of tension, disposition stabilisers, and temperament problems. BDNF Met/Met presented in transgenic mice showed expanded tension related practices that are uninvolved with serotonin, particular serotonin reuptake inhibitor inhibitors through BDNF lacking mice showed forcefulness and uneasiness dynamic yield to stressors. This connotes that BDNF is concerned with the balance of nervousness related issues. Partner degree SNP (single nucleotide polymorphism) in the BDNF cistron correlates with tension and discouragement problems. The human BDNF gene variant that results in an amendment from essential amino acid to a vital amino acid in prodomain of BDNF supermolecule in 66th position results in decreased activity-based secretion of BDNF and is said to increase conditions toward medical speciality disorders like bipolar disorder, anxiety-related disorder and depression (Kunugi *et al* 2001, Chen *et al* 2004). Anxiety is a feeling of a person once subjected to a unique setting that a genetic component may influence. Mice with BDNF Met/Met showed elevated pulse and mirrored increased anxiety level and indifferent response to antidepressants.

Music is found to be helpful in prompting emotional changes. It has been speculated that paying attention to music can cut anxiety levels. Melodic boosts in masses initiate different areas of the cerebrum that are identified with feelings. These regions epitomise the separate cortex, nerve centre, hippocampus, foremost cortex, and amygdala (Chikahisa *et al* 2006). The component of the anxiolytic effect of music stays dull. However, the music stimuli in young mice will increase the BDNF level but cannot manage the nerve growth factors in varied regions and the neural structure and hippocampus. It has been conjointly discovered that music exposure to prenatal mice will alter the brain's BDNF levels and intracellular signalling. Music exposure elicits the anxiolytic effect on BDNF Met/Met injected mice, as shown in figure 7.6. Anxiolytic studies had been carried out on mice with BDNF and without BDNF. It has been reported that there is no vital distinction in locomotive activity in each management and mice with BDNF; however, it has been discovered that there is anxiety behaviour. Experiments were perennial with music exposure, and results have shown reduced anxiety behaviour, specifically in mice with BDNF Met/Met.

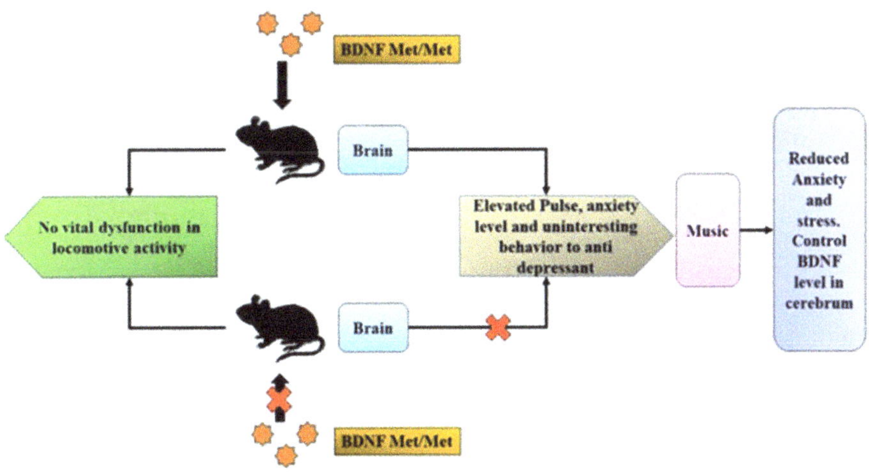

Figure 7.6. Music listening enhances cognitive recovery and mood after middle cerebral artery stroke.

Music openness does not exclusively regulate the BDNF courier RNA and protein levels in a few locales of the mind but conjointly improves the TrkB mRNA level inside the cerebrum. Many studies have suggested that exposure to music features a therapeutic intervention. Music exposure helps in reducing pain, stress, and anxiety levels in patients, pregnant women, people with traumatic brain injury, AD, etc (Li *et al* 2010).

During initial recovery weeks and months from stroke, the brain can bear substantial plastic changes that might be exaggerated by stimulation contributed by the setting. It has been determined that post-stroke motor and sensory system environmental enhancement, virtual environment, peripheral pricking, and electrical animal tissue are well-tried to help enhance motor recovery. Intermodal stimulation and visual, olfactory, and exteroception stimuli together with an enriched environment enhance psychological features and motor recovery better than an enriched environment alone (Maegele *et al* 2005). In various studies, it has been observed that an enriched sound environment promotes the higher functioning of auditory cortical functions and additionally learning and memory. Animal studies have shown that a stimulating and happy environment can boost the rate of brain healing after a stroke. Music stimulates the bilateral brain regions involved in memory, cognition, motor activities, emotional processing, and attention in humans. Music has been shown to improve cognitive function in both healthy and ill patients (Bhattacharya *et al* 2001).

Music is the most potentexteroception stimulation in the case of humans. Listening could be an advanced method for the brain that activates the psychological feature and emotional parts of distinct neural networks. Recent studies of brain imaging have shown that neural activity correlates with being attentive to music way on the far side of the cognitive cortical area, which involves an intensive bilateral network of parietal, frontal, temporal, and neural structure which are related to processing, memory, motor functions, and emotions processing (Janata *et al* 2002). Music listening additionally helps in reducing anxiety, pain, and stress levels in bodily diseases like dyslexia, AD, somatic diseases, coronary artery disease, sclerosis and traumatic brain damage. According to cognitive studies, exposure to music enhances communication skills in healthy people and clinical patients. In stroke rehabilitation, elements of music are used as physiotherapy to patients to improve their speech and motor functions. The brain's middle cerebral artery is responsible for music processing. It has been claimed that, in addition to stimulating emotional and cognitive networks, music also activates perilesional and healthy brain regions, which in general display heightened excitability and flexibility during the sensitive recovery phase, increasing and speeding up the recovery process. Listening to music with lyrics activates the brain bilaterally, which aids in the rehabilitation process after a unilateral stroke better than listening to only spoken material, which affects the left hemisphere, as shown in figure 7.7 (Khalfa *et al* 2002).

During the post-stroke healing phase, listening to musing regularly improves cognitive function and reduces depression. Music listening is linked to a more upbeat

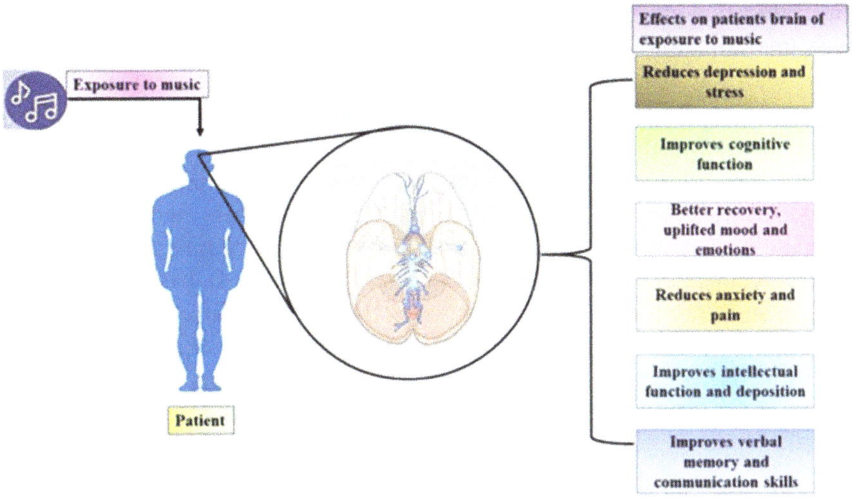

Figure 7.7. Music and speech listening enhance the recovery of early sensory processing after stroke.

and less gloomy mood, implying that it copes with the emotional stress brought on by psychological disease and hence aids recovery (Särkämö *et al* 2008).

The current circumstance is loaded with acoustic sound from various sources and containing superposition properties. It is an exceptionally complicated undertaking for the mind to sort out this scattered climate. It is a mind-boggling convention for the cerebrum to measure, store and screen an enormous measure of hearable data. Auricular tangible memory is an exact memory portrayal of the hearable climate, which is dependable for a few minutes and is the underlying advance in social event approaching data to the memory framework. It is significant for vocal perception and dynamic memory assignments where friendly hearable data is should have been handled throughout some undefined time frame (Cowan 1988). Hearable tangible memory capacities by change in the explicit ERP (integrity index of the cerebrum) part called MMN. Mismatch memory may be a prompt response to the resistance of associate degree exteroception constancy reminiscent of an unaccustomed modification in an acoustic feature of monotonous sound, generally returning ahead concerning 200 ms from the start of onset. Even when an individual is not responding to activity sounds neglecting accuracy, MMN is active and has sensible test–retest reliability. Thus, it is appropriate for the early auditory recovery of clinical patients (Kujala *et al* 2001).

Environmental incitement is an imperative angle in moulding our cerebrum. Creatures concentrated on revealed that advanced climate invigorates inciting plastic changes including biochemical boundaries, neurogenesis, stress alleviation, diminishing torment, further developing mastering and relational abilities. Steady openness to music actuates the broad neural organisation in the hearable cortex and upgrades learning, memory, and neuronal versatility in the mind (Van Praag *et al* 2000). Multimodal incitement additionally assists with working on intellectual and engine recuperation in harmed rodent cerebrums. Various creature studies have demonstrated that improving the climate and hearable incitement upgrades cerebrum recuperation and mind pliancy in different levels, improving hearable memory working, learning, and preparing. In people, complex hearable incitements like music showed an upgraded recuperation rate from mind harm. It has been seen that steady openness to music and discourse incitement in the recuperation stage after centre cerebral conduit stroke can improve intellectual capacity and disposition (Särkämö *et al* 2008). Music listening works on verbal memory and centred consideration recuperation better than an audiobook recording and non-tuning in, and prevented wretchedness and confused temperament. It has been proven that listening to music or an audiobook increases the rate of recuperation. Patients who listened to music or an audiobook in the clinic had a higher frequency of MMNm, or early sensory processing, intellectual, and mental functioning in the right cerebral half of the globe than patients not presented with any hearable incitement (Särkämö *et al* 2010).

7.6 Hyperhomocysteinemia and its influence on spatial memory

Improved degrees of homocysteine are connected with an expanded danger of Alzheimer's infection in elder people. Hyperhomocysteinemia and dementia are the reason and signs of AD. A trial was performed with hyperhomocysteinemic rodents utilising MWM to investigate spatial memory of rodents in hippocampal DG LTP in sedative rats. It has been accounted for that hyperhomocysteinemia debilitates spatial memory and long-term potential (LTP) in the rodent hippocampus. The synapsin I, a synapsin vesicle protein that is answerable for synapse discharge, is diminished in hyperhomocysteinemic rodents. Hypercysteinemia essentially reduces the declaration of N-Methyl D-Aspartate receptor and postsynaptic density 95 protein (Jiang 2011).

Most of the populace over 65 are susceptible to dementia. Dementias altogether influence scholarly abilities overall and now and again gradually influences language as it were. Essential Progressive Aphasia (PPA) is frontotemporal cerebrum brokenness that separates itself from various perspectives, including the diminished potential to measure and produce syntactically correct sentences, defective understanding abilities, or failures of memory to review word meaning. This makes it incapable of reviewing words in discussion and settling on choices to describe items and pictures. In ongoing investigations, it has been seen that the phonologically based methodology is gainful for no expressive aphasia while the clarification-based methodology benefits explicit aphasia patients. A semantically based methodology helped patients in further developing learning and aided in forestalling mistakes while learning. It additionally has been demonstrated that intercession likewise further develops relational abilities in patients with dementia with dependable and quantifiable impacts in mind (Jokel *et al* 2011).

Post-stroke cognitive impairment (PSCI) shows distinctively in various periods of stroke. Structuring the administration of stroke forecast of longitudinal intellectual execution assumes a significant part. Patients with PSCI have been seen with more noteworthy pre-stroke hypersensitivity (Kandiah *et al* 2011). Schizophrenia is connected with composite inadequacy of neuroscholarly working, including learning, consideration, memory, leader working, and scholarly handling work. Intellectual harm is an known component of schizophrenia that is available at the beginning of affliction and remains in patient manifestations changes. Intellectual harm is regularly an impediment to social recuperation and visualises dull, clinical results in schizophrenia patients (Bilder *et al* 2000).

BDNF has a place with the neurotrophin family, which is one of the classes of development factors. Mind inferred neurotrophic factors assume an indispensable part in movement subordinate neuroplasticity liable for principal learning and memory in the hippocampus (Poo 2001). In various animal studies, it had been accounted for that hindrance of BDNF emission by influencing the elevation of antisense BDNF thwarts spatial learning and memory. BDNF assumes a vital part in both long-term potentiation and late-stage potentiation. It has been revealed that BDNF levels are very low in patients experiencing scholarly decay related issues, including Alzheimer's sickness, gentle intellectual harm, and Huntington's disease. Conversely, a higher convergence of BDNF is related to better neurophysiological execution in these illnesses. In addition, flowing BDNF is a biomarker of memory and general scholarly movement in human adults (Komulainen *et al* 2008).

In an investigation of repeatable battery for assessing physiological status (RBANS) and serum BDNF in schizophrenia patients versus wellbeing controls, the BDNF levels are observed to be altogether lower in patients than in sound people. Scholarly or intellectual scores in every one of the five sublevels are essentially lower in patients with the exception of visuospatial and constructional files than in ordinary sound controls. BDNF was observed to be related to quick memory and engaged with the pathophysiology of schizophrenia (Tan *et al* 2005, Zhang *et al* 2012).

7.7 Speech and language disorder

Discourse and language are normal formative challenges in adolescence. It very well may be regarded as a secondary difficulty, i.e., it is accounted for by essential conditions like a chemical imbalance, hearing, weakness, general formative challenges, social or passionate hardships or neurological harm and not attributed to some condition other than as essential troubles (Law *et al* 1999). On average, 6% of kids have discourse and language challenges with a critical extent of primary difficulty. By and large, there is an overlapping of immediate trouble with deferred/disorder. This overlapping of primary difficulties and deferred/disorders are heterogenous. These challenges are determined or transient and are available as cluttered discourse, language, expressive or responsive language hardships, or a combination. There are not many examinations about the cause of essential language delay/disorder (Whitehurst *et al* 1991).

In several cases, studies revealed having joined entirely different parts incorporating otitis hereditary elements, financial difficulties, physiological condition difficulties and oral motor. Primary speech and language difficulties are a major concern to those working in child development and have research implications for child–parent cases that may have an adverse result on college achievements or social, emotional and activity problems (Aram and Nation 1980). These difficulties continue in youngsters for a long time, relying upon individual family and society they could be long-term or short-term.

Primary speech and language intervention may take different forms:

1. Didactical (direct coaching of linguistic behaviour).
2. Naturalistic (teaching the child to reply effectively to the linguistic demands on the environment).
3. Hybrid (a combination of didactical and naturalistic) (Law *et al* 2000).

7.8 Effect of BDNF dis-regulation on polymorphism

The effect of APOE (apolipoprotein E) and BDNF (brain-derived neurotrophic factor) Val66Mat polymorphisms, either individually or together, with older individual cognitive function is reported here. In some previous investigations, non-pathological cognitive function disruption does not always occur due to APOE polymorphisms (Jorm *et al* 2007). Furthermore, hippocampal morphology is also affected by BDNF polymorphisms and their function, and its association with cognitive function has not been found. Hippocampal morphology impairment and accumulation of abnormal AD-like pathology is observed in the case of APOE ε4 inheritance (Espeseth *et al* 2008, Ready *et al* 2011). On the other hand, APOE ε2 inheritors have neurological benefits and protection against AD-like accumulation (Suri *et al* 2013). Some study suggests a lower cognitive function in APOE ε4 allele inherited individual. Similarly, BDNF is one of the primary growth factors responsible for neuron growth, viability and maintenance. Met variant of the Val66Met human polymorphism is thought to be accountable for reducing BDNF secretion at the synapse, leading to decreased hippocampal volume (Bath and Lee 2006). Reports on the effects of BDNF polymorphism on cognitive memory have a contradictory view (Gong *et al* 2012, Laing *et al* 2012), as shown in figure 7.8.

For these studies, 433 healthy older adults were selected between 50 and 79 years. They were subjected to comprehensive neuropsychological assessments to measure episodic memory (EM), executive function, language processing and walking memory. Three main hypotheses were examined in this paper. First, APOE ε2 is responsible for better cognitive function, whereas APOE ε4 is associated with inferior cognitive function. The second is that Val homozygotes of BDNF are important and strongly linked with cognitive function compared to Met carriers. The third and last hypothesis is that combining the effect of APOE ε2/BDNF Val carriers has the highest cognitive function, and APOE ε4/BDNF Met carrier has the lowest. The participants did not have dementia and its side effects and were in good physical and psychological condition (Ward *et al* 2014).

Out of the 433 participants, 11 participants had APOE ε2/ε4 genotype so they were excluded from the study. Genotype data suggested an APOE genotype distribution of 11.11% ε2 carrier, 32.5% ε4 carrier and 56.4% ε3 homozygote. The BDNF Val66Mat genotype allele distribution was 33% Met carrier and 67% Val

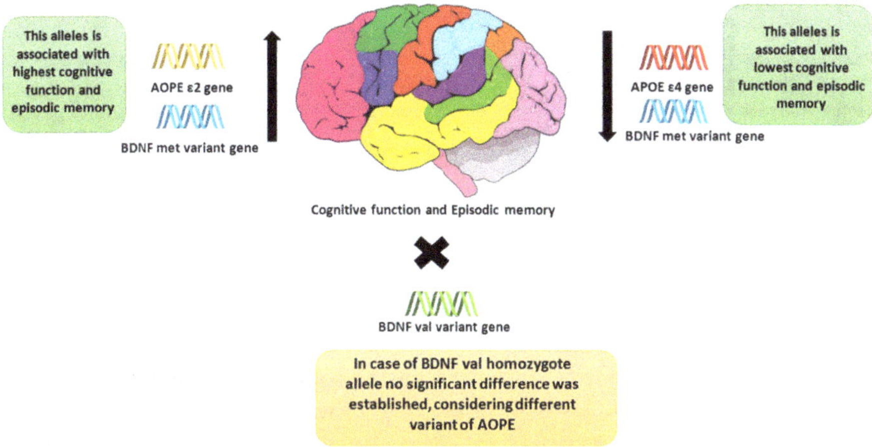

Figure 7.8. Influence of APOE and BDNF polymorphism on cognitive function.

homozygote. Using univariate ANCOVAs, the significance between BDNF gene and education year was measured, and it was found that the number of years in education was higher in the case of BDNF Met carrier than in BDNF Val homozygotes. When both APOE and BDNF were considered, the education covariates showed a considerable relationship with each cognitive domain, while the age covariate was related with a few. The univariate ANCOVA did not show any enormous consequences for the mental environment when the qualities were taken autonomously. When examining gene–gene interaction using ANCOVA was done, significant APOE and BDNF effect was found for EM. When only BDNF Val homozygotes were considered, there was no difference in EM resulting from both variances of APOE. But in the case of BDNF Met carriers, a significant relationship was found between APOE genotype and the EM scores. The least squares deference post-hoc found that APOE ε2 and BDNF Met carriers had more EM scores than APOE ε4 carriers or homozygotes ε3 (Ward *et al* 2014).

Their first and second hypotheses predicted that both the different genotypes individually affecting the cognitive function were not proved, but their third hypothesis was partially supported where APOE ε4/BDNF Met alleles are connected with the lowest mean EM performance. However, higher activity was found in the case of APOE ε2/BDNF Met carrier. The predicted EM performance in variation APOE gene was found to be only variable in the case of BDNF Met allele (Ward *et al* 2014).

Beta-amyloid (Aβ) accumulation results in memory decline and leads to AD (Villemagne *et al* 2013). This paper examined the role of APOE (apolipoprotein E)ε4 + and ε4- as well as BDNF Val homozygote and Met carrier in moderating Aβ associated memory decline.

This study aims to find out the potential interaction and relation between Aβ, APOE and BDNF polymorphism. Aβ neuroimaging was done on 333 healthy adults

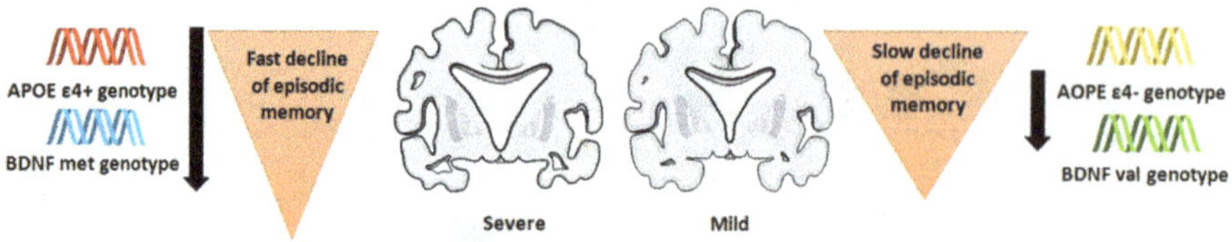

Figure 7.9. Influence of APOE and BDNF polymorphism in response to β—an amyloid accumulation (preclinical Alzheimer).

having a mean age of 70 years. The neuropsychological test was conducted at 18, 36, and 54 months (Lim *et al* 2015).

Individuals having Aβ+ ε4+ showed a faster cognitive decline over 54 months when compared to Aβ- ε4- across all domains. However, Aβ+ ε4- individuals only decrease verbal episodic memory (EM) (Lim *et al* 2015). In addition, no significant difference was found between Aβ- ε4- and Aβ- ε4+ groups (Lee *et al* 2012, Verghese *et al* 2013).

Participants showing ε4+/BDNF Met genotype among the Aβ+ individuals have a significantly faster language, verbal and visual EM decline compared to ε4-/BDNF Val/Val, over the 54 months. This finding states that at least two genetic loci are associated with Aβ related cognitive decline (Lim *et al* 2015). Aβ+ ε4+/BDNF Met individuals are expected to have significant clinical memory decline by three years, however, for Aβ+ ε4+/BDNF Val it will take around ten years to achieve this degree of impairment (Lim *et al* 2015). Aβ- and Aβ+ ε4- groups, including both the BDNF gene individuals, had shown very little memory impairment over the 54 months (as shown in figure 7.9). High Aβ accumulation suggests the start of pre-clinical AD, but the variation also indicates that other factors play a role. These results suggest that the APOE ε4 allele is a significant genetic risk factor (Jedynak *et al* 2012).

Individual carrier ε4 APOE alleles having low Aβ accumulation have no significant memory impairment, which indicates that both ε4 alleles, as well as higher Aβ accumulation, is responsible for memory decline (Hudry *et al* 2013).

Some studies reported that reduction of BDNF is significantly associated with major depression disorder in patients (MDD), which makes BDNF a biomarker for MDD (Duman and Monteggia 2006, Castrén *et al* 2007). Therefore, the objective of this study is to find out the association of BDNF levels at periphery upon anxiety and depression-like behaviour, along with chronic unpredictable stress (CUS)/anhedonia (Yalcin *et al* 2008), elevated plus maze (EPM), forced swim test (FST) (Duman *et al* 2007) and novelty induced hypophagia (NIH). In addition, hippocampal neurogenesis, extracellular signal-regulated kinase (ERK) and CAMP response element-binding protein (CREB) were examined to identify any antidepressant-like role of BDNF on the brain.

To fulfil this objective, recombinant BDNF was administrated peripherally to C57BL/6 and BALB/C mice, male (8–10 weeks), with the help of an osmotic mini-pump subcutaneously over a period of 14 days. BALB/C mice were used for CUS, and for the rest of the experiment, C57BL/6 was used (Schmidt and Duman 2010). The decrease in immobility during the FST session gives the efficiency of the antidepressants. So, the immobile time spent by the mice after receiving different peripheral BDNF doses was measured and using one-way ANOVA, it was imparted that there is a significant effect of the treatment. Reduction in latency in drinking alleviated milk in NIH depicts the involvement of chronic antidepressants; that is why this was used to measure the effect of regular antidepressants in the case of administrated BDNF (Dulawa *et al* 2004). A two-way ANOVA showed a significant relationship between the treatment and condition.

Chronic administration of antidepressants induces behavioural deficits on the CUS model upon sucrose consumption (Willner 1997). This phenomenon was used to see the effect of BDNF administration, and an ANOVA analysis (two-way) gave remarkable interaction between therapy and stress. In response to the antidepressant proliferation of neurons in the adult hippocampus, it depends on BDNF-TrkBsignalling (Li *et al* 2008). So, to decide the impact of administrated BDNF on the growth of the neurons, BrdU was also given. All Brdu+ cells were taken into computation, at the prefrontal cortex and dentate gyrus, of the mice administered with BDNF (Banasr and Duman 2007). No difference was found in cell numbers between BDNF administrated subjects and controls. But survival rate of immature neurons was significantly increased after BDNF treatment.

The ERK and CREB proteins levels were determined using western blot analysis of hippocampus, and β-actin was taken as control protein. After administering peripheral BDNF significant increase in the ERK and CREB (along with their active form) levels was revealed using an unpaired t-test. So, in general, in FST, increased mobility was observed after administration of peripheral BDNF; not only that, but effects of CUS were reduced upon sucrose consumption; NIH test showed decreased latency and increased time spent in EPM. Furthermore, peripheral BDNF administration also increased hippocampal neurogenesis and elevated pCREB and pERK expression in adult mice (as shown in figure 7.10). All this observation suggests that administration of peripheral BDNF has a similar effect to administration of antidepressants. To conclude, the results and observations from this paper indicate that BDNF is a biomarker for MDD; it is also useful for behaviour and neurogenesis (Schmidt and Duman 2010).

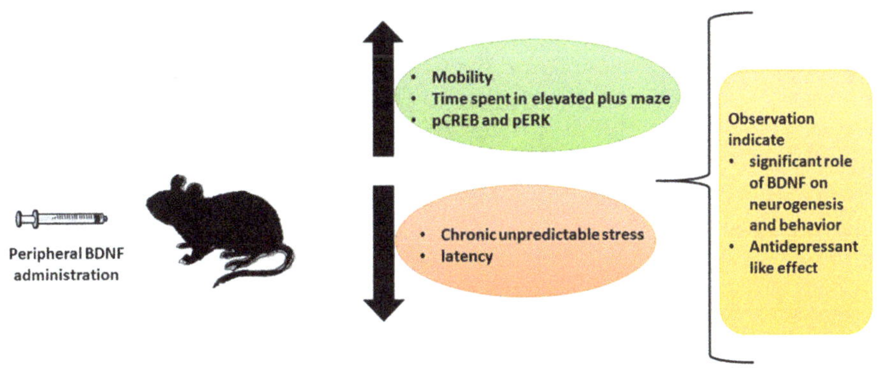

Figure 7.10. Effects of peripheral BDNF administration in cellular and behavioural models.

Motor experience and motor training can start physiological pliancy in the essential motor cortex. Transcranial magnetic stimulation (TMS) helps identify and understand the changes occurring in the motor cortex, like enhancing corticospinal output and reorganising movement representation, due to motor training (Pascual-Leone *et al* 1995, Classen *et al* 1998). The objective of this study is to compare the intensity of these cortex plasticities due to motor training in subjects having val66met polymorphism in the BDNF gene (Egan *et al* 2003, Klintsova *et al* 2004), with issues having normal BDNF gene with the help of TMS. They discovered no essential contrast in the corticospinal yield or motor map region in Val and Met subjects. Be that as it may, after a concise motor training period, the corticospinal yield was improved, and the map region was expanded generally in Val/Val when contrasted with Val/Met or Met/Met people (Kleim *et al* 2006).

These results suggest that Val/Mat and Mat/Mat BDNF genotype individuals may not differ in their basal state from the Val/Val BDNF genotype, but they respond differently towards behaviorally driven neural activity. Met polymorphism shows a reduction in neural activity due to stimulation. This study also supports *in vitro* studies previously done by others, which indicates that the BDNF Met allele does not influence BDNF emission, yet they have diminished BDNF discharge in light of neuronal incitement when contrasted with the typical BDNF Val allele (Kleim *et al* 2006).

It is known that BDNF inhibits food intake, and disruption in its level have been shown to increase food intake and obesity in rodent models (Snider 1994, Rios *et al* 2001). This study reports an 8-year-old girl mainly suffering from hyperactivity, hyperphagia, impaired cognitive function and severe obesity. This individual was found to have a nucleotide chromosomal inversion, 46, XX, inv (II) (p13p15.3), in the place which is believed to have the BDNF gene (Gül *et al* 2002, Borg *et al* 2005).

At the time of birth, the patient faced breathing abnormalities and started gaining weight from the age of 4 months; they also had delayed speech and language development. The patient had extreme hyperactivity from early childhood. The hyperphagia was also confirmed by 18-MJ ad minimum of two meals given after fasting overnight. The patient had fasting hyperinsulinemia but had average blood glucose and had normal thyroid function, lipid profile, and insulin-like growth factor-1 concentration. She showed general impairment of IQ, which is comparable to TrkB mutation (Gray *et al* 2006).

The genotype of the patient for the BNDF was heterozygous with Val66Met polymorphism. However, in the peripheral lymphocytes, monoallelic expression of the BDNF gene was observed. The BDNF concentration in serum was less compared with other BMI matched subjects (Gray *et al* 2006). This haploinsufficiency for BDNF was also responsible for increased food consumption, hyperactivity, acute obesity and cognitive disorder. This case proves the association of BDNF protein with the body's homeostasis and cognitive function (Friedel *et al* 2005). It was checked that the platelets count of the individual did not justify the lower concentration of BDNF in serum; that is the only factor that impacts serum levels of BDNF in the subject (El-Gharbawy *et al* 2006).

7.9 Case study

Previous studies have shown that language recovery is enhanced using tDCS (transcranial direct current stimulation) (Flöel *et al* 2008, Baker *et al* 2010). In addition, it has been suggested that the level of BDNF might have a role to play in the mechanism involved in the working of tDCS on synaptic connectivity (Pilc 2010). But all of these language studies are conducted using unihemispheric stimulation.

This study investigates the effect of tDCS on the bihemispheric of aphasic patients' language recovery and checks the difference in the amount of different BNDF serum levels. For this study, seven aphasic persons participated in intensive language therapy (Gersner *et al* 2011). The conduction of the therapy was done in two different conditions, first the actual bihemispheric stimulation over the left and right Broca's area and a sham condition (Marangolo *et al* 2014).The observation in the stimulated participant showed repossession of three different dialect tasks: picture description, verb and noun naming, significantly. However, in sham conditions, the results were not significant (Marangolo *et al* 2014). Furthermore, after the tDCS stimulation, no significant difference was found in the BDNF level (Gedge *et al* 2012).

However, a useful relationship was established between BDNF level and verb naming task results in real stimulation conditions. Therefore, this study concludes that the bihemispherict DCS method may act as a potential method to recover language in chronic aphasia (Marangolo *et al* 2014), as shown in figure 7.11.

This review aims to determine the effectiveness of the speech and language intervention method, in children and adolescents, for primary speech and language delay using systematical randomised controlled trials (RCTs). To perform the statical analysis, various relevant articles were considered and different essential databases like the Cochrane Controlled Trials Register, EMBASE, MEDLINE, etc. Only children or adolescents were considered for this study; the oldest participants were fifteen-year-old (Law *et al* 2007). Children whose problem was because of stuttering or were described as learned disarticulation were excluded from this study. In addition, any intervention responsible for the functioning of either expressive or

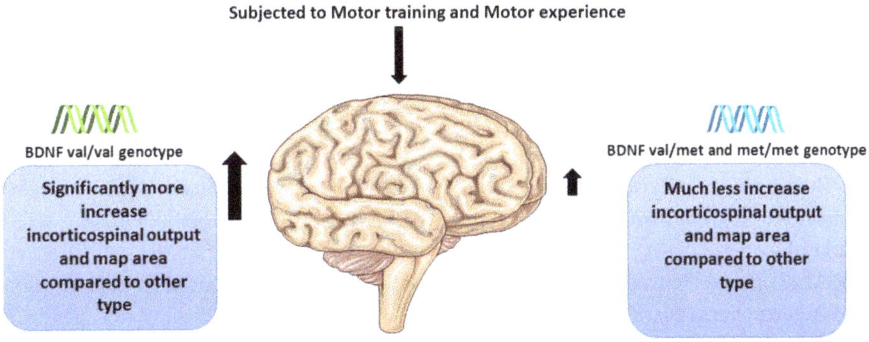

Figure 7.11. Response to motor training in a subject having different BDNF polymorphism.

receptive phonology or expressive or receptive syntax was considered (Law *et al* 2000).

Mainly three types of comparisons were investigated, first intervention comparison to healthy children undergoing delayed treatment or with no treatment condition. Secondly, intervention compared to healthy children who are provided with cognitive therapy or speech and language therapy treatment, which does not focus on the area of interest of the study. Third, intervention is compared with traditional treatment approaches in speech and language therapy (where intervention is considered experimental treatment). For example, stimulation is given by parents versus clinicians.

The overall outcome measurement was done in three different levels. First, considering the target for intervention which improved the targeted speech. Secondly, overall language functioning and phonological language maturity were considered. Finally, the broader language functioning, in which parents informed the betterment of language, also included (Law *et al* 2003). A total of 25 studies were used for this analysis. The results suggest that children with vocabulary or phonological difficulties had effective speech and language therapy outcomes. But in the case of children with continuous problems effectiveness of the interventions was not established. Regarding expression syntax intervention, the mixed finding was reported. Results for administered intervention by a clinician or trained parents had no significant difference. Similarly, no significant difference was found between group and individual intervention (Law *et al* 2003).

References

Agster K L and Burwell R D 2013 Hippocampal and subicular efferents and afferents of the perirhinal, postrhinal, and entorhinal cortices of the rat *Behav. Brain Res.* **254** 50–64

Angelucci F *et al* 2007 Investigating the neurobiology of music: brain-derived neurotrophic factor modulation in the hippocampus of young adult mice *Behav. Pharmacol.* **18** 491–6

Aram D M and Nation J E 1980 Preschool language disorders and subsequent language and academic difficulties *J. Commun. Disorders* **13** 159–70

Baker J M, Rorden C and Fridriksson J 2010 Using transcranial direct-current stimulation to treat stroke patients with aphasia *Stroke* **41** 1229–36

Banasr M and Duman R S 2007 Regulation of neurogenesis and gliogenesis by stress and antidepressant treatment *CNS Neurol. Disord. Drug Targets* **6** 311–20

Bath K G and Lee F S 2006 Variant BDNF (Val66Met) impact on brain structure and function *Cogn. Affect. Behav. Neurosci.* **6** 79–85

Bhattacharya J, Petsche H and Pereda E 2001 Interdependencies in the spontaneous EEG while listening to music *Int. J. Psychophysiol.* **42** 287–301

Biffo S, Offenhauser N, Carter B D and Barde Y A 1995 Selective binding and internalisation by truncated receptors restrict the availability of BDNF during development *Development* **121** 2461–70

Bilder R M *et al* 2000 Neuropsychology of first-episode schizophrenia: initial characterisation and clinical correlates *Am. J. Psych.* **157** 549–59

Borg K, Stankiewicz P, Bocian E, Kruczek A, Obersztyn E, Lupski J R and Mazurczak T 2005 Molecular analysis of a constitutional complex genome rearrangement with 11 breakpoints involving chromosomes 3, 11, 12, and 21 and a ~ 0.5-Mb submicroscopic deletion in a patient with mild mental retardation *Human Genet.* **118** 267–75

Boyle P A *et al* 2010 Effect of a purpose in life on risk of incident Alzheimer disease and mild cognitive impairment in community-dwelling older persons *Arch. Gen. Psych.* **67** 304–10

Buchler N G *et al* 2011 Effects of repetition on associative recognition in young and older adults: item and associative strengthening *Psychol. Aging* **26** 111–26

Castrén E, Võikar V and Rantamäki T 2007 Role of neurotrophic factors in depression *Curr. Opin. Pharmacol.* **7** 18–21

Chen Z Y, Patel P D, Sant G, Meng C X, Teng K K, Hempstead B L and Lee F S 2004 Variant brain-derived neurotrophic factor (BDNF)(Met66) alters the intracellular trafficking and activity-dependent secretion of wild-type BDNF in neurosecretory cells and cortical neurons *J. Neurosci.* **24** 4401–11

Chikahisa S *et al* 2006 Exposure to music in the perinatal period enhances learning performance and alters BDNF/TrkB signaling in mice as adults *Behav. Brain Res.* **169** 312–19

Chikahisa S, Sei H, Morishima M, Sano A, Kitaoka K, Nakaya Y and Morita Y 2006 Exposure to music in the perinatal period enhances learning performance and alters BDNF/TrkB signaling in mice as adults *Behav. Brain Res.* **169** 312–19

Clarke J R *et al* 2010 Plastic modifications induced by object recognition memory processing *Proc. Natl Acad. Sci. USA* **107** 2652–7

Classen J, Liepert J, Wise S P, Hallett M and Cohen L G 1998 Rapid plasticity of human cortical movement representation induced by practice *J. Neurophysiol.* **79** 1117–23

Cowan N 1988 Evolving conceptions of memory storage, selective attention, and their mutual constraints within the human information-processing system *Psychol. Bullet.* **104** 163

Ding Q, Ying Z and Gómez-Pinilla F 2011 Exercise influences hippocampal plasticity by modulating brain-derived neurotrophic factor processing *Neuroscience* **192** 773–80

Dulawa S C, Holick K A, Gundersen B and Hen R 2004 Effects of chronic fluoxetine in animal models of anxiety and depression *Neuropsychopharmacol.* **29** 1321–30

Duman R S and Monteggia L M 2006 A neurotrophic model for stress-related mood disorders *Biol. Psychiatry* **59** 1116–27

Duman C H, Schlesinger L, Kodama M, Russell D S and Duman R S 2007 A role for MAP kinase signaling in behavioral models of depression and antidepressant treatment *Biol. Psychiatry* **61** 661–70

Egan M F *et al* 2003 The BDNF val66met polymorphism affects activity-dependent secretion of BDNF and human memory and hippocampal function *Cell* **112** 257–69

El-Gharbawy A H, Adler-Wailes D C, Mirch M C, Theim K R, Ranzenhofer L, Tanofsky-Kraff M and Yanovski J A 2006 Serum brain-derived neurotrophic factor concentrations in lean and overweight children and adolescents *J. Clin. Endocrinol. Metab.* **91** 3548–52

Enderby P and Emerson J 1996 Speech and language therapy: does it work? *Brit. Med. J.* **312** 1655–8

Espeseth T, Westlye L T, Fjell A M, Walhovd K B, Rootwelt H and Reinvang I 2008 Accelerated age-related cortical thinning in healthy carriers of apolipoprotein E ε4 *Neurobiol. Aging* **29** 329–40

Flöel A, Rösser N, Michka O, Knecht S and Breitenstein C 2008 Noninvasive brain stimulation improves language learning *J. Cogn. Neurosci.* **20** 1415–22

Friedel S *et al* 2005 Mutation screen of the brain derived neurotrophic factor gene (BDNF): identification of several genetic variants and association studies in patients with obesity, eating disorders, and attention-deficit/hyperactivity disorder *Am. J. Med. Genet.* B **132** 96–9

Gard T *et al* 2014 Fluid intelligence and brain functional organisation in aging yoga and meditation practitioners *Front. Aging Neurosci.* **6** 1–12

Gedge L, Beaudoin A, Lazowski L, du Toit R, Jokic R and Milev R 2012 Effects of electroconvulsive therapy and repetitive transcranial magnetic stimulation on serum brain-derived neurotrophic factor levels in patients with depression *Front. Psych.* **3** 12

Gersner R, Kravetz E, Feil J, Pell G and Zangen A 2011 Long-term effects of repetitive transcranial magnetic stimulation on markers for neuroplasticity: differential outcomes in anesthetized and awake animals *J. Neurosci.* **31** 7521–6

Gong P, Zheng Z, Chi W, Lei X, Wu X, Chen D, Zhang K, Zheng A, Gao X and Zhang F 2012 An association study of the genetic polymorphisms in 13 neural plasticity-related genes with semantic and episodic memories *J. Mol. Neurosci.* **46** 352–61

Gour N *et al* 2014 Functional connectivity changes differ in early and late-onset Alzheimer's disease *Human Brain Mapping* **35** 2978–94

Gray J *et al* 2006 Hyperphagia, severe obesity, impaired cognitive function, and hyperactivity associated with functional loss of one copy of the brain-derived neurotrophic factor (BDNF) gene *Diabetes* **55** 3366–71

Gül D, Oğur G, Tunca Y and Ozcan O 2002 Third case of WAGR syndrome with severe obesity and constitutional deletion of chromosome (11)(p12p14) *Am. J. Med. Genet.* **107** 70–1

Heldt S A *et al* 2007 Hippocampus-specific deletion of BDNF in adult mice impairs spatial memory and extinction of aversive memories *Mol. Psychiatry* **12** 656–70

Hne T K 2012 Great men and large numbers: undertheorising a history of mass killing *Contemp. Euro. Hist.* **21** 133–43

Hudry E *et al* 2013 Gene transfer of human Apoe isoforms results in differential modulation of amyloid deposition and neurotoxicity in mouse brain *Sci. Transl. Med.* **5** 212ra161

Janata P, Tillmann B and Bharucha J J 2002 Listening to polyphonic music recruits domain-general attention and working memory circuits *Cogn. Affect. Behav. Neurosci.* **2** 121–40

Jedynak B M, Lang A, Liu B, Katz E, Zhang Y, Wyman B T, Raunig D, Jedynak C P, Caffo B and Prince J LAlzheimer's Disease Neuroimaging Initiative 2012 A computational neurodegenerative disease progression score: method and results with the Alzheimer's disease neuroimaging initiative cohort *Neuroimage* **63** 1478–86

Jiang X 2011 P4-145: Hyperhomocysteinemia impairs spatial memory and inhibits long-term potentiation (LTP) by modulation synapse-associated proteins in rat brain *Alzheimer's Dement.* **7** S754

Jokel R, Anderson N, Black S, Rochon E, Freedman M, Chow T and Tang-Wai D 2011 P4-146: neuroplasticity in dementia following langauge intervention: illusion of possibliity *Alzheimer's Dement.* **7** S754–5

Jorm A F, Mather K A, Butterworth P, Anstey K J, Christensen H and Easteal S 2007 APOE genotype and cognitive functioning in a large age-stratified population sample *Neuropsychology* **21** 1

Kaiser N C *et al* 2012 Neuropsychological and neuroimaging markers in early versus late-onset Alzheimer's disease *Am. J. Alzheimer Dis. Other Dement.* **27** 520–9

Kalpouzos G *et al* 2005 Working memory and FDG-PET dissociate early and late onset Alzheimer disease patients *J. Neurol.* **252** 548–58

Kandiah N, Ting Y, Wiryasaputra L, Chew I and Yih-Yian S 2011 Deep subcortical white matter disease is a major risk factor for late post stroke cognitive impairment *Alzheimer. Dement.* **4** S755–6

Khalfa S, Isabelle P, Jean-Pierre B and Manon R 2002 Event-related skin conductance responses to musical emotions in humans *Neurosci. Lett.* **328** 145–9

Kleim J A, Chan S, Pringle E, Schallert K, Procaccio V, Jimenez R and Cramer S C 2006 BDNF val66met polymorphism is associated with modified experience-dependent plasticity in human motor cortex *Nat. Neurosci.* **9** 735–7

Klintsova A Y, Dickson E, Yoshida R and Greenough W T 2004 Altered expression of BDNF and its high-affinity receptor TrkB in response to complex motor learning and moderate exercise *Brain Res.* **1028** 92–104

Komulainen P, Pedersen M, Hänninen T, Bruunsgaard H, Lakka T A, Kivipelto M, Hassinen M, Rauramaa T H, Pedersen B K and Rauramaa R 2008 BDNF is a novel marker of cognitive function in ageing women: the DR's EXTRA Study *Neurobiol. Learn. Mem.* **90** 596–603

Korte M *et al* 1995 Hippocampal long-term potentiation is impaired in mice lacking brain-derived neurotrophic factor *Proc. Natl Acad. Sci. USA* **92** 8856–60

Kottke F J 1965 Medical education for comprehensive medical care. *Arch. Phys. Med. Rehab.* **46** 349–53

Kujala T, Karma K, Ceponiene R, Belitz S, Turkkila P, Tervaniemi M and Näätänen R 2001 Plastic neural changes and reading improvement caused by audiovisual training in reading-impaired children *Proc. Natl Acad. Sci.* **98** 10509–14

Kunugi H, Ueki A, Otsuka M, Isse K, Hirasawa H, Kato N, Nabika T, Kobayashi S and Nanko S 2001 A novel polymorphism of the brain-derived neurotrophic factor (BDNF) gene associated with late-onset Alzheimer's disease *Mol. Psychiatry* **6** 83–6

Law J 1997 Evaluating intervention for language impaired children: a review of the literature *Int. J. Lang. Commun. Disord.* **32** 1–14

Law J, Boyle J, Harris F, Harkness A and Nye C 1998 Screening for speech and language delay: a systematic review of the literature *Report* Database of Abstracts of Reviews of Effects (DARE): Quality Assessed Reviews

Law J, Kot A and Barnett G 1999 A comparison of two methods of providing intervention to three-year-old children with expressive/receptive language impairment *Unpublished Report* City University London

Law J, Boyle J, Harris F, Harkness A and Nye C 2000 Prevalence and natural history of primary speech and language delay: findings from a systematic review of the literature *Int. J. Lang. Commun. Disorders* **35** 165–88

Law J, Boyle J, Harris F, Harkness A and Nye C 2000 Prevalence and natural history of primary speech and language delay: findings from a systematic review of the literature *Int. J. Lang. Commun. Disord.* **35** 165–88

Law J, Garrett Z and Nye C 2003 Speech and language therapy interventions for children with primary speech and language delay or disorder *Cochrane Database Syst. Rev.* CD004110

Law J, Garrett Z and Nye C 2007 Intervenciones de terapia del habla y ellenguaje para niños con retraso o trastornoprimario del habla y ellenguaje *Report* Recuperado de (http://update-software.com)

Laing K R, Mitchell D, Wersching H, Czira M E, Berger K and Baune B T 2012 Brain-derived neurotrophic factor (BDNF) gene: a gender-specific role in cognitive function during normal cognitive aging of the MEMO-study? *Age* **34** 1011–22

Lee C D, Tse W, Smith J D and Landreth G E 2012 Apolipoprotein E promotes β-amyloid trafficking and degradation by modulating microglial cholesterol levels *J. Biol. Chem.* **287** 2032–44

Li Y, Luikart B W, Birnbaum S, Chen J, Kwon C H, Kernie S G, Bassel-Duby R and Parada L F 2008 TrkB regulates hippocampal neurogenesis and governs sensitivity to antidepressive treatment *Neuron* **59** 399–412

Li W J, Yu H, Yang J M, Gao J, Jiang H, Feng M, Zhao Y X and Chen Z Y 2010 Anxiolytic effect of music exposure on BDNFMet/Met transgenic mice *Brain Res.* **1347** 71–9

Lim Y Y *et al* 2015 APOE and BDNF polymorphisms moderate amyloid β-related cognitive decline in preclinical Alzheimer's disease *Mol. Psychiatry* **20** 1322–8

Maegele M *et al* 2005 Reversal of neuromotor and cognitive dysfunction in an enriched environment combined with multimodal early onset stimulation after traumatic brain injury in rats *J. Neurotrauma* **22** 772–82

Marangolo P, Fiori V, Gelfo F, Shofany J, Razzano C, Caltagirone C and Angelucci F 2014 BihemispherictDCS enhances language recovery but does not alter BDNF levels in chronic aphasic patients *Restor. Neurol. Neurosci.* **32** 367–79

Morris M C *et al* 2014 O2-02-04: mind diet score more predictive than dash or mediterranean diet scores *Alzheimer Demen.* **10** P166

Nantais K M and Schellenberg E G 1999 The Mozart effect: an artifact of preference *Psychol. Sci.* **10** 370–3

Neeper S A *et al* 1995 Exercise and brain neurotrophins *Nature* 109

Newberg A B *et al* 2010 Meditation effects on cognitive function and cerebral blood flow in subjects with memory loss: a preliminary study *J. Alzheimer Dis.* **20** 517–26

Novkovic T, Mittmann T and Manahan-Vaughan D 2015 BDNF contributes to the facilitation of hippocampal synaptic plasticity and learning enabled by environmental enrichment *Hippocampus* **25** 1–15

Ossenkoppele R *et al* 2015 Cerebrospinal fluid biomarkers and cerebral atrophy in distinct clinical variants of probable Alzheimer's disease *Neurobiol. Aging* **36** 2340–7

Pascual-Leone A, Nguyet D, Cohen L G, Brasil-Neto J P, Cammarota A and Hallett M 1995 Modulation of muscle responses evoked by transcranial magnetic stimulation during the acquisition of new fine motor skills *J. Neurophysiol.* **74** 1037–45

Pievani M *et al* 2013 Striatal morphology in early-onset and late-onset Alzheimer's disease: A preliminary study *Neurobiol. Aging* **34** 1728–39

Pilc J 2010 The effect of physical activity on the brain derived neurotrophic factor: from animal to human studies *J. Physiol. Pharmacol.* **61** 533–41

Poo M M 2001 Neurotrophins as synaptic modulators *Nat. Rev. Neurosci.* **2** 24–32

Ready R E, Baran B, Chaudhry M, Schatz K, Gordon J and Spencer R M C 2011 Apolipoprotein E-e4, processing speed, and white matter volume in a genetically enriched sample of midlife adults *Am. J. Alzheimer's Dis. Other Dement.* **26** 463–8

Rios M, Fan G, Fekete C, Kelly J, Bates B, Kuehn R, Lechan R M and Jaenisch R 2001 Conditional deletion of brain-derived neurotrophic factor in the postnatal brain leads to obesity and hyperactivity *Mol. Endocrinol.* **15** 1748–57

Riverol M and López O L 2011 Biomarkers in Alzheimer's disease *Front. Neurol.* **2** 46

Sakata K *et al* 2013 Role of activity-dependent BDNF expression in hippocampal-prefrontal cortical regulation of behavioral perseverance *Proc. Natl Acad. Sci. USA* **110** 15103–8

Särkämö T *et al* 2008 Music listening enhances cognitive recovery and mood after middle cerebral artery stroke *Brain* **131** 866–76

Särkämö T *et al* 2010 Music and speech listening enhance the recovery of early sensory processing after stroke *J. Cogn. Neurosci.* **22** 2716–27

Schmidt H D and Duman R S 2010 Peripheral BDNF produces antidepressant-like effects in cellular and behavioral models *Neuropsychopharmacol.* **35** 2378–91

Sheardova K *et al* 2017 [P3–564]: The effect of spirituality/religiosity on regional brain atrophy in subjects at risk of Alzheimer disease: three-year follow-up data from Czech brain aging study *Alzheimer Demen.* **13** P1195

Snider W D 1994 Functions of the neurotrophins during nervous system development: what the knockouts are teaching us *Cell* **77** 627–38

Suri S, Heise V, Trachtenberg A J and Mackay C E 2013 The forgotten APOE allele: a review of the evidence and suggested mechanisms for the protective effect of APOE ε2 *Neurosci. Biobehav. Revi.* **37** 2878–86

Tan Y L, Zhou D F, Cao L Y, Zou Y Z and Zhang X Y 2005 Decreased BDNF in serum of patients with chronic schizophrenia on long-term treatment with antipsychotics *Neurosci. Lett.* **382** 27–32

Van Praag H, Kempermann G and Gage F H 2000 Neural consequences of enviromental enrichment *Nat. Rev. Neurosci.* **1** 191–8

van der Flier W M *et al* 2011 Early-onset versus late-onset Alzheimer's disease: the case of the missing APOE ε4 allele *Lancet Neurol.* **10** 280–8

Verghese P B, Castellano J M, Garai K, Wang Y, Jiang H, Shah A, Bu G, Frieden C and Holtzman D M 2013 ApoE influences amyloid-β (Aβ) clearance despite minimal apoE/Aβ association in physiological conditions *Proc. Natl Acad. Sci.* **110** E1807–16

Villemagne V L *et al* 2013 Australian Imaging Biomarkers and Lifestyle (AIBL) Research Group. Amyloid β deposition, neurodegeneration, and cognitive decline in sporadic Alzheimer's disease: a prospective cohort study *Lancet Neurol* **12** 357–67

Voss M W *et al* 2013 Bridging animal and human models of exercise-induced brain plasticity *Trends Cognit. Sci.* **17** 525–44

Ward D D, Summers M J, Saunders N L, Janssen P, Stuart K E and Vickers J C 2014 APOE and BDNF Val66Met polymorphisms combine to influence episodic memory function in older adults *Behav. Brain Res.* **271** 309–15

Whitehurst G J, Arnold D S, Smith M, Fischel J E, Lonigan C J and Valdez-Menchaca M C 1991 Family history in developmental expressive language delay *J. Speech, Lang. Hear. Res.* **34** 1150–7

Willner P 1997 Validity, reliability and utility of the chronic mild stress model of depression: a 10-year review and evaluation *Psychopharmacol.* **134** 319–29

Yalcin I, Belzung C and Surget A 2008 Mouse strain differences in the unpredictable chronic mild stress: a four-antidepressant survey *Behav. Brain Res.* **193** 140–3

Yang H *et al* 2016 Neurochemical and neuroanatomical plasticity following memory training and yoga interventions in older adults with mild cognitive impairment *Front. Aging Neurosci.* **8** 1–9

Zhang X Y, Liang J, Xiu M H, De Yang F, Kosten T A and Kosten T R 2012 Low BDNF is associated with cognitive impairment in chronic patients with schizophrenia *Psychopharmacology* **222** 277–84

Chapter 8

Brain engineering mechanics for cognitive modeling

Arindam Bit, Khemraj Deshmukh and Shashikanta Tarai

Lab-on-a-chip (LOC) is a hybrid technology that enables the insight of integrating diverse technologies together on a single platform. The flow process of LOC is indicated in figure 8.1, which gives an insight into the production process of the LOC. To make the insight practical, microfluidics and nanofluidics play a crucial role. An integrative study that culminates in understanding the behaviour of fluids through the micro-channels and engineering the microminuscule devices that contain chambers and tunnels through which fluid flow is limited is called microfluidics. This science and technology phenomena deal with the fluids where fluids act very contrarily on the micrometric gauge compared to their everyday behaviour. Microfluidic systems are optimum in the management of small cell counts. Dynamically organized methods are used for metered cell payloads with high spatial precision (Dinh *et al* 2013).

8.1 Microfluidic chip-based neuronal modelling

In recent years various focused microfluidic cell culture strategies and techniques have aided manoeuvring axonal outgrowth (Peyrin *et al* 2011). Axon guidance in neuronal networks in amalgamation with the position of the soma is attained by sailing through several approaches but not without numerous encounters to enable quality guidance of axons (Yamada *et al* 2016). Microfluidics continues to evolve inspired by the precision-based results and outcomes from the analysis methods such as high-performance liquid chromatography (HPLC) and capillary electrophoresis (CE), even with a very small sample input, as in figure 8.1 (Dinh *et al* 2013).

8.1.1 Technological interventions on neuronal cultures

Understanding the human nervous system and its organizational perspective requires a deep insight into the neural pathways' operational knowledge. The scientific

doi:10.1088/978-0-7503-3383-2ch8

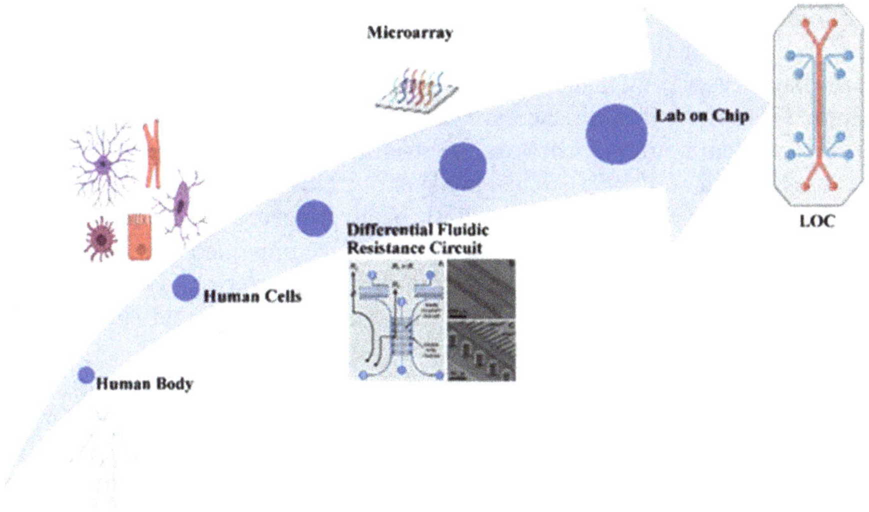

Figure 8.1. Lab-on-chip procedural flow.

community makes daunting efforts to gain breakthroughs about brain and neural degenerations. A group of scientists proposed a microfluidic system that enabled the modernization of oriented neuronal networks that related numerous diverse neuron populations with an established preface of predefined connection framework and a dedicated spanned network branching across numerous cellular subcubicles. The noteworthy mentioning of this innovation is the incorporation of the asymmetrical micro-channels that can be intriguing and direct the axons in a single direction creating a separation amongst two or more individual chambers (Peyrin *et al* 2011).

Professor Ayako Yamada and his team members suggested an 'in-Mold Patterning' (iMP) based neuronal culture technique, which enabled axo-somatic cubicles for on-chip processes. They concluded that the iMP methodology not only exhibited superior guidance efficiency, but it also had an undue advantage over the other techniques such as micro-contact printing (μCP) and micro-grooves (μGro). Furthermore, the study also indicated the significance of oriented neuronal networks with controlled connectivity for research in neuro-computational perspective and studies about neurogenerative mechanisms (Yamada *et al* 2016).

Ngoc-Duy Dinh and their team of scientists created a microfluidic construction by the method of minimalistic neuronal co-cultures. They presented a compartmentalized neuron arraying (CA) microfluidic circuit to design and deliver the neuronal networks with the assistance of nominal cellular inputs significantly less than the existing mechanisms. The team achieved the method jointly with microfluidics, which diligently handles the single-cell and biomaterial modelling for the enduring conservation of neuronal activities. The proposed microfluidic circuits based on differential flow principles enabled arraying neurons with the help of consistent cubicles with single-cell precision. Along with this, efficient fluid isolation methods proposed are used for local chemical or biological disturbances of networked neuronal co-cultures (Dinh *et al* 2013).

Striatum activity is driven primarily by excitatory connections originating from various expanses of the cerebral cortex, including sensory, motor, and associative regions that project principally through glutamatergic projections ipsilateral to the striatum. This results in a directed system in which cortical fibres originating from layer V pyramidal neurons penetrate the striatum and 'en passant' connect striatal dendrites (Kincaid *et al* 1998). Thus, pre-synaptic clustering along striatal dendrites and striatal neuron maturation were both being triggered by cortical fibre reconnection on striatal dendrites in our system. This is accompanied by an increase in the complexity of striatal dendritic arborization, PSD95 clustering, and dendritic spine formation. These findings are consistent with earlier research that suggests cortical neurons play a role in striatal differentiation (Segal *et al* 2003).

When axons are not tightly concentrated, they preferentially form at the boundaries of the grooves on the bottom surface along the sidewalls, as indicated by the arrowheads, rather than on the groove walls, as previously disclosed (Béduer *et al* 2013). Additionally, if the microstructures have a sufficiently high aspect ratio (usually >1), axons or cell bodies somewhere at the bottom of the microstructures are shielded from shear stress inside the microfluidic channel. Shear stress can cause phenotypic or viability changes in cells, but neurons are particularly vulnerable in this regard (Morel *et al* 2012).

The crucial channel present in the microfluidic neuronal array allows for concurrent neuronal arrangement in the microfluidic neuron arraying system, which is completely distinct from the previous versions of the co-culture systems, which needed the cell ventilation properties adhesion and flattening before the incorporation of second layers of cells to it (Frimat *et al* 2011). However, the microfluidic arrangement imposes fluid stress for a short period. Also, direct entrapment in microscale openings (without using different microcurrents) causes extreme deformation of the cell body, leading to cell death. Therefore, these systems are not suitable for culturing neurons but can be used well for short-term single-cell electrophysiology (Ionescu-Zanetti *et al* 2005).

8.1.2 Architectures for a functional LOC

In a research study, the oriented neuronal networks, basically the primary cortical neurons and the striatal neurons, were reconstructed using axon diodes. The research outcome indicated that the cortical fibres approaching from the emitting cavity endorse striatal differentiation *in vitro* in the reception cavity. The oriented and completely established cortico-striatal neuronal synapses are permitted to reconstruct themselves by the system, making the post-synaptic neurons much more functionally connected to the glutamatergic cortical fibres. After establishing the functional synaptic connections, the synchronization and the striatal differentiation stimulation are initiated for the neural activities. Thus, the axon diode plays a very vital role in tracing the direction of the neuronal pathways, not only pioneering a classic revolution in further studies about neuronal culture platforms (Peyrin *et al* 2011).

A group of researchers defined a method that integrates the utilization of a novel detachable partition and iMP, enabling the placement of soma separated from the axon guidance outlines resulting in a hybrid mechanism including chemical and mechanical properties of cell positioning signs for the neurons. The results suggested that in-mould patterning (iMP) delivered improvement in axon confinement efficiency in the gain up to 100 on the tracks, delivering a completely accessible on-chip axon array. On the other hand, with reference to the fabrication perspective, iMP does not possess technologies which are complex and multifaceted aspect when compared with others such as micro-grooves (μGro) and micro-contact printing (μCP). iMP will therefore open new avenues for the construction of complex and precisely controlled neural networks (Yamada *et al* 2016).

A novel approach *in situ* patterning method connecting plasma tracing with water masking is established and utilized to mediate bonded biomaterials with the microfluid stratagem. A microfluidic neuron arraying technique is implemented to formulate arrays by establishing contact with heterotypic single-cell co-cultures. The neuronal array established with single-cell precision is an outcome of the differential resistance fluidic circuit. The spatial organization is maintained due to the biomaterial pattern, which promotes and guides the neurite (Dinh *et al* 2013).

8.2 Brain tissue mechanics

Our brain has been the most intriguing part of our system, and hence it is considered a subject of substantial research for comprehending its operation and mannerisms. Recent research is mostly dedicated to chemical substances and vital processes in the brain and the electrical properties of biological cells and tissues in the nervous system. In this study, conventional mechanical principles such as distortion, strain, stress, and distention play a very important part in attuning the structure and operation of the brain. Hence acumen in mathematical operations, fluid and bio-mechanisms, the study of eyes and nervous system abnormality, and spinal cord and spinal column abnormality is required to address the brain-related issues such as oedema in the cerebral area, brain distortion classified by lack of normal convolutions (folds) in the cerebral cortex and an abnormally small head (microcephaly), an abnormal buildup of fluid in the ventricles (cavities) deep within the brain, surgery for removal of part of your skull (to relieve pressure due to brain trauma), abnormalities in the spinal cord, shaken baby syndrome and growth of the tumors. Mechanical projecting can become the main instrument in the analysis of the above-mentioned pathologies. Study about mechanical attributes of tissue structure (white matter) of the brain within a particular parametric situation is carried out. Magnetic resonance elastography (Kruse *et al* 2008, Sack *et al* 2008) has emerged as an incipient new technique to describe the mechanical attributes of live brain tissues. It is a brain imaging technique that is non-invasive and operates by projecting shear waves to tissue, capturing the proliferating waves and extricating the result with the help of computational algorithms (Hamhaber *et al* 2010, Johnson *et al* 2013). The fundamental importance of brain mechanics lies in the fact that it includes extraordinary scales ranging from extremely soft (for neurosurgery) to extremely hard (skull) and extremely fast (with brain trauma or TBI) to extremely slow (brain development). Brain abnormalities such as swelling in cerebral tissue (brain edema) require the help of electrochemistry, which is a result of several brain abnormalities such as infection, strokes and trauma, as due to injury or concussion discrepancy in electric ion and particles is caused and electrochemical impacts are important for maintaining the equilibrium of stress, fluids and tissues structure in the brain. Like TBI, the shaken baby syndrome is explained by cranial aspects such as bleeding in the retina, bleeding in the subdural area, and encephalopathy biomechanical notions of rotational acceleration and bridging vein tear has been recognized. Also, it is evident from recent research that the cortical folding and gyrification during developmental stages of the brain can be explained through methodical and statistical mechanical modeling (Budday *et al* 2014). The regulating mechanisms of mechanical factors have been proven to be of utmost significance in structural aspects of the brain due to their analytical and statistical approaches to identify physiological, pathological and gynogenesis abnormalities, which can help diagnose and manage neurological disorders like mental retardation, autism, epilepsy and schizoaffective disorders. Hence, the current study clearly shows that support of solid, fluid, electromechanical, and electrochemical dimensions of mechanics holds a very important place in identifying and managing cerebral structural and operational abnormality. This study provides an opportunity for future growth in facilitating complete knowledge about physiology and pathophysiology of the brain with the help of brain mechanics.

8.2.1 Brain tissue biomechanics

Knowing how the loading/kinematic constraints implemented to the organ boundary equates into local stress–strain circumstance inside the tissue spectrum is difficult since the brain is a massively complicated body part accommodating various 'substructure components', e.g., brainstem, cerebellum, thalamus, cerebral cortex, corpus callosum, each affiliated with slightly varying mechanical properties (Arbogast and Margulies 1998). The current investigation is part of a collaborative endeavour to clarify a few of the main impacts of primary blast on the CNS, and it is an initial step towards building a prediction model for the reaction of brain tissue across a wide span of strains and strain rates (Moore *et al* 2009). This research is a first step toward creating a rigorous empirical dataset and upgraded analytical approaches that will be used to facilitate a range of therapeutic uses and unravel mechanically regulated mechanisms resulting in traumatic brain damage. The experimental procedure involved posthumous examination of sixteen 6- to 18-month-old swine brains. The transverse displacements, axial data (force and displacement) and lateral deformation images were taken. The basic characteristics of the tissue response to the uniaxial compression loading procedure were discovered to be similar across all examined samples. The Tamura study's (virgin) loading response at a straining rate of 1 s^{-1} showed to be in good accordance with the present report's findings. Even though extracellular fluid diffusion and associated transport processes have previously been acknowledged to play an important role in neural activity (Nicholson 2001), the poroelastic method has gained just a quick glimpse in the brain tissue biomechanics field. The research procedures used in this work allowed for acquiring a vast, reliable pool of biomechanical data collected *in vitro* on large brain specimens at bounded stresses (0%–50%) in the low to moderate strain rate range (0.01–1 s^{-1}). The scientific assessment of the tissue response during unloading was critical in determining elastic and viscoelastic processes' relative impact on total tissue resilience to deform. Because these factors were determined during the modelling stage, the resultant model could predict tissue behaviour at strain rates beyond the initial range upon which the fit was conducted. The recent research is merely the initial part of developing a model capable of providing correct estimates for tissue response throughout random strain experiences. Early findings appear to show that if a specimen was deformed at a certain rate, it became 'conditioned' for deformity at that rate as well as at lesser rates, but it will still demonstrate further conditioning if evaluated at greater rates later on. Further research that might change the sequence of the loading segments might also give helpful validation data for a model that accounts for conditioning impacts. The suggested modelling approach well captures the major characteristics of the extreme strain-tissue response as evaluated in uniaxial contraction and expansion. An initial fit of the model to the unconditioned (initial loading ramp) tissue-response was performed at low to high deformation rates (0.01–3000 s^{-1}). The proposed formulation is still quite generic and may simulate tissue responses over a wider range of strain rates. With adjusted materials properties, the suggested model covers the main characteristics of the unconditioned loading response of brain tissue throughout a strain rate span of 0.01 to 3000 s^{-1}. Providing an appropriate constitutive law to describe brain tissue response is critical for assessing local levels of strain, stress, and strain rate linked with prospective injurious processes. The suggested model is the primary step in achieving this objective. The constituent model shown here efficiently apprehends the advanced structures underlying the tissue response (hysteresis, nonlinearities, volumetric compliance, short- and long-time behaviours) over four orders of strain rate magnitude (0.01–10 s^{-1}) and up to 50 percentile nominal strain with a limited quantity of material parameters. A subsequent step will be to evaluate the model's ability to anticipate material reaction during diverse types of deformation. Finally, the present composition does not explain the observed conditioning effects, where the initial loading ramp was linked with a much more rigid tissue response.

8.2.2 Cortical complexity of the brain in the presence of secondary irregularities

Knowledge of the relationship among neural connections, grey matter volume, surface morphology, and, eventually, the behaviour might significantly impact how we identify, categorise, measure, and cure neurological diseases. Latest developments in neurological imaging have shed light on the phenomena of brain folding at various sizes (Luhmann *et al* 2009). Folding events caused by compacting pressures in layered material have applications in a variety of disciplines. Compressive stresses can be generated by external events such as pressure and internal processes such as growth (Yin and Chen 2011). Numerous investigations, usually theoretically or quantitatively, tackle the crucial circumstances for primary and secondary disturbances in multilayer media. It was recently demonstrated, via indentation studies on the newly removed brain, that the stiffness difference across grey and white matter is significantly lower, practically on order. This study aims to investigate secondary folding events for physiologically relevant stiffness differences less than 100 and biologically relevant growth extremes much beyond the elastic limit. Previous research has suggested how fundamental disturbances of a developing grey matter layer on a developing white matter substrate cause consistent creasing patterns. Secondary disturbances that develop after the first instability point are the subject of this paper. The continuum model of differential growth was used to investigate secondary folding events. This model describes a wide range of folding events in animal brains, with a morphogenetically developing grey matter layer and a stretch-induced increasing white matter substrate. It describes not only just the creation of periodic, sinusoidal creases but also the appearance of uneven, complicated folds. When the growth-induced tension in the brain reaches a certain level, it discharges its tension by folding into a regular sinusoidal shape. The model ignores the spatial limitation of the cranium and believes that brain growth is largely restricted by subcortical tissue. This results in a sinusoidal-shaped main folding arrangement. It is demonstrated here that the sinusoidal solution diverges into uneven secondary forms with continued development at the start of primary folding. These secondary forms explain the cortex's intricacies in subsequent growth, childhood, and adolescence (Naidich *et al* 2012). According to the findings, the second unstable threshold for a completely elastic substrate is largely unaffected by the stiffness ratio. Nevertheless, with a developing substrate, the necessary development to produce the second disturbance rises as the stiffness ratio increases. Stretch-induced subcortical expansion, caused by axon's adaptation to mechanical stretch, was found to act as a stabilizer of the folding process: the quicker the axons react to mechanical stress, the steadier the primary sinusoidal structure and the less probable the onset of secondary disruptions. The folding patterns imply that the cortical layer's continued development causes secondary disturbances, which explains the growing cortical sophistication with ageing. According to the findings, secondary folding events such as period-doubling and period-tripling lead to a somewhat more complicated exterior look. Hence, this research explained that the relationship among neuronal connectivity, cortical thickness, surface structure, and behaviour significantly influences the investigation, categorizations, and management of neurological abnormality.

8.3 Mechanical characteristics of brain tissue

Nowadays, the functionality, as well as the shape of the brain, can be changed by the mechanics. We can make a protocol for identifying brain damage with the help of a computational model. The current study gives the knowledge to rebuild the brain model and acquire the status of the brain for deferent loading conditions. For our study, we collected tissue from 10 different persons' brains via a postmortem performed time duration within 24 h. The subjects are between 54 and 81 of age. After collecting brain tissue, magnetic resonance imaging (MRI) and diffusion tensor imaging (DTI) were performed.

Pre-conditioning conditions occurred when new loads replaced loads or load value was stepped up from old ones. It is found that during the first and second loading conditions, the hysteresis portion mechanical flexibility fell. This hysteresis portion was maximum drop during the first and second load condition in comparison and tension compared to shear. Our result indicates that no brain tissue was damaged during the pre-conditioning situation, but some of the brain tissue was corrigible. We also find that during load conditions, no variation was found in the dominion of mechanical direction. The result also indicates that the tissue obtained from the brain was isotropic. These brain tissues help us to develop a more accurate model for computational analysis. We also conclude that mechanical directional change occurs more in grey matter as compared to white matter. We found that in a particular region of the brain area, mechanical properties were changed. Comparing the mechanical response of specimens of both corpus callosum and cortex gives us softness and hardness responses, respectively. As compared to other brain regions, cortical grey matter exhibits maximum rigid reaction. The grey matter result for basal ganglia and white matter result for corona radiate was mirrored. For collected tissue, stress hysteresis area was maximum in white matter compared to grey matter (van Dommelen *et al* 2010). The above result compared with tissue collected from the bovine brain. Higher viscosity was obtained for white matter as compared to grey matter for the same tissue.

By joining the indentation test and histological staining, we can develop a relationship between mechanical properties and brain microstructure (Koser *et al* 2015). The hardness of the mouse's spinal cord somehow matched up the area of cell centre and plane repenetration of the cell. Time and mechanical test chain span was a major factor in altering brain-related tissue's mechanical properties. The above observable things are independent of the sample collected by human age and gender. Overestimate shear modulus was calculated with the help of compression test, while underestimate had the shear and tension tested modulus. In our study, computational software formulated three strain energy functions using finite element analysis and collected observational data under load conditions.

The value of shear can be stepped up by combining the different loading conditions and axial tension's step-up value. Therefore, these experiments provide an insightful conclusion of human brain tissue under a combination of compression–tension called combined loading. To capture the response of brain-related tissue under combined load conditions, we use the Ogden model (Mihai *et al* 2015). However, all these studies were performed in *in vitro* conditions which is a major drawback of the above experiments. Furthermore, the above experiments were performed at room temperature, which is another drawback because external temperature affects brain-related tissue's mechanical properties. One thing noted is that the above study was not suitable to find out the influences of age, gender and disease on mechanical parameters.

8.3.1 Brain tissue modelling: hyperplastic model

A constitutive equation is used to establish the relationship from stress to strain in the mechanical response of the biological system (Holzapfel *et al* 2000).

The microstructure of brain tissue was not operated by the collagen and elastin fibre, and these properties indicate how brain tissue was different from the other soft tissue. The combination of compression and shear is called elastic shear, whose value increased while increasing the axial compression, and very little improvement occurs while increasing the tension value. Hyperplastic incompressible based Ogden model gave a good response for single as well as multiple loading. The conclusion found based on the obtained result helped us with forecasting the response of brain cells under different load conditions such as tension, compression and combinational arrangements. It is crucial to estimate the mechanical task of the brain for calculating the stresses of the mind. The above task was only performed in *in vitro* conditions. The Ogden type model's performance was better than other models available to us to optimize the mechanical response of brain, and these models are Neo-Hookean, mooney-RiVlin, Gung, Gent and murine brain tissue models.

The experimental result indicates the brain tissue shows tension–compression inequality for the combined form of finite shear and axial distortion. These phenomena show by the increase of the shear stress as well axial compression. Under a minimum shear, tissue related to the murine brain shows the value of shear modulus increase when we boost the value of axial compression, but the value of shear modulus was saturated for increased value of axial tension (Mihai *et al* 2015). A minimum variation on stress for a huge amount of shear value could be measured by the one-term Ogden model when the model was only operated in the quasi time-independent elastic behaviour and neglecting the material properties like viscoelasticity and poroelasticity. The first model was known as Ogden-term with two parameters. The two parameters can be derived by calculating all the related data for nonlinear shear modules for minimum shear deformation. These data can be calculated from the experiments. After that, the data calibration for minimum shear stress along with axial tension and compression was made. An inaccurate result for a big amount of shear deformation was obtained. It is also seen that an inversely proportional relationship has been found between compression and nonlinear elastic modulus under heavy shear. But these relationships were shoving opposite relations for tension. Four parameters based models were developed, called three terms Ogden model. This type of model shows the different results for the multiple load condition (Budday *et al* 2015).

- No variation has been found in the result for various tension and compression and large shear for brain tissue.
- The huge shear governs the constant value obtained for elastic action for different tension and compression range values.

The above model proposed by us is hyperplastic, and these models are continuously updated from data obtained by the experiments followed by the finite simple shear superposed for a different axial tension and compression value. The purpose of these models was to focus on the effect of nonlinear shear on tissue response under huge distortion.

8.3.2 Mechanics of brain development

Surface morphology of the brain can be done by the mechanical modelling of the growth of the brain of any living animal. Brain pattern generation can depend heavily on the depth of the cortical and subcortical thickness and their stiffness. Factors for build-up of the grey matter, such as width, softness, moderate formation of layers, etc, raises the cortical folding and decreases the Gyral wavelength and vice versa. The brain dimension is directly proportional to mammals' size of mammals but cortical thickness was independent of the size of mammals. This developed model indicates that inside all mammals, the area of absolute gyral wavelength was constant. However, the relative gyral wavelength was proportional to the size of mammals; this model also gives some information about pathological disorders linked with the thin cortex and lissencephaly associated with the fatty convoluted cortex. Thus, we can identify the mind disorder by clearing the concept of phenomena of cortical folding in a period of brain development.

The proposed model can give a rapid response for any change of cortical width. The developed model also gives the proportional relationship between intersulcal distance and cortical diameter (Yi and Wu 2020). So we can eliminate the evolution of folding completely by the thickened cortex. In other words, we can say that gyral wavelength can be altered by the cortical thickness and cortical thickness, which was the main factor influencing the folding and surface pattern. In the above statement, cortical thickness influences the different parameters. Now cortical thickness was altered by the stiffness ratio obtained from the cortex and subcortex, and it is measured by in third root. The cortical stiffness is smaller than the order of quantity, but it is higher than the subcortical stiffness. Literature shows that the stiffness difference is 50 percentile. Now we can say that the stiffness ratio is responsible for changing the surface pattern. But a small amount of stiffness ratio was not driven by the folding mechanism and pattern disorder. The critical premise is part of analytical studies, and these premises are used to establish the relationship between critical wavelength, the time constant of development and rate of subcortical growth (Soza *et al* 2005). If the disorder has a foundation on the rapid development of cortical, it creates flexibility on a subcortex that was earlier a solid-like structure, so that axon was disabled to acknowledge. The phenomenon rapidly increases the cortical area's pressure, which is responsible for the strike of the secondary fold. Absolute gravel wavelength was not altering when the brain size increased and uniform cortical thickness, but relative gyral wavelength was increased when brain size increased.

The above analytical and computational model gives detailed information about mammalian brain growth with the following limitation.

1. For developing the model, the topology of the skull was not considered because simulation results indicate that skull is not necessary to provoke gyrification. But from various literature, the skull is a key element for cortical folding (Nie *et al* 2010).
2. Constitutive conduct was considered to be quasi incompressible, although it was found to be fully compressible.
3. The flexibility response of the brain was calculated by the Neo Hookean isotropic, but the characterization of anisotropic material was very difficult.

8.4 Modeling of clinical brain

Nonlinear field theory and theory of finite growth of a living brain system has been developed with a growing inner core and outer surface. It has been found that intelligence and cortical gyrification positively correlate (Luders *et al* 2008). On the other hand, the surface morphology of the brain is responsible for malformation like poly-microgyria and disorders like schizophrenia and autism. The main point is that all these abnormalities start from the early embryo development stage (Raybaud *et al* 2013), leading to various pathologies (Raybaud and Widjaja 2011). Furthermore, it was recently found that the mechanical microenvironment inside the head has important moles regarding cortical folding patterns (Li *et al* 2012).

The hypothesis of initiating cortical folding by axon pull on the cortex (Van 1997) was disproven (Xu *et al* 2010). Currently, the differential growth between the slow-growing inner core and fast-growing surface layer results in the cortical folds (Ronan *et al* 2014). They create a mechanical model for differential growth to imitate cortical folding in the growing human brain (Budday *et al* 2014). As mechanically driven growth can justify gyral wavelength and patterns (Bayly *et al* 2013), they hypothesize that improper cortical and subcortical growth initiates abnormalities in the morphology of the human brain.

Compared to the MRI images of preterm neonates at 27, 29 and 32 weeks of gestation, the human brain and the simulated brain slices showed similar growth progression. However, a 65% increase in volume at 29 weeks and shallow sulci formation was observed. More prominent sulci were seen in week 29, along with a 76% increase in volume. By the 32nd week volume is doubled and sulci have significant depth (Budday *et al* 2014), cellular differentiation, proliferation, and migration are responsible for the cortical growth because of which it varies significantly. In the case of cortical growth rate below a critical value, it is compensated by fast grade sub-cortical growth, due to which a smooth surface is obtained by suppressing gyrification.

Similarly, cortical growth above the critical value decreases the subcortical growth leading to increased elastic volume stretch, resulting in shallow sulci. The initial cortical thickness of the human brain varies. The growth of both cortex and subcortex decreases by increasing the initial cortical thickness, leading to reduced axonal tension and less localized deformation patterns in the subcortex. All the information leads to the understanding of the cortical folding mechanism, which directly impacts neurological disorders like epilepsy, autism, and schizophrenia. The simulation may be a useful tool to diagnose and treat these neurological disorders (Budday *et al* 2014).

8.4.1 Axon growth in the presence of mechanosensing events

The axons' development and extension have a well-defined pathway in nervous system development. This axon development depends on the chemical signal and the mechanical environment (Chan and Odde 2008). It was found that these mechanical signals are a valid regulator far mural neural development. For the study, they use

Xenopus retinal ganglion cell (RGC) axon for *in vitro* study and Xenopus embryonic brain for *in vivo* study.

The Axon Xenopus laevis optic pathway is believed to be regulated by slit1, slit2 and Semaphorin 3A (Sema 3A) (Atkinson-Leadbeater *et al* 2010) expression chemically. The *in vitro* study of Xenopus RGC revealed that with different substrate stiffness (Koch *et al* 2012), the normal developing activity of axon like branching pattern, neural growth patterns, neuronal traction forces and neurite extension is significantly affected. To determine that *in vitro* mechano-sensitivity assays were performed, two different substrate stiffnesses of 1 and 0.1 kPa were taken, which approximately imitate the stiffness of the upper and lower parts of brain tissue (Franze *et al* 2009), having similar chemical environments. Using Sholl analysis, the axon's growth was larger in care of the stiffer substrate suggesting its mechano-sensitivity.

The neuro mechano-sensitivity depends on stretch-activated ion channels (Franze *et al* 2009), which help the neurons to detect the stiffness of the substrate, so removing the ion channels will result in similar neural growth despite different substrate stiffness phenotype. Piezo1 is a known mechanically activated cation channel (Coste *et al* 2010) involved in neural developing cascades, as piezo1 is present in the axon environment. Spider venom peptide GsMTX4 was used to block the activity of piezo1 (Gottlieb and Sachs 2012), which showed axon growth on the stiff surface compared to control in scattering, indicating that axon growth on the stiff surface compared to control mechanosensitive ion channels are an important aspect of mechanosensing in Xenopus RGCs (Koser *et al* 2016).

For *in vivo* study, atomic force microscopy (AFM) was used to study the local tissue stiffeness of the developing brain. Tissue stiffness was heterogeneously distributed and had a stiffness gradient perpendicular to the direction and growth of RGC axons. Stiffness gradient directs the axon development, and the axons tend to grow towards the soft tissue. These stiffness gradients are imposed by mechanical signals demonstrated by cell culture and stiffness gradient incorporation (Koser *et al* 2016). CNS tissue stiffness is due to the extracellular matrix present along with the neuron cells. The main component of ECM in the developing brain is chondroitin sulphate (CS) proteoglycans (Walz *et al* 2002). The CS-treated brain was used to develop differential stiffeners *in vivo*. Softening of brains results in dispersed axons with lost trajectory and decreased directionality. All these suggest that neuronal growth significantly depends on the local tissue stiffness of the developing brain.

8.4.2 Decompressive craniectomy modelling of brain

Brain swelling caused due to traumatic brain injury (TBI) can result in increased intracranial pressure (ICP) that can lead to severe brain damage and death. To reduce the ICP using a surgical procedure, decompressive craniectomy (DC) is used (Kolias *et al* 2013). In the DC procedure, part of the skull is removed to relieve the pressure by expanding the brain outside the skull (Timofeev *et al* 2012). But the effectiveness of the treatment is a variable (Sahuquillo 2006). Therefore, the clinical case of decompressive craniectomy and hyperelastic finite element models was

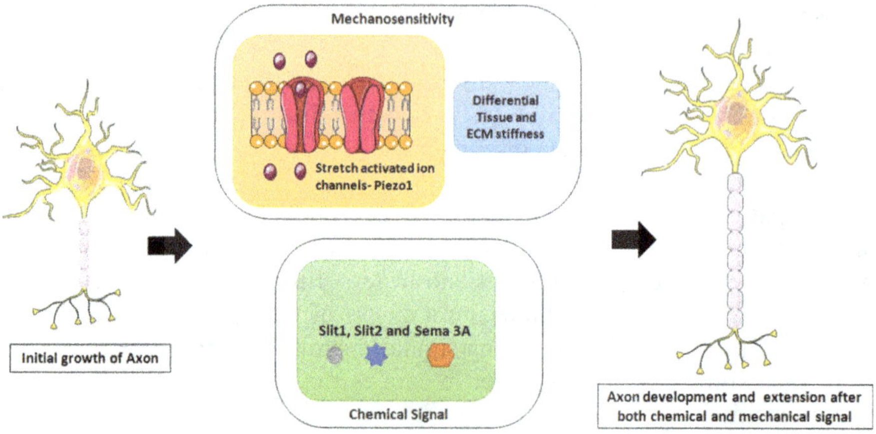

Figure 8.2. Axon growth and extension due to both chemical and mechanical signals.

developed with a realistic geometry using critical shear strain value. In addition, the volume of brain tissue damage was calculated.

Even if the model geometry is not similar to the skull, the risk of damage will still be similar for the clinical situation. The results confirm that it is less likely to have tissue damage if a larger craniectomy opening is performed due to high strains present after the DC procedure. Using the hyperelastic finite element model, potential brain tissue damage can be predicted by calculating brain tissue volume exceeding a critical shear strain. With an increase in herniated volume, maximum bulge displacement increases; however, it decreases in the increased craniectomy area. The region below the brain surface has a maximum shear strain, increasing herniation volume while decreasing with craniectomy diameter.

The dura provides effective protection, due to which details of the craniectomy edge are not considered. In the case of volume of highly sheared material, the craniectomy in the realistic model varies with the real craniectomy areas with more damaged volume than expected. In total, the developed model provides complete biomechanical guidance for DC, as shown in figure 8.2 (Fletcher *et al* 2016).

8.5 Axonal stiffness and clinical brain

Accidents can result in traumatic brain damage, resulting in persistent brain injury (health concerns) or even death. The Brain Injury Criteria are used to determine the likelihood of a TBI when mechanical load is applied. For traumatic brain criteria, the global head kinematics head injury criterion is now employed. Recent developments include new methodologies, such as tissue-based injury criteria, based on finite element design at a smaller scale. The HIC approach is based on global head kinematics, although brain injury happens at the cellular level, and it is also based on experimental data that only considers anterior-posterior load application while ignoring head angular acceleration (Cloots *et al* 2008).

Injury methodologies and loading parameters can be discriminated in three-dimensional finite element head models. However, inhomogeneous geometry, these finite element head models portray heterogeneous, complicated anatomy. To achieve a complicated level of brain function, heterogeneous morphology increases cortical surface geometry. By eliminating convolutions of the cerebral cortex, the most recent models incorporate ventricles and invaginations of the duramater. As a result, stress and strain predictions are inaccurate. The use of brain damage criteria is prohibited due to the shortcomings of numerical models (Al-Bsharat *et al* 1999).

In vivo and *in vitro*, investigations are used to predict tissue-level criteria. For correct criteria, these models must incorporate a full description of the cerebrum's biomechanical behaviour, including its morphological complexity (Bain and Meaney 2000). Two-dimensional finite element models are employed with precise geometries of various sections of the cerebral cortex and contrasted to homogeneous morphology to examine the biomechanical implications of morphological complexity in the cerebral cortex. Stress is observed to be enhanced by a factor of two in the diverse morphology of the cerebral cortex, according to loading conditions obtained by simulation.

8.5.1 Brain stiffness and myelin content

Neuronal development and illness are influenced by brain stiffness. However, various species, brains, and even different areas of the same brain have been shown to have dramatically varying stiffness values. The cause of the reported brain stiffness value changes is currently unknown. The mechanical environment and stimulation have been shown to aid neuronal growth and illness. Magnetic resonance elastography can quantify regional and temporal stiffness fluctuations in the human brain, which aids in characterizing the mechanical environment *in vivo* and non-invasively. Magnetic resonance elastography has recently been proven to be effective. Magnetic resonance elastography has recently been utilized to link changes in brain stiffness to degeneration in chronic neurological illnesses, although the specific mechanism of these stiffness fluctuations remains unknown (Weickenmeier *et al* 2016).

An outer grey matter layer comprises neuronal cell bodies, dendrites, unmyelinated axons, an inner white matter core of astrocytes, oligodendrocytes, microglia, and a dense network of myelinated axons that make up the brain. Myelin promotes electrical function while simultaneously insulating signal transmission. Around week 14 of pregnancy, myelination reaches its most advanced stage, corresponding to an infant's rapid development during the first year. Demyelination, or the creation of a faulty myelin sheath, occurs due to genetic alterations linked to leukodystrophies. In addition, several autoimmune disorders are characterized by demyelination (Chew *et al* 2013).

The most reliable, durable, and repeatable method for determining the mechanical behaviour of the brain is indentation testing. Only the human brain can be probed *in vivo* using tissue identification. However, it has lately been utilized to explore diverse regions of the brain's white and grey matter with high fidelity and resolution. According to research conducted utilizing atomic force microscopy on several brain areas, Grey matter is twice as rigid as white matter. Grey matter is one-third softer than white matter in pigs and lambs when it comes to tissue identification. Grey and white matter appear to be indistinguishable in humans according to magnetic resonance elastography. According to magnetic resonance elastography, grey and white matter are indistinguishable in humans and animals on a whole organ level. The concentration of myelin sheath increases the stiffness of the white matter of the brain. The white matter myelin content has a density gradient, with lower myelin content in the anterior region and higher myelin content in the posterior region (Braak *et al* 2004).

8.5.2 Microtubule polymerization and axonal degeneration

Axonal injury is a symptom of trauma caused by a physical blow to the head. The actual mechanism of axonal injury, however, remains uncertain. Neurons are the building blocks of communication, and their axon protrusions, which connect other neuron cells, are long and slender. These axons are made up of longitudinal microtubules surrounded by the actin cortex and can be up to 1 m long. Actin is cross-linked with spectrin and myosin, whereas dynein and taw are cross-linked with dynein and dynein. As previously documented, a constant force is present in the axon, which is necessary for axon physiology. Axonal elongation and towed growth are caused by mild or moderate strains, whereas high forces cause axonal damage and diffuse axonal injury. The beginning of mechanical stresses in the axon is aided by crosslinks between individual microtubules and actin filaments. These crosslinks are extremely active, constantly attaching to, detaching from, pulling on, and pushing the axon cytoskeleton. Understanding the biology of axons relies heavily on computational simulation. Exact models that depict axons as distinct microtubules and crosslinks are used in current and most recent models, providing insight into the axon's static and dynamic responses, crosslink outcomes, microtubule breakage, and gene expression (Bell 1978, Spires-Jones *et al* 2009).

With the typical finite element method, the computational framework directly captures the dynamic nature of crosslinks. This permits any chemical mechanism to crosslink microtubules in the axon through a broad and modular interface. Axonal models are made up of continuous microtubule polymerization and depolymerization networks that dynamically remove and reattach crosslinked proteins. Physical forces acting on axons cause their attachment dissociation. Physical forces operating on axons involve molecular-level mechanisms related to crosslinking, microtubule dynamics, and stiffness damage, as shown in figure 8.3 (de Rooij and Kuhl 2018).

8.6 Viscoelastic and rheological models of brain tissue

Susceptibility of the human brain towards numerous loading cases, shear, compression and tension in a time-reliant manner is presented here to understand the rheology of four different regions of the human brain: cortex, basal ganglia, corona radiata, corpus callosum by characterising and calibrating the family of finite viscoelastic Ogden-type models for multiple/mixed loading parameters. Moreover, comprehending the rheology of the human brain will aid in precise modelling of brain behaviour during disease and development and predict outcomes of

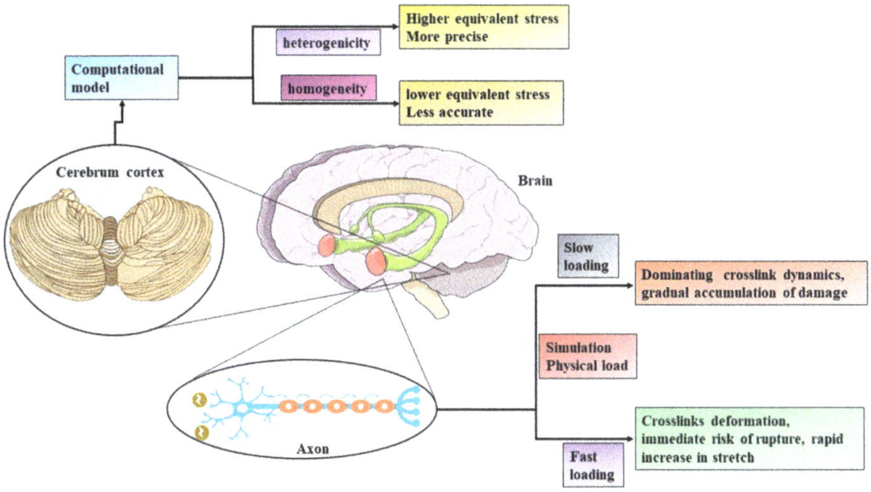

Figure 8.3. Influence of microtubule polymerization on axonal degeneration process.

neurosurgical procedures, notify brain wound benchmark, and upgrade the layout of protective mechanisms.

Accurate rheological modelling demands qualitative and quantitative understanding of loading mode-specific, time-dependent material response (Miller and Chinzei 2002). Furthermore, the brain tissue exhibits non-linear behaviour for quasi-static loading rates, whereas the linear viscoelastic parameter is observed under single loading modes (with finite strains) (Budday *et al* 2017). Nevertheless, random loading conditions with finite strains are not well characterized for the human brain. Therefore, the objective here is to perform simple shear, unconfined compression, tension, and stress relaxation in shear and compression with simultaneous calibration in a time-dependent fashion with established finite strain. This nonlinear, viscoelastic built-in platform apprehends the stimuli to brain tissue under numerous loading scenarios. Also, contradictory observations for regional stiffness variation are presumed to be time-dependent (Budday *et al* 2017); the cortical grey matter was reportedly stiffer than white matter and vice-versa. Budday *et al* harvested small homogenous specimens from brain regions: an outer grey matter of cortex (GMC), the inner gray matter of basal ganglia (BG), the white matter of corona radiate (CR), the white matter of corpus callosum (CC) to systematically compare the region-specific elastic and viscous material parameters to characterize brain across space and time ultimately; by adopting a nonlinear approach to characterize large deformability of brain tissue by multiplicatively decomposing the deformation gradient into elastic and inelastic parts, additively decompose free energy function into equilibrium and non-equilibrium parts. Various physical parameters like fluid motion within solid cell network and extracellular matrix establish a poroelastic behaviour while the viscoelastic behaviour is triggered during intracellular interactions between cytoplasm, nucleus and membrane (Franceschini *et al* 2006). Thus, the poroelastic/viscoelastic origin of time-dependent rheology of brain tissue is associated with various timescales and physical parameters.

Budday *et al* analysed data from 58 samples: 13 from, 15 from BG, 19 from CR, 11 from CC; by mounting them in a triaxial testing device followed by hydrating with PBS and final testing. The authors performed a sequence of different loading modes, shear, compression, and tension for each specimen. And five different tests were conducted (to calibrate): simple shear, unconfined compression, tension, shear relaxation, and compression relaxation. The outcome indicates that the simplest model with only one viscoelasticity mode and five material parameters naturally captures the essential features of brain tissue, i.e., its characteristic nonlinearity, pre-conditioning, hysteresis, and tension-compression asymmetry as well as increasing the number of viscoelastic modes improves the agreement between model and experiment, especially across entire relaxation regime (Budday *et al* 2017). Suggesting, two cycles of pre-conditioning decrease the grey matter stiffness by a factor of three, while the white matter stiffness remains almost identical.

Here, the rheology of brain tissue via a family of limited viscoelastic Ogden-type models has been determined along with characterizing their parameters for multiple loading modes in four different regions of the brain. Simultaneously the authors identified a single parameter set (for shear, compression, tension, shear relaxation, and compression relaxation loading), which is critical for computational simulations when loading is naturally mixed-mode. Furthermore, in grey matter regions, a marked sensitivity to pre-conditioning was observed, suggesting that in certain brain regions, at certain loading rates, additional time-dependent effects like poroelasticity could play a non-negligible role, as shown in figure 8.4. Overall, the study will improve the simulations of human brain development with the ultimate goal to enhance personalized treatment planning.

The model was calibrated for two different parameter sets: unconditioned response (left bar graph) using first loading cycle; conditioned response (right) using third loading cycle. Four different regions of the brain were used: C: Cortex;

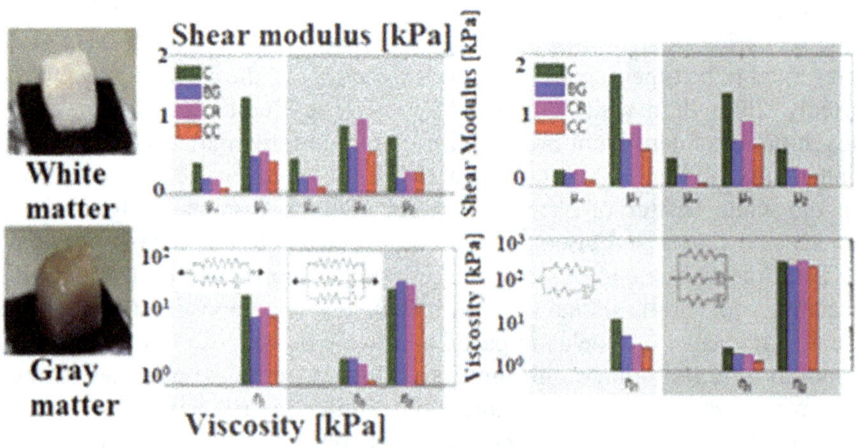

Figure 8.4. Shows quantification of susceptibility of the ultrasoft human brain towards arbitrary loading conditions.

BG: Basal Ganglia; CR: Corona Radiata; CC: Corpus Callosum. The bar graph here clearly indicates that unconditioned tissue was stiffer when compared to conditioned tissue in all four different brain regions. Also, the grey matter stiffness of the cortex varied by almost a factor of three in between 0.65 and 0.24 kPa, whereas the white matter of corona radiata varied only marginally between 0.29 and 0.25 kPa. Therefore, these data display that even after calibration of both parameter sets with the same stress relaxation experiment, larger slow time constants in conditioned response were observed compared to unconditioned response, suggesting that cyclic experiments have a pronounced effect on viscoelastic parameter identification.

8.6.1 Viscoelastic modeling of brain tissue

To model, the characteristic nonlinearity, conditioning, hysteresis, and tension-compression asymmetry of the human brain, a finite viscoelastic Ogden model with six material parameters—an elastic stiffness, two viscoelastic stiffness, a nonlinearity parameter, and two viscous time constants—are used to predict behaviour under random loading rates. Unlike conventional model parameters, the model was calibrated under shear, shear relaxation, compression, compression relaxation, and tension for four different brain regions: cortex, basal ganglia, corona radiata, and corpus callosum. The outcome of such an experiment can improve the accuracy of human brain simulations in health and disease.

Human brain tissue exhibits ultrasoft mechanical behaviour (nonlinear and hysteric) even for relatively small strains and quasi-static loading rates (Miller and Chinzei 2002, Budday *et al* 2017a), where both time-dependent and time-independent characteristics show regional variations (Budday *et al* 2017a, 2017b). Therefore, designing appropriate experiments to accurately identify material parameters and a mathematical model to capture time-dependent tissue response at finite strains is key to establishing realistic constitutive brain models. Moreover, imprecise results upon using animal models like porcine or bovine (being structurally similar to human brain) is inevitable (Budday *et al* 2015). Unlike prior time-dependent mechanical behaviour research limited to linear viscoelastic properties at small strains, the advanced approaches characterize the time-dependent behavior using a Prony series (Miller and Chinzei 2002, Budday *et al* 2015). But when actual strain history was considered, the Prony series made poor predictions of porcine brain experiments; indicating that material parameters identified for single loading mode do not necessarily represent constitutive behaviour under random loading cases (Miller and Chinzei 2002). The objective here is to systematically analyze time-dependent effects under different loading conditions to predict a probable methodology at a cellular level by focusing on viscoelasticity modeling to address porous effects caused by CSF (~80% of total brain mass) held in solid networks of cells and ECM to discriminate between the different mechanism that triggers time-dependent effects, Budday *et al* (2017) provided individual parameter sets for the unconditioned and conditioned tissue response.

Data shows unconditioned white and grey matter were equally stiff, whereas conditioned grey matter was three times stiffer than the white matter. Also, the pair of unconditioned viscous time constants was greater in the grey matter tissue of the brain when compared to the white matter. These rheological differences suggest different porosity between both tissues, having direct implications on improving the accuracy of human brain simulations in health and disease. Moreover, these data can be rationalized with underlying tissue microstructure: CR consists of a sparsely crosslinked network of myelinated axons, whereas the cortex is made of a densely connected dendrite network that traps the fluid phase inside the tissue. Overall, the findings bolster the assumption involving the rheology of brain tissue that is identified by at least two different time scales: one associated with poroelastic crosstalk of solid and fluid phases within the tissue, and the other is related to the viscoelastic behaviour of solid skeleton itself. These parameter sets can be widely used for finite simulations with a software package that features Ogden type models at finite deformations. Budday *et al*'s finite viscoelastic model might be applicable to simulate the brain's response at moderate to long time scales with applications in neurodevelopment, neuro-oncology, neurosurgery, and neurodegeneration.

8.7 Conclusion

The microstructural disparity between mammalian outer grey matter (encompassing cell bodies, dendrites, and unmyelinated axons) and the inner core of white matter (encompassing primarily myelinated axons); plays an indispensable role in neurodevelopment. Whilst the rheological attribution of the brain is eminent, the mechanical features of grey and white matter are not well identified. Authors devised a rugged, safe, easy-to-use, and repeatable technique to probe and inquire fresh mammalian brain specimens using flat-punch indentation. This technique mitigates the adhesion effect and naturally minimizes consequences of borderline, desiccation, swelling, and structural degradation besides maintaining intact mechanical characteristics. Overall regional variations between tissues can help in diagnosing neurological disorders and neurodevelopment.

The brain embedded inside the skull is isolated from its mechanical environment (Miller 2011); thus, the major focus is shifted more towards the electrical aspect and less towards the mechanical characteristics of brain tissue (Chatelin *et al* 2010). But a broad array of development disorders represents the involvement of mechanical factors like abnormal CSF accumulation and reduced/increased brain folding, to name a few, as shown by the research of Bayly *et al* (2014). Neuromechanics exhibits a strong interest in fast loading regimes associated with a dynamic phenomenon like extreme loading rate induced intracranial damage leading to permanent loss of function. Contrastingly, neurodevelopment exhibits a slow loading regime associated with quasi-static phenomenon with prolonged time of weeks/months like in cortical folding where compressive forces between grey matter layer and white matter substrate cause structural instabilities and induce surface buckling (Budday *et al* 2014). Understanding the mathematical modelling of time-scale phenomena and distinct materials that drive neurodevelopment and trigger morphological abnormalities is critical to understand the rheological differences between grey and white matter tissues. Chatelin *et al*'s (2010) research for fifty long years offered immense novel findings plus an understanding of 'whole' brain tissue, but as a result of incompatible construction of specimens, duration of post-mortem and testing states the individual rheology is poorly implied and deciphered. To address this imbalance, Budday and the team adopted a novel method to quantify mechanical properties of tissues by systematically probing the sensitivity to indenter diameter, loading time, holding time, and duration of post-mortem to ultimately explain that indention continually gives rise to rugged proportions and dimensions that implies that white matter tissue is nearly one third stiffer relative to the grey matter tissue.

Observable data suggests that white matter displays higher maximum indentation forces and steeper indentation curves than grey matter; differences in stiffness are microstructurally plausible. White matter primarily consists of myelinated axons that act as a network of biopolymer filaments, while grey matter is largely composed of cell bodies. Furthermore, in contrast to the prior conception that considered biofilaments non-load-bearing under applied pressure (compression), a recent study indicates that biofilaments remarkably bestow towards the compressive load-carrying ability of soft tissues. Therefore, the display of large regional deformations, viscoelastic property and temporal variations can altogether decipher underlying rheological dissimilarity, ultimately assisting in diagnosis, manipulation, and mechanical phenomenon during neurodevelopment, including polymicrogyria, brachycephaly, and hydrocephalus.

References

Al-Bsharat A S, Hardy W N, Yang K H, Khalil T B, Tashman S and King A I 1999 Brain/skull relative displacement magnitude due to blunt head impact: new experimental data and model (No. 99SC22) *SAE Technical Paper*

Arbogast K B and Margulies S S 1998 Material characterization of the brainstem from oscillatory shear tests *J. Biomech.* **31** 801–7

Atkinson-Leadbeater K, Bertolesi G E, Hehr C L, Webber C A, Cechmanek P B and McFarlane S 2010 Dynamic expression of axon guidance cues required for optic tract development is controlled by fibroblast growth factor signaling *J. Neurosci.* **30** 685–93

Bain A C and Meaney D F 2000 Tissue-level thresholds for axonal damage in an experimental model of central nervous system white matter injury *J. Biomech. Eng.* **122** 615–22

Bayly P V, Okamoto R J, Xu G, Shi Y and Taber L A 2013 A cortical folding model incorporating stress-dependent growth explains gyral wavelengths and stress patterns in the developing brain *Phys. Biol.* **10** 016005

Bayly P V, Taber L A and Kroenke C D 2014 Mechanical forces in cerebral cortical folding: a review of measurements and models *J. Mech. Behav. Biomed. Mater.* **29** 568–81

Bell G I 1978 Models for the specific adhesion of cells to cells *Science* **200** 618–27

Béduer A *et al* 2013 Investigation of the competition between cell/surface and cell/cell interactions during neuronal cell culture on a micro-engineered surface *Macromol. Biosci.* **13** 1546–55

Braak H, Ghebremedhin E, Rüb U, Bratzke H and Del Tredici K 2004 Stages in the development of Parkinson's disease-related pathology *Cell Tissue Res.* **318** 121–34

Budday S, Steinmann P and Kuhl E 2014 The role of mechanics during brain development *J. Mech. Phys. Solids* **72** 75–92

Budday S, Nay R, de Rooij R, Steinmann P, Wyrobek T, Ovaert T C and Kuhl E 2015 Mechanical properties of gray and white matter brain tissue by indentation *J. Mech. Behav. Biomed. Mater.* **46** 318–30

Budday S *et al* 2017a Mechanical characterization of human brain tissue *Acta Biomater.* **48** 319–40

Budday S, Sommer G, Haybaeck J, Steinmann P, Holzapfel G A and Kuhl E 2017b Rheological characterization of human brain tissue *Acta Biomater.* **60** 315–29

Budday S *et al* 2017 Mechanical characterization of human brain tissue *Acta Biomater.* **48** 319–40

Budday S, Steinmann P and Kuhl E 2015 Secondary instabilities modulate cortical complexity in the mammalian brain *Philos. Mag.* **95** 3244–56

Budday S, Raybaud C and Kuhl E 2014 A mechanical model predicts morphological abnormalities in the developing human brain *Sci. Rep.* **4** 1–7

Budday S *et al* 2015 Mechanical properties of gray and white matter brain tissue by indentation *J. Mech. Behav. Biomed. Mater.* **46** 318–30

Chan C E and Odde D J 2008 Traction dynamics of filopodia on compliant substrates *Science* **322** 1687–91

Chatelin S, Constantinesco A and Willinger R 2010 Fifty years of brain tissue mechanical testing: from *in vitro* to *in vivo* investigations *Biorheology* **47** 255–76

Chew L J, Fusar-Poli P and Schmitz T 2013 Oligodendroglial alterations and the role of microglia in white matter injury: relevance to schizophrenia *Develop. Neurosci.* **35** 102–29

Cloots R J H, Gervaise H M T, Van Dommelen J A W and Geers M G D 2008 Biomechanics of traumatic brain injury: influences of the morphologic heterogeneities of the cerebral cortex *Ann. Biomed. Eng.* **36** 1203

Coste B, Mathur J, Schmidt M, Earley T J, Ranade S, Petrus M J, Dubin A E and Patapoutian A 2010 Piezo1 and Piezo2 are essential components of distinct mechanically activated cation channels *Science* **330** 55–60

de Rooij R and Kuhl E 2018 Microtubule polymerization and cross-link dynamics explain axonal stiffness and damage *Biophys. J.* **114** 201–12

Dinh N D *et al* 2013 Microfluidic construction of minimalistic neuronal co-cultures *Lab Chip* **13** 1402–12

Franceschini G, Bigoni D, Regitnig P and Holzapfel G A 2006 Brain tissue deforms similarly to filled elastomers and follows consolidation theory *J. Mech. Phys. Solids* **54** 2592–620

Franze K *et al* 2009 Neurite branch retraction is caused by a threshold-dependent mechanical impact *Biophys. J.* **97** 1883–90

Frimat J P *et al* 2011 A microfluidic array with cellular valving for single cell co-culture *Lab Chip* **11** 231–7

Fletcher T L, Wirthl B, Kolias A G, Adams H, Hutchinson P J and Sutcliffe M P 2016 Modelling of brain deformation after decompressive craniectomy *Ann. Biomed. Eng.* **44** 3495–509

Gottlieb P A and Sachs F 2012 Piezo1: properties of a cation selective mechanical channel *Channels* **6** 214–19

Hamhaber U, Klatt D, Papazoglou S, Hollmann M, Stadler J, Sack I, Bernarding J and Braun J 2010 *In vivo* magnetic resonance elastography of human brain at 7 T and 1.5 T *J. Magn. Reson. Imaging* **32** 577–83

Holzapfel G A, Gasser T C and Ogden R W 2000 A new constitutive framework for arterial wall mechanics and a comparative study of material models *J. Elast.* **61** 1–48

Ionescu-Zanetti C *et al* 2005 Mammalian electrophysiology on a microfluidic platform *Proc. Natl Acad. Sci. USA* **102** 9112–17

Johnson C L, McGarry M D, Gharibans A A, Weaver J B, Paulsen K D, Wang H, Olivero W C, Sutton B P and Georgiadis J G 2013 Local mechanical properties of white matter structures in the human brain *Neuroimage* **79** 145–52

Kincaid A E, Zheng T and Wilson C J 1998 Connectivity and convergence of single corticostriatal axons *J. Neurosci.* **18** 4722–31

Koch D, Rosoff W J, Jiang J, Geller H M and Urbach J S 2012 Strength in the periphery: growth cone biomechanics and substrate rigidity response in peripheral and central nervous system neurons *Biophys. J.* **102** 452–60

Kolias A G, Kirkpatrick P J and Hutchinson P J 2013 Decompressive craniectomy: past, present and future *Nat. Rev. Neurol.* **9** 405–15

Koser D E *et al* 2016 Mechanosensing is critical for axon growth in the developing brain *Nat. Neurosci.* **19** 1592–8

Koser D E *et al* 2015 CNS cell distribution and axon orientation determine local spinal cord mechanical properties *Biophys. J.* **108** 2137–47

Kruse S A, Rose G H, Glaser K J, Manduca A, Felmlee J P, Jack C R Jr and Ehman R L 2008 Magnetic resonance elastography of the brain *Neuroimage* **39** 231–7

Li B, Cao Y P, Feng X Q and Gao H 2012 Mechanics of morphological instabilities and surface wrinkling in soft materials: a review *Soft Matter* **8** 5728–45

Luders E, Narr K L, Bilder R M, Szeszko P R, Gurbani M N, Hamilton L, Toga A W and Gaser C 2008 Mapping the relationship between cortical convolution and intelligence: effects of gender *Cereb. Cortex* **18** 2019–26

Luhmann H J, Kilb W and Hanganu-Opatz I L 2009 Subplate cells: amplifiers of neuronal activity in the developing cerebral cortex *Front. Neuroanat.* **3** 19

Mihai L A *et al* 2015 A comparison of hyperelastic constitutive models applicable to brain and fat tissues *J. R. Soc. Interface* **12** 20150486

Miller K and Chinzei K 2002 Mechanical properties of brain tissue in tension *J. Biomech.* **35** 483–90

Miller K (ed) 2011 *Biomechanics of the Brain* (New York: Springer) pp 111–36

Moore D F, Jérusalem A, Nyein M, Noels L, Jaffee M S and Radovitzky R A 2009 Computational biology—modeling of primary blast effects on the central nervous system *Neuroimage* **47** T10–20

Morel M *et al* 2012 Amplification and temporal filtering during gradient sensing by nerve growth cones probed with a microfluidic assay *Biophys. J.* **103** 1648–56

Naidich T P, Castillo M, Cha S and Smirniotopoulos J G 2012 *Imaging of the Brain: Expert Radiology Series* (Beijing: Elsevier)

Nicholson C 2001 Diffusion and related transport mechanisms in brain tissue *Rep. Prog. Phys.* **64** 815

Nie J *et al* 2010 A computational model of cerebral cortex folding *J. Theor. Biol.* **264** 467–78

Peyrin J M *et al* 2011 Axon diodes for the reconstruction of oriented neuronal networks in microfluidic chambers *Lab Chip* **11** 3663–73

Raybaud C, Ahmad T, Rastegar N, Shroff M and Al Nassar M 2013 The premature brain: developmental and lesional anatomy *Neuroradiology* **55** 23–40

Raybaud C and Widjaja E 2011 Development and dysgenesis of the cerebral cortex: malformations of cortical development *Neuroimag. Clin.* **21** 483–543

Ronan L, Voets N, Rua C, Alexander-Bloch A, Hough M, Mackay C, Crow T J, James A, Giedd J N and Fletcher P C 2014 Differential tangential expansion as a mechanism for cortical gyrification *Cereb. Cortex* **24** 2219–28

Sack I, Beierbach B, Hamhaber U, Klatt D and Braun J 2008 Non-invasive measurement of brain viscoelasticity using magnetic resonance elastography *NMR Biomed.* **21** 265–71

Sahuquillo J 2006 Decompressive craniectomy for the treatment of refractory high intracranial pressure in traumatic brain injury *Cochrane Database Syst. Rev.* CD003983

Segal M, Greenberger V and Korkotian E 2003 Formation of dendritic spines in cultured striatal neurons depends on excitatory afferent activity *Eur. J. Neurosci.* **17** 2573–85

Soza G *et al* 2005 Determination of the elasticity parameters of brain tissue with combined simulation and registration *Int. J. Med. Rob. Comput. Assist. Surg.* **01** 87

Spires-Jones T L, Stoothoff W H, de Calignon A, Jones P B and Hyman B T 2009 Tau pathophysiology in neurodegeneration: a tangled issue *Trends Neurosci.* **32** 150–9

Timofeev I, Santarius T, Kolias A G and Hutchinson P J A 2012 Decompressive craniectomy—operative technique and perioperative care *Advances and Technical Standards in Neurosurgery* (Vienna: Springer) pp 115–36

van Dommelen J A W *et al* 2010 Mechanical properties of brain tissue by indentation: Interregional variation *J. Mech. Behav. Biomed. Mater.* **3** 158–66

Van E D C 1997 A tension-based theory of morphogenesis and compact wiring in the central nervous system *Nature* **385** 313–18

Walz A, Anderson R B, Irie A, Chien C B and Holt C E 2002 Chondroitin sulfate disrupts axon pathfinding in the optic tract and alters growth cone dynamics *J. Neurobiol.* **53** 330–42

Weickenmeier J, de Rooij R, Budday S, Steinmann P, Ovaert T C and Kuhl E 2016 Brain stiffness increases with myelin content *Acta Biomater.* **42** 265–72

Xu G, Knutsen A K, Dikranian K, Kroenke C D, Bayly P V and Taber L A 2010 Axons pull on the brain, but tension does not drive cortical folding *J. Biomech. Eng.* **132** 1–8

Yamada A *et al* 2016 In-mold patterning and actionable axo-somatic compartmentalization for on-chip neuron culture *Lab Chip* **16** 2059–68

Yi M and Wu X 2020 Dynamics of charged particles around a magnetically deformed Schwarzschild black hole *Phys. Scr.* **95** 085008

Yin J and Chen X 2011 Buckling patterns of thin films on compliant substrates: the effect of plasticity *J. Phys. D: Appl. Phys.* **44** 045401

IOP Publishing

Neurocognitive Perspectives of Prosocial and Positive Emotional Behaviours

Theory to application

Shashikanta Tarai and Arindam Bit

Chapter 9

Processing of prosocial language and its impact on human brain: electroencephalographic study in the frequency domain

Shashikanta Tarai and Arindam Bit

Prosocial communicative behaviours improve human relationships, cooperation, harmony and peace. In language, using prosocial words such as caring, helping, sharing, devoting and contributing to others has a beneficial and utilitarian effect. However, the value judgments of accepting, adapting and rejecting in prosocial communicative behaviours have not been studied in psycho- and neurolinguistics. Using the electroencephalographic (EEG) technique, we investigated and examined the band-frequencies of the delta, theta and beta, and the event-related potential (ERP) mechanisms of prosocial positive and unsocial negative communicate-behaviours during the processing of grammatically correct and incorrect English sentences. Early delta frequencies (1–4 Hz) displayed a high power spectrum in the prefrontal, frontal and temporal regions of brain during the processing of unsocial-negative sentences. However, the theta band frequencies (4–7 Hz) revealed a higher power-spectra for grammatically wrong than right sentences in the prefrontal lobes. Thus, prosocial communicative behaviours facilitate the neurocognitive mechanisms to perceive and comprehend the grammaticality of a language.

9.1 Introduction

Humans are prosocial-cooperative species (Henrich and Muthukrishna 2021). Human cognition and language have a socio-communicative capacity to promote intra-group prosocial behaviour to minimise excessive violent, aggressive and unsocial behaviours (Hare 2017). In contrast to unsocial interactions, prosociality refers to positive but possibly selfishly driven activities (Eisenberg *et al* 1983). Aggressive or unsocial behaviour has been defined as behaviour that causes physical

doi:10.1088/978-0-7503-3383-2ch9

or emotional harm to another person (Kitts 2006, Obsuth *et al* 2015, Krahé 2020). For example, stealing intra-group resources without informing others is considered corruption, part of unsocial action (Rand *et al* 2009). On the other hand, prosocial behaviour refers to activities that seem to have a positive social impact (Eisenberg *et al* 2014). For example, we consider the prosocial behaviours and actions such as to give, help, be kind, cooperate, friendship, etc, as an essential element of giving that consistently contributes to establishing a stable relationship, intra-group harmony, collective identity and reconciliation (de Waal 2000, Ripley and Worthington 2002, Tyler and Blader 2003, DeCremer and Tyler 2004). Moreover, people who are accustomed to helping gain more benefit because the action or event-help enhances a great sense of moral values in helpers' lives, advances self-judgment and evaluation, proliferates in a positive mood, and establishes social-cooperation and integration (Midlarsky 1991). Also, caregivers who care about others get to have greater self-efficacy, self-worth, self-esteem and self-respect (Crocker 2008). Prosociality and kindness are collectively gratifying and rewarding forever (Keltner *et al* 2014). These cultural values of generosity, hospitality and service are essential to reduce world-wide unsocial activities like violence, terror and wars (Triandis 1978).

9.1.1 Linguistic root of prosociality

The study of Wispe (1972) has defined the word 'prosocial behaviour' to distinguish it from 'unsocial or pro-self behaviour.' The majority of these researches have mainly emphasised non-linguistic pro- and antisocial behaviours. Feeding a hungry child, helping a stranger, or calming a distressed friend are all examples of voluntary activities to promote the well-being of others (Gross *et al* 2017). Premature comprehension of prosociality occurs early and has significant consequences for societal actions (Spinrad *et al* 2006). When making choices, unsocial is optimistic and determined to optimise self-centeredness; prosocial actions, on the other hand, are more trustworthy and able to comply while they follow social standards (Lambert *et al* 2017). Prosocialists optimise net wealth allocation between themselves and others whilst limiting their distance (Haruno and Frith 2010). On the other hand, individuals who devote all of their resources to themselves without thinking about others have widened the difference between self and others (Haruno and Frith 2010). For example, the gap between self and others suppresses the notion of collectiveness when the participants attend their group rituals and food sharing ceremony (Gurven 2004, Henrich *et al* 2004). This research indicates that an individual with kindness and prosociality is either governed by the top-down control in overriding self-interest actions or has suppressed the neural activities that represent self-interested impulses to combat any antipathy, aggression and other socially undesirable actions (Haidt 2001, Knoch and Fehr 2007). Most of these prosocial and unsocial behaviours, actions and events are stored, processed, and transmitted through language. Though language aids in decoding others' prosocial and unsocial behaviour, prosocial behaviour directly improves communicative and relational skills of collaboration and harmony. A cooperative form of communication emerges through language to test the false belief and understanding (Wellman *et al* 2011, Lane *et al* 2013, Mink *et al* 2014).

Our prosocial behaviours are rooted in linguistic capabilities and superior cognitive abilities (Wrangham 2019). Most linguistic or cognitive unsocial traits like exploiting, lying, stealing and cheating others can quickly be suppressed by using prosocial, positive and persuasive language and resourceful tactics to fool or satisfy us (McNally *et al* 2012, McNally and Jackson 2013, Boyd and Mathew 2015). The development of countless sociality, which overrides the unsocial and aggression, opens a path of cooperative communication systems. Therefore, when children's ability to perceive language and converse better improves, they tend more to be involved and engaged in prosocial behaviour (Girard *et al* 2017). Earlier communicative and ethnographic studies have found a strong association between language and prosocial behaviours throughout children's developmental phases (Ensor and Hughes 2005, Rhee *et al* 2013). Humans domesticate the language to facilitate cultural cognition, cooperation, and technology (Pagel 2012, Somel *et al* 2013). During the unprecedented COVID-19 pandemic, the public or community health and well-being messages often use prosocial words and persuasive tones to minimise the isolated negative attitudes and behaviours (Heffner *et al* 2021). When conveying the prosocial significance, the verbal means of communication like words and phrases are more descriptive and have a more extensive semantic network than non-verbal means of communication like voice and tone (Pennebaker and King 1999, Newman *et al* 2003). Any effects on inner- and emotional awareness are attributed to the processing of loving-kindness language and the language of love and goodwill (Lee 2013, Nowak and Coakley 2013, Gilbert 2016, Williams *et al* 2018).

9.1.2 Use of prosocial language in political discourse

In contrast to the positive words like hope, help and harmony, the negative words like hate, hurt and harm, augment the unsociality at the cost of suppressing prosociability (Oxford and Curtis 2021). A friendly and prosocial demeanour is considered in interpersonal conversation for raising social acceptance (Newman *et al* 2003, Cohn *et al* 2004, Fiske *et al* 2007, Kacewicz *et al* 2014, Dale *et al* 2020). It is observed that the use of the first-person singular pronoun 'I' may create a distance between leader and voters (exclusion); thereby, it may decrease overall public approval. However, the use of the first-person plural pronoun 'we' may increase the voters' approval and positive sentiment on casting their votes in favour of the leader, as our analysis of the political textual speech of Hillary Clinton and Donald Trump shows in figure 9.1.

This type of prosocial communication style has always created a favourable impact on listeners or readers minds (McLeod and Owens 2004, Von Hippel and Trivers 2011) because prosocial aspects of communication are linked with health, well-being and happiness (Sapolsky 2005). This result has recently been attributed to the US Congress's poor public support due to a lack of prosocial language in debates. As a whole, using prosocial terms like solidarity, aid, and compassion helps people and governments win mutual acceptance and encouragement (Jansari *et al* 2000). Furthermore, the language of prosocial forecasts the public's opinion in

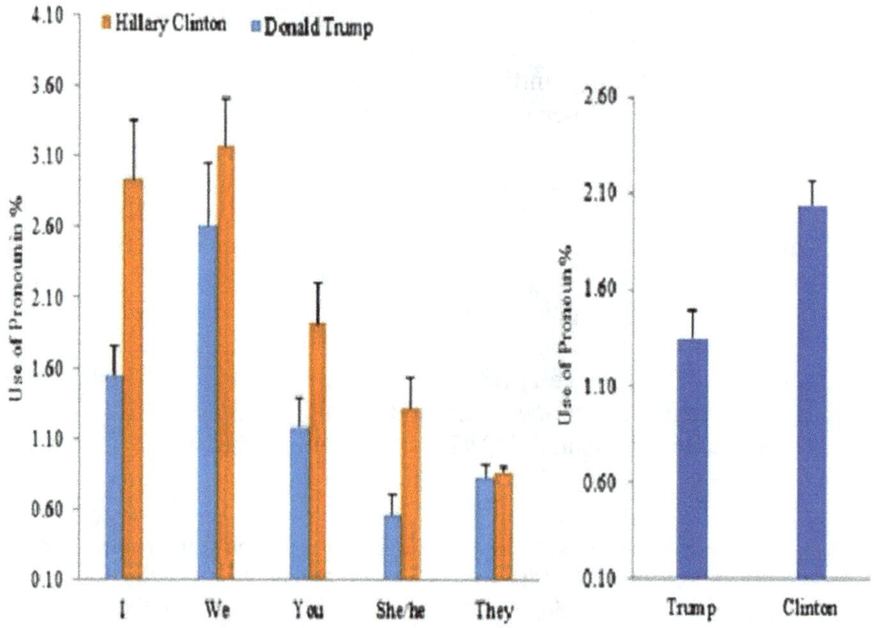

Figure 9.1. The higher frequency of first-singular pronoun 'I' in the case of Clinton than Donald Trump.

making a judgement or verdict (Dixon 2013, Frimer *et al* 2015). The analysis of Donald Trump and Hillary Clinton (from March to July 2016) reveals that they often use persuasive, prosocial and positive language to gain social approval during the Presidential election. Clinton used the modal auxiliary 'can' more than Trump. In contrast, Trump used the modal auxiliary 'will' more than Clinton, as figure 9.2 shows. Moreover, Clinton used more pronouns than Trump. These types of language use facilitate public approval and disapproval during the election. However, the prediction of acceptance and rejection in pro- or antisocial words has never been examined in the area of neuro-linguistic or neuroscience of language.

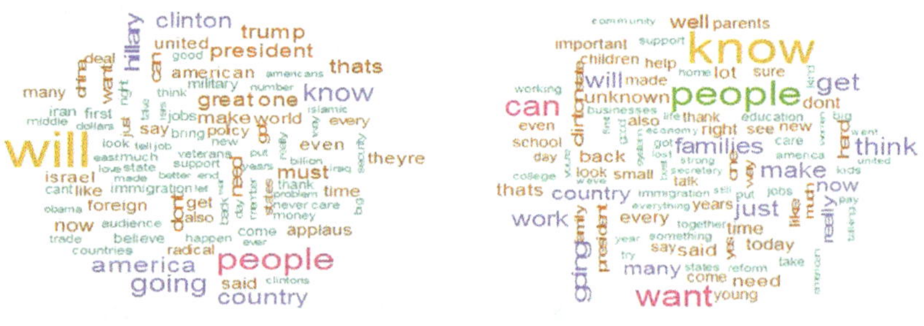

Figure 9.2. Political speech determines differences in terms of the use of modal auxiliary 'will', which was higher for Donald Trump than Hillary Clinton.

9.1.3 Processing of prosocial behaviours in the human brain

Many studies using functional near-infrared spectroscopy (fNIRS), functional magnetic resonance imaging (fMRI) and electroencephalographic (EEG) techniques have explored the regions of the brain that involve the processing of prosocial moral and unsocial immoral behaviours and actions (Yamada *et al* 2011, Hu *et al* 2017, Jie *et al* 2019a, 2019b, Pletti *et al* 2019, Descorbeth *et al* 2020, Hackel *et al* 2020, Jie *et al* 2021). For example, using the functional neuroimaging techniques, a study has found two regions of the brain, such as the ventromedial prefrontal cortex (vmPFC) and the dorsolateral prefrontal cortex (dlPFC), are associated with the executive function and evaluation during any choice or decision-making. When university students played an excellent public game with an option to follow either cooperative or selfish norms, participants with prosocial, communal norms showed higher activation in vmPFC than dlPFC areas. However, the participants with selfish criteria revealed higher activation in dlPFC than vmPFC areas (Zhu *et al* 2014, Hackel *et al* 2020). More extensive connectivity between dlPFC and vmPFC was observed when participants violated the groups or cooperative norms (Carter and Van Veen 2007, Hare *et al* 2009). Prosocial behaviours and collaborative activities were strongly associated with the temporoparietal regions of the brain. The ventromedial prefrontal cortex (vmPFC) is also associated with evaluating emotional judgment and prosocial value-based anticipation of decision-making (Satpute and Lieberman 2006, Lebreton *et al* 2009, Hutcherson *et al* 2012). The anticipated and expected value of prosociality is processed in the vmPFC regions of the brain (Rangel and Hare 2010, Levy and Glimcher 2012). Moreover, the ventromedial prefrontal cortex integrates the neuro-computation during cooperative decisions or referring to collective intentions of others while receiving neurocognitive inputs from the learning experience, memory and attention (Cooper *et al* 2010, Pärnamets *et al* 2020).

9.1.4 Empathy and counter-empathy facilitates human communication

Like cooperation, empathy is prosocial behaviours and altruistic activities that facilitate communicative interaction in a social context (Yamada *et al* 2011). The neurocognitive mechanisms of empathy for ingroup members are conversed to those mechanisms and regions brain involved in antipathy towards outgroup members (Takahashi *et al* 2009, Dvash *et al* 2010, Hein *et al* 2010). For example, the counter empathetic response of a revengeful act is processed in the nucleus accumbens areas instead of the brain areas, i.e., the anterior cingulate cortex is devoted to empathy (Singer *et al* 2006, Takahashi *et al* 2009). The nuclear accumbens area showed high activation when participants did not help outgroup members. However, when participants helped ingroup members, the anterior insula showed high activation (Hein *et al* 2010). ERP studies have found that the processing of counter empathy occurs much later than empathetic processing (Yamada *et al* 2011, Feng *et al* 2016, Luo *et al* 2018, Jie *et al* 2019b, Fan *et al* 2021). Using the perception-action model paradigms proposed by Jie *et al* (2019a) study has shown that facial expression induces the empathic response (de Greck *et al* 2012a, 2012b) when participants perceive others' emotional faces feel their emotions (Decety and Grèzes 2006).

9.1.5 ERP studies on prosocial behaviours

Social value orientation (SVO) refers to honesty-humility predicting a person's prosocial behaviours (Van Lange 2000, Li *et al* 2013, Hilbig *et al* 2014, Yang *et al* 2014). For instance, individuals with social values preferring competition and individualism have pro-self-attitudes, whereas individuals denoting social cooperation, joint attention, and equality orientation have a robust prosocial attitude (Joireman and Duell 2005, Stouten *et al* 2005). Therefore, individuals' prosocial and pro-self attitudes differ based on cooperation and competition, respectively (Van Lange 2000, Bieleke *et al* 2017). Usually, the pro-self individuals solitarily care for their own or self-interests without looking at others interests. However, prosocial individuals always prefer interests and outcomes that benefit themselves and others (Murphy and Ackermann 2014). These behavioural results of SVO are replicated in the fMRI studies, which reveal higher activation in the amygdala regions for prosocial than pro-self-judgement (Haruno and Frith 2010). The pro-self actions are processed in the medial prefrontal cortex (Declerck *et al* 2014, Christopoulos and King-Casas 2015, Yang *et al* 2015). Analysing the time course of the brain activities, an ERP study has shown that three components such as feed-back related negativity (FRN), P300 and the late positive complex (LPC), are associated with the outcomes linked with others and self (Scheepers and Derks 2016, Hu *et al* 2017). FRN and P300 processed the prosocial effects, whereas the pro-self-outcome is processed in the late positive component (LPC). The moral content of prosociality is detected in the early components such as N1, EPN, N2 and the late positive potential (LPP) (Gan *et al* 2016, Gui *et al* 2016). Moreover, the amplitudes of early negativity of N1 or EPN are larger for prosocial than unsocial actions both in adults and children (Yoder and Decety 2014, Cowell and Decety 2015, Leuthold *et al* 2015). Prosocial scenes are processed in the early harmful components (Schupp *et al* 2003, Weinberg and Hajcak 2010). The N2 component is more significant for unsocial than prosocial action displayed by children (Yoder and Decety 2014, Decety and Cowell 2018). The LPP (350–420 ms) is stated to be higher for positive, moral and prosocial actions than negative, immoral and unsocial actions in the midline parietal and occipital lobes (Hajcak *et al* 2010, Yoder and Decety 2014, Cowell and Decety 2015, Gui *et al* 2016). Most of these studies have found that the moral-self of prosociality is implicitly and automatically processed in the early component within 100 ms. The moral-self is explicitly processed in the LPP component at 400 ms (Lapsley and Narvaez 2004, Schupp *et al* 2004).

In addition to EEG and fMRI findings, some biological studies have focused on many neurotransmitters and genetic traits of prosocial and unsocial behaviours, revealing the neurohormones and neuropeptides that regulate prosocial actions (Kuepper *et al* 2010, Montoya *et al* 2012). However, serotonin, testosterone, and oxytocin control unsocial behaviours (Hare 2017). Prosocial behaviours are transmitted through neurotransmitters like dopamine (Reuter *et al* 2011), serotonin (Crockett *et al* 2010) and oxytocin (Kogan *et al* 2011). Avoiding harm and violent behaviour or aggression and enhancing prosocial activities largely depend on exogenous serotonin (Crockett *et al* 2010, De Dreu and Kret 2016). The unsocial behaviours activate and improve the prefrontal cortex via the dorsolateral neural pathways, primarily involved in controlling executive function and cognitive regulation and cost-benefit scrutiny or profit-loss analysis (Miller and Cohen 2001, Lambert *et al* 2017). Contrarily, prosocial behaviours have more activity in the frontal and temporal regions of the brain (Schaich Borg *et al* 2006). These regions of the brain are involved during routine moral judgements and conformity. Prosocial attitude is linked with the increased neural activity in the prefrontal areas (Knoch and Fehr 2007, Haruno and Frith 2010), whereas the pro-self behaviours are processed in the insula or amygdala regions (Adolphs *et al* 2002, Sanfey *et al* 2003, Tabibnia *et al* 2008). These results imply that prosocial behaviour helps us to organise spontaneous thought and decision making.

9.1.6 Aim of the current chapter

This chapter examines how pro- and antisocial or unsocial words are computed and processed in our brains. We have described the results obtained from previous multiple studies, including our reflections in the domain of prosocial language. In this chapter, the neuroscience literature on the processing of (a) prosocial, cooperative sentences, (b) unsocial or antisocial non-cooperative sentences, (c) grammatically correct, and (d) incorrect English sentences has been analysed to understand the neurocognitive or neural computational mechanisms in the frequency domain. Previously, the early behavioural processing of prosociality is predicted by anticipating the prosocial actions and communication through language, which are always affirmative and consistent to human experience and learning. For inaccurate and grammatically incorrect sentences, the adult bilingual participants may predict and anticipate the prosocial words that may need fewer neural resources than unsocial or antisocial words in sentences. As a result, prosocial words would be detected far more quickly than unsocial or antisocial negative words. Unsocial words might have more significant and enhanced neural amplitudes than prosocial and positive words because prosocial words demand more considerable behavioural benefit with less effort during early childhood understanding. Considering the negative emotional word processing in the previous research, the current chapter predicts that unsocial words may be processed in the tempro-parietal areas because of the manipulation of prosocial language stimuli.

Further, a hemisphere asymmetry effect can be found, resulting in hemisphere segregation of prosocial positive and unsocial or negative words. However, an fMRI study has proposed that prosocial, cooperative behaviours tend to elicit higher activity in vmPFC and dlPFC regions (Hackel *et al* 2020). This activation hypothesis of vmPFC and dlPFC may be strongly linked with the study findings on the perception of moral or prosocial judgments as in the study of Jie *et al* (2021), Descorbeth *et al* (2020), and Schaich Borg *et al* (2006) proposed a similar kind of neural activation hypothesis. According to these studies, the medial frontal, temporal and parietal regions would be shown to have more activation during the processing of moral or prosocial intention or action values as compared to immoral or unsocial intention or action values. Studies have also hypothesised that the computation of negative emotion in the paralimbic regions such as the amygdala, temporal lobe and prefrontal cortex would processing the negative unsocial actions or intentions (Mesulam 2000, Miller and Cohen 2001). However, the prosocial, moral, and positive choice would be linked with the central executive and cognitive system's partial and lateral brain regions (Greene *et al* 2004). In this regard, the current chapter intends to examine the cognitive neural mechanisms of prosocial positive and unsocial negative words when the selected participants processed grammatically incorrect and correct sentences with the terms. This chapter may widen our understanding of cognitive neural mechanisms of prosociality and unsociability in the domain of language processing. The knowledge of neural mechanisms of prosocial and unsocial aspects of language can provide scientific and rational evidence on the processing of language acquisition, learning and teaching that can regulate emotional reactions and enhance human happiness and social stability.

9.2 EEG and behavioural methods

9.2.1 Sampling technique and sample size

Most of the behavioural, EEG and fMRI experimental designs used the purposive and value judgment sample technique to select the participants for the studies. For instance, the study of Jie *et al* (2021) that investigated unsocial or counter-empathetic behaviours by employing the fMRI technique estimated the sample size of 38 participants. This number of samples is adequate and purposed enough to find a significant result. They also equally consider the gender representation of participants (e.g., F = 19, M = 19) to avoid any suggestion of gender-biased development. At the time of selection of participants, the age, including other social and physical parameters such as education, profession and vision, need to be controlled for getting adequate unbiased results. In this regard, the study of Descorbeth *et al* (2020) has recruited participants from different socioeconomic backgrounds to test how the neural mechanisms of prosocial dialogue varied across social strata. In their study, they used to have a total of 78 participants (M = 39, F = 38). As part of ethical guidelines, the experimenter was used to inform the objective of the experiments to all participants before the commencement of the experiment. Most of the participants had normal vision and no complaint of neurological, pathological and psychological disorders. Before the investigation, they provided a written consent declaration that they had no objection to participating in the experiment. Our investigations involved both bilingual (English and Hindi) 11 healthy and right-handed participants. From our study, one participant was disqualified, resulting in low behavioural accuracy (49%). Participants willingly agreed to take part in the experiment and provided a written consent form for their participation.

9.2.2 Materials and stimuli composition

Prosocial positive and unsocial negative words were used at the sentence level to comprise the stimuli. The place of the target words was in the fifth position of the sentences. Sentences were manipulated with grammar to write correct and incorrect sentences. We compiled a list of prosocial words using a database of 425 terms, including 127 terms used by Frimer *et al* (2015). Additionally, we employed a semantic value judgment task following a 7 likert point scale to represent higher to lower socialistic words (pro or anti) in a judge task. To determine the meaning of 425 words, ten participants were asked to judge whether they were prosocial or unsocial in terms of importance. The words rated for neutral, i.e., neither prosocial nor unsocial meaning were considered as neutral words; those neutral words were excluded from the experiment. In total, 50 prosocial words with high ratings were picked to project the target stimulus for the EEG experiments.

Another 50 unsocial words were chosen to compose the sentences for conducting the experiments. The simplest structure employing determiner, nouns, verbs and objects were used to construct the sentences. Most of these target words were picked based on the syllabic systems (1–5) to maintain and ensure the equal length of word uniformity and minimise any processing effects caused by different syllable counts. The words in the sentences were used in black colour English letters with 24 font sizes. After the target words (prosocial/unsocial), the sentences' grammar was altered, particularly the English tense indicators, to build grammatically incorrect statements. The stimuli were separated into two groups: grammatically accurate ($N = 100$) and inaccurate ($N = 100$). Each sentence was made up of six words that were arranged in random order. A short sentence in figure 9.3 shows a diagram of how stimuli were represented to the participants.

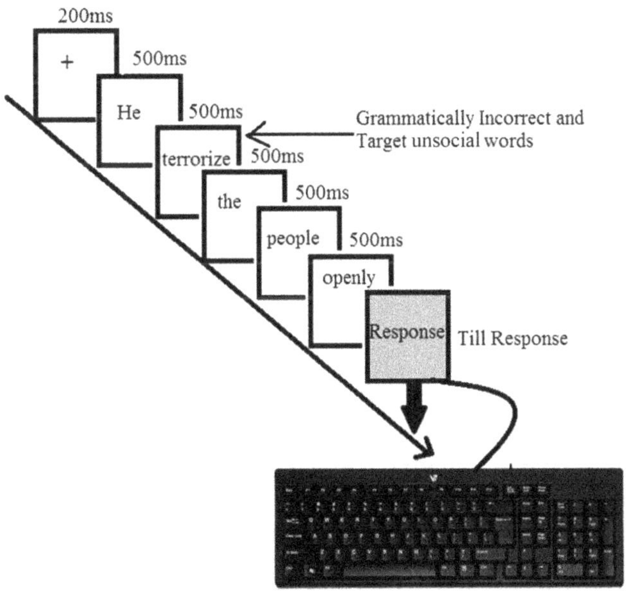

Figure 9.3. Trial structure and timeline of prosocial and unsocial grammatically correct and incorrect sentences are presented systematically. Each word is presented within the time limit of 500 ms.

9.2.3 Stimuli presentation and experimental procedures

The sentences were presented and appeared separately on a 17-inch screen LCD (5.0 version) using 'super lab' software. Participants were sat comfortably in a sound-mitigated compartment facing the LCD monitor. Words of each sentence appeared on the screen one by one. However, the complete meaning of a sentence was clear to the participants at the end of the last word. Each word from the sentence appeared for 600 ms with a period of 300 ms. At the end of each sentence, a black screen was displayed to alert the participants to accomplish the experimental task (e.g., whether the sentential trial was grammatically incorrect or correct). Written consent was taken from the participants to keep their personal information and demographic profile confidential as per the Institutional Ethical Guidelines.

We instructed the participants to read and comprehend the meaning of words in sentences. Additionally, they were asked to assess the grammatical errors of the sentences. Subsequently, their behavioural responses were recorded and captured when they were asked to respond by using the key 'N' for grammatically incorrect and 'Y' for correct sentences of English. We asked participants to respond to the sentential stimuli as soon as possible with high accuracy. A training session comprising ten sentences was piloted separately to get familiar with the response task. None of the sentential stimuli was repeated in this experiment. These experimental designs and stimulus representations were used to test the neuro-cognitive mechanisms of prosocial and unsocial words at the level of sentences. Previously, this design was tested in the context of moral-pleasant and immoral-unpleasant judgment (Moll *et al* 2002, Heekeren *et al* 2003). Participants were asked to judge or evaluate whether moral actions were suitable or unsuitable (Heekeren *et al* 2003, Greene *et al* 2004). The cognitive processing of moral values related to scenarios like killing, letting die, rape, theft, and lying can be captured to determine prosocial and unsocial behaviours. Most of these moral scenarios were compared with non-moral or immoral scenarios to find out demanding and less demanding neurocognitive mechanisms. Participants were categorically asked to execute an action that may or may not be appropriate with the scenarios.

9.2.4 Behavioral and EEG data acquisition

Behavioural and EEG data were collected from each participant. Behavioural data referring to behavioural response time in ms and accuracy in percentile were measured and captured across all trials. The 10–14 channels were used for recording the EEG signals, as shown in figure 9.4.

The electrode cap, power lab, and lab-chart software designed by AD Instrument Company were set up to capture the EEG signals. The connectivity between electrode cap and scalp in terms of impedance was checked using a UFI machine, preserved under 5 kHz. EEG signals were persistently captured at a sample rate of 100 Hz with an online band frequency ranging from 0.1 to 50 Hz. An earlobe electrode was used to reference all EEG channels, as in the montage given in figure 9.4.

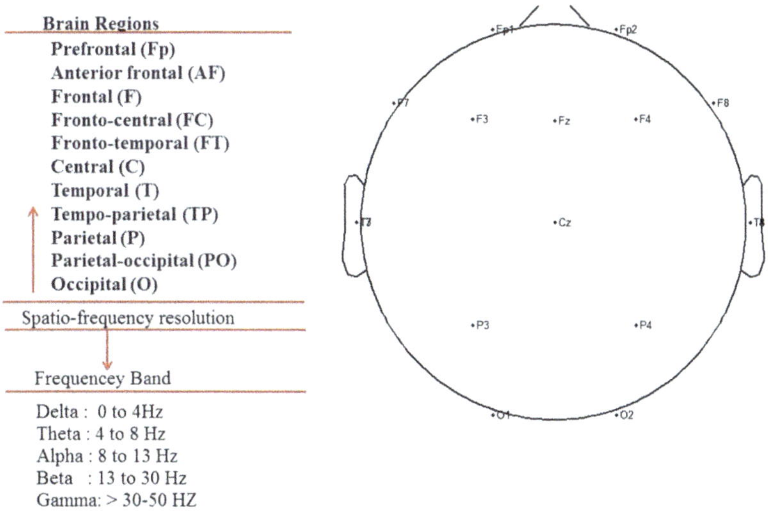

Figure 9.4. The spatio-frequency resolutions of EEG frequency bands such as delta, theta, alpha, beta and gamma are analyzed concerning the montage of 10–14 channels.

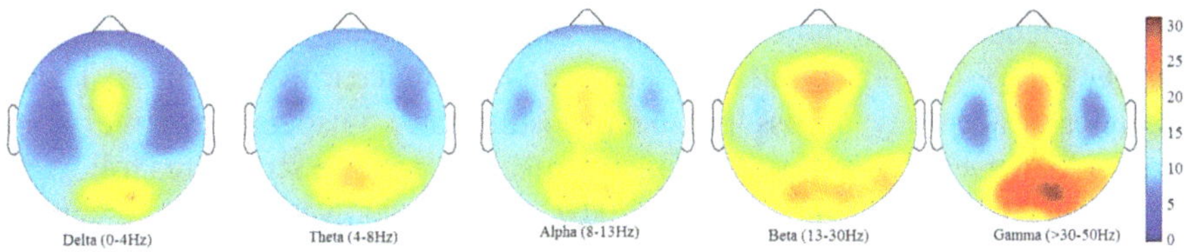

Figure 9.5. The representative topo-map of the brain classifies band-frequencies from low to high comprising delta, theta, alpha, beta and gamma.

9.2.5 EEG raw signals filtering and analysing

The essential EEG singles were segmented and averaged out concerning the experimental conditions. Mean average EEG signals, which were segmented, were time-locked by following positive-prosocial, negative-antisocial correct and incorrect sentences. Off-line EEG signals were filtered out to avoid ocular and muscle artefacts by using a band-pass frequency ranging from 0.1 to 50 Hz. The baseline segmented EEG signals covering the entire presentation timeline of each stimulus, i.e., a time window consisting of the minus 100 ms before the stimulus and the plus 600 ms after the stimulus, was calculated and measured to quantify the artefact-free data from correct trials. We visualised the change in the ERP and frequencies of EEG waveforms from lower to higher that differed throughout the brain regions concerning several band frequencies comprising: delta ranging from 0 to 4 Hz, theta ranging from 4 to 8 Hz, alpha ranging from 8 to 13 Hz, and beta ranging from 13 to 40 Hz. After the baseline segmentation, the mean average EEG signals were presented to visualise the peak of amplitudes considering the brain regions as a variable (figure 9.5).

The mean amplitudes (μV) of segmented EEG signals were collected across four experimental variables and conditions: grammatically incorrect and correct sentences with pro- and antisocial words. The statistical inferences from EEG frequencies were drawn by computing a two-way ANOVA, two words (unsocial, prosocial) and two sentence types (grammatically incorrect, correct). The mean amplitudes were classified and calculated across the brain regions using the time and frequency domain analysis techniques and different frequency bands of EEG signals. We analysed the band frequencies in the flowing areas: anterior-frontal (AF), prefrontal (PF), frontal (F), frontotemporal (FT), temporal (T), tempro-central (TC), central (C), centro-parietal (CP), parieto-occipital (PO) and occipital (O) regions, and the regions are classified according to montage in figure 9.4. The Tukey post-hoc test was utilised for factorial comparisons, with a significance probability value ($p < 0.05$) with 95% confidential measures. The change and modulation of EEG signals were visualised before and after the early and late ERP amplitudes (μV), found at each distinct band-frequency.

9.3 Behavioral and EEG results

9.3.1 Participants' response accuracy (RA) and time (RT) results

Participants responded correctly across trials. RA (%) of correct sentences with pro- and anti-social was higher (M = 84.6, SD = 9.9) than incorrect sentences with pro- and anti-social (M = 52.6, SD = 13.9) words. We observed the significant main-effect of sentences (grammatically correct versus incorrect; $p = 0.006$), demonstrating higher RA (%) for grammatically accurate than inaccurate sentences. There was no significant accuracy across prosocial-positive and unsocial-negative words in sentences. However, there was a significant effect in sentence structures following the sentence's words and grammar ($p = 0.01$), which showed higher accuracy for prosocial words with accurate sentences than inaccurate ones. No significant variation was found across in/correct sentences with unsocial-negative words. Post-hoc analysis using Tukey procedures did not reveal any significant variation across in/accurate sentences with unsocial-negative words, but it showed significant variations of in/accurate trials with prosocial and positive words ($p = 0.001$). Overall, the in/correct sentences with prosocial words were found effective as compared to unsocial words. Most of these interpretations advocated that prosocial and positive words had a noteworthy influence on language computation.

In RT (ms), there was a significant main effect across pro- and antisocial words ($p = 0.001$), exhibiting faster response to prosocial words than antisocial ones. It indicates a quick involuntary and ultra-first response to prosocial and positive words in English, as shown in figure 9.6. There was furthermore a robust variable effect of mean response time (RT) between incorrect and correct sentences ($p = 0.005$), resulting in quicker response (ms) for grammatically accurate than wrong sentences, as depicted in figure 9.6. Additionally, the statistical computation showed significant ($p = 0.05$) two-way ANOVA results between two levels of words (prosocial-positive, antisocial-negative) and two levels of sentences (incorrect and correct), suggesting higher RT (ms) for grammatically correct than wrong ones with antisocial-negative words. In this experiment, participants quickly determined the incorrect sentences associated with prosocial-positive words rather than antisocial-negative ones. Post-hoc analysis using Tukey procedures showed a significant variable effect in grammatically incorrect and

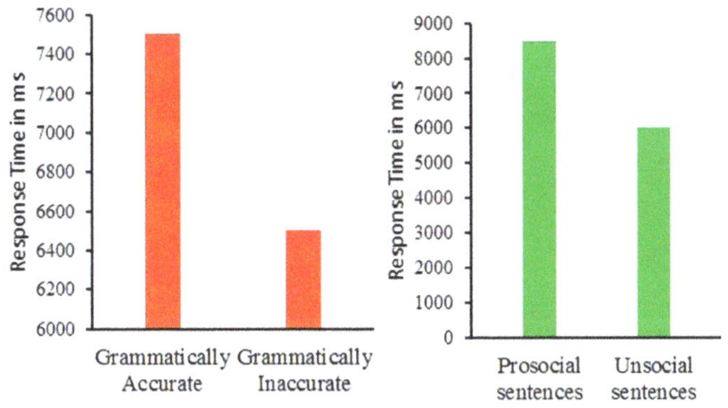

Figure 9.6. The response time of grammatically accurate and inaccurate sentences are presented along with prosocial and unsocial sentences.

correct sentences with unsocial-negative words ($p = 0.0008$), but there was no significant variation in trials with positive words. Furthermore, the interaction effect between grammatically inaccurate or wrong sentences with two levels of terms was substantial ($p = 0.006$), revealing the slower response to incorrect sentences with negative words than positive words. It demonstrates that the prosocial-positive words and antisocial-negative words interfered with the task-bound computation of grammatically wrong and right sentences in English.

9.3.2 EEG results

Signals of EEG were segmented and classified in four band-frequencies: (i) delta: 0–4 Hz; (ii) theta: 4–8 Hz; (iii) alpha: 8–13 Hz; and (iv) beta: 13–40 Hz. We examined the EEG signals based on bands and established a substantial and systematic frequency difference across experimental stimulus conditions in low and high band-frequencies. Only those bands with significant changes received an extensive description in the current study. Power spectrum of EEG signals was presented only in response to prosocial-positive and antisocial-negative stimuli at 1–4 Hz in the left-right hemispheric side of prefrontal and frontal (Fp1 and Fp2; F1 and F2) regions of the brain, as in the topo-map of the brain shown in figure 9.7. Regardless of the grammatical form of sentences, antisocial-negative words had a greater grand mean of EEG power magnitudes (0.120 μν) in prefrontal and frontal regions, whereas prosocial stimuli had a lower mean of power magnitudes (0.020 μν) in these regions. The high and low power-spectrums for antisocial-negative and prosocial-positive words that were processed in our brain by following the grammatical judgment task (correct versus incorrect) were captured and measured in the topo-map of the brain, as depicted in figure 9.7. When participants processed antisocial-negative words, the right side of frontal, temporal and temporoparietal and occipital regions showed high magnitudes of power-spectrum. These neurocognitive mechanisms and processing effects of antisocial-negative terms were directly associated with the longer behavioural duration (ms) development. However, when the participants processed prosocial-positive stimuli, the frontal part of the brain showed higher power-spectrum in a very restricted manner.

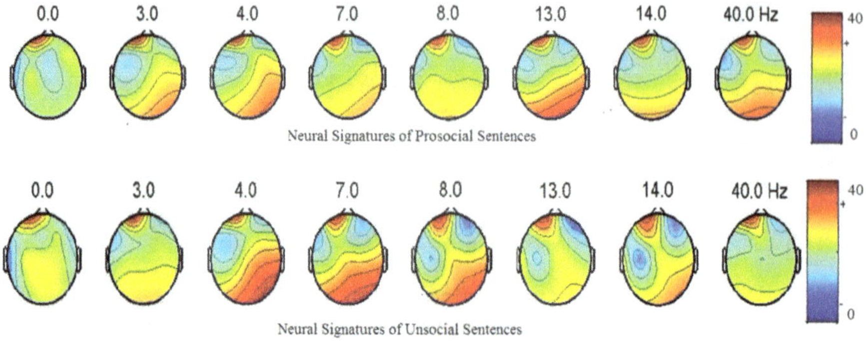

Figure 9.7. The topo-maps of the brain covering the range of frequencies (from 0 to 40 Hz) delta, theta, alpha, beta and gamma are measured during the processing of prosocial and unsocial sentences.

Even the power spectrums of delta-frequency (1–4 Hz) were substantially decreased for prosocial-positive words. This reduction of delta-frequency band for prosocial words indicates a neural shift from unsocial to prosocial effects when our brain shifts from conscious voluntary to the unconscious, involuntary processing. In this sense, our statistical inferences support the idea that the unsocial-negative words demand more considerable cognitive resources when these require a conscious voluntary-neural effort during processing.

Further, our statistical result demonstrates the change in the power-spectrum of delta frequency spanning from 1 to 4 Hz for the prosocial-positive and antisocial-negative words in the parietal and occipital lobes of the brain, revealing more significant frequencies for unsocial rather than prosocial sentences ($p = 0.01$). The grand average of delta-band frequency showed the early positive peak P100, which was observed for unsocial words after 100 ms of onset of the stimulus. However, the P200 positive peak was higher for prosocial than unsocial words at around 200 ms. This is followed by N400, a negative deflection ranging from 300 to 400 ms time windows that were higher for unsocial than prosocial words. This harmful delta wave dislocation concerning time windows was illustrated in the power-spectrum EEG wave-plot. The prefrontal portion of the brain had a greater degree of stimulation and computation induced EEG response, which had been expanded to the frontal region with more excellent delta movements. Correct sentences elicited extraordinary heights of stimulus-evoked activity and calculation in the right hemispheric side of the occipital lobe, but the erroneous sentences produced a similar amount of activity in the left hemispheric sides of the lobe. The average of EEG signal delta waves showed higher activation in the occipital regions conforming to the incorrect (0.125 $\mu\nu$) and correct (0.025 $\mu\nu$) sentences. Our highly significant impact ($p = 0.05$) of the grammatical judgment task (whether the sentences are grammatically correct or incorrect) supported this fact. In these brain regions, we did not catch any robust ($p = 1$) interaction result between prosocial-positive and unsocial-negative on the one hand and correct and incorrect sentences on the other.

EEG band of theta activity ranging the frequency from 4 to 7 Hz showed higher activation in the prefrontal regions of the brain for incorrect than correct sentences irrespective of positive-prosocial and negative-unsocial sentences. Furthermore, the grammatically incorrect sentences exhibited greater evoked power-spectra that increased from the prefrontal regions (low-theta activity) to the brain's frontal (high-theta activity) regions. Thus, a greater degree of cognitive ability and high neural resources were required to process erroneous sentences. Similarly, the mean delta frequency of EEG signals collected in the frontal area of the brain revealed a greater magnitude of power spectra (0.015 μν) for wrong or erroneous sentences than right (0.010 μν) ones. In addition, our numerical data demonstrated a robust effect ($p = 0.007$) of grammatically incorrect and correct sentences, which implies that our brain demands higher neurocognitive resources for grammatically incorrect or erroneous than correct or right sentences in the frontal (F) and temporal (T) and frontotemporal (FT) areas of the brain.

We also found the beta band-frequencies ranging from 13 to 40 Hz linked with incorrect and correct sentences regardless of unsocial-negative and prosocial-positive sentences. The spectral density for in/correct sentences is displayed in the topo-map of the brain regions. The right sides of the prefrontal, frontal and occipital areas demonstrate the higher beta-band activity, which was engaged with the computation of incorrect sentences. However, the correct-accurate penalties (0.020 μν) processed in the left side of the frontal and prefrontal lobes of the brain. This beta activity was also high for the grammatically incorrect and inaccurate sentences (0.050 μν) in the right-side of anterior-frontal regions of the brain, indicating a greater cognitive resource demand for inaccurate than accurate sentences. As a result, the grammatical judgment task referring to incorrect and correct sentences was substantial and robust ($p = 0.01$) in the brain's prefrontal and anterior frontal areas.

In the higher order of beta-band frequency ranging from 13 to 40 Hz, we found a robust interaction effect between words (prosocial-positive, unsocial-negative words) and grammar (incorrect, correct). The high power-spectral density of beta-band was amplified in the prefrontal area of the cortex when prosocial-positive words were associated with grammatically correct or accurate sentences. A large area of the right-side of tempo-parietal (TP), parietal (P), and occipital (O) regions showed more extensive activations in terms of neuro-cognitive sources for understanding incorrect or erroneous sentences, which is linked with prosocial-positive words. Grammatically correct-accurate sentences with unsocial words needed more brain efforts in the tempro-parietal (TP), parietal (P) and occipital (O) regions. However, the grammatically inaccurate sentences needed more neural, cognitive resources in the brain's prefrontal (PF) and frontal (F) regions. The incorrect or grammatically wrong sentences with unsocial-negative words were processed in the frontal (F) lobe.

Moreover, the unsocial-negative or antisocial words are computed mainly in the frontal lobe of the brain. As a result, a two-way ANOVA of beta-band frequencies between grammar (incorrect, correct) of the sentence and the presence of words (prosocial-positive, antisocial-negative) showed a considerable effect ($p = 0.05$), defining higher power spectra for unsocial-negative incorrect than prosocial-positive incorrect sentences in the frontal (F), temporal (T) and frontotemporal (FT) regions of the brain. These resultant descriptions are also reflected in the time-domain statistical analysis in which the prosocial incorrect sentences showed a lower magnitude of power-spectra than unsocial-negative words used in sentences.

9.4 Discussion and interpretation of results

This chapter examined how prosocial positive and antisocial negative words are processed in our brains when we read incorrect and correct English sentences. Employing the frequency-domain techniques and analysis procedures, we identified the neurocognitive mechanisms of the brain during the processing of prosocial positive and antisocial negative words by establishing behavioural response time and accuracy results with EEG frequency and time domain effect. Our results revealed that participants performed the grammatical task accurately. They were very much quicker to perceive and recognise the positive prosocial language than unsocial negative words by considering automatic, involuntary processing and computation of prosocial positive words, as it was observed in the processing of negative and positive emotional language (Kanske and Kotz 2007, Estes and Verges 2008, Palazova *et al* 2009). In the emotional recognition task, positive, happy words have a robust processing advantage over negative sad or angry words. In the grammatical judgment task, the current chapter described that joyful words were computed earlier, but the positive prosocial words were also computed quicker than negative unsocial words. According to semantic network theory, the faster or earlier perception and understanding of positive prosocial words are thoroughly grounded with the temporary memory distribution, the wide allotment of socio-pragmatic and semantic linkage of the human brain (Collins and Loftus 1975, Hertrich *et al* 2020). Therefore, positive prosocial language was memorised and remembered faster with less effort than unsocial negative language. This evidence is corroborated with the observations of earlier literature about the processing of pleasant or happy words that are evoked more regularly and commonly than unpleasant or sad words (Kissler *et al* 2009). Considering the grammatical judgment task, we found that participants took more time to compute the incorrect sentences associated with unsocial negative words than prosocial positive words. From the point of accuracy (%), participants recognised the correct sentences with prosocial positive words more accurately than unsocial negative words. Further, the grammatically incorrect and correct sentences interacted with prosocial words, reducing the accuracy for incorrect sentences than correct ones. These findings suggest that the interference of pragmatic and semantic forms of language like prosocial positive and unsocial negative forms is automatic and involuntary when the goal or task of the experiment is to predict grammatically correct and incorrect sentences.

From the neurocognitive point of view, we interpret that the grammatical comprehension of English, as a second language in India, is influenced by prosocial positive words in sentences. Sentences with prosocial positive words have a profound impact and faster computation than unsocial negative words in our brain, even whether the sentences are right or wrong according to grammatical judgment. Prosocial positive words demand minimum neurocognitive resources with involuntary behavioural efforts, whereas unsocial negative words require maximum neurocognitive resources with voluntary behavioural effort. This is evidenced in our delta band frequency-domain results, suggesting a higher power spectrum of delta ranging from 1 to 4 Hz for unsocial negative sentences than positive prosocial ones. Delta band frequency was higher for unsocial words in the right side of temporal (T), Parietal (P) and occipital (O) areas of the brain. However, the high band frequencies ranging from 4 to 7 Hz and beta fluctuating from 13 to 40 Hz showed more prominent oscillation for grammatically incorrect or wrong than correct sentences in anterior-frontal, prefrontal and frontal regions of the brain. These observations are reinforced by the notion that ungrammatical sentences have a greater elicited perspective than grammatical ones at the low-theta band frequencies ranging from 3.5 to 5 Hz (Roehm *et al* 2004). In terms of regions of interest (ROI), this chapter proposes that syntactic comprehension, especially the processing of grammatical errors, are computed in the anterior-frontal and frontotemporal areas of the brain, which is consistent with the results of prior research (Vandenberghe *et al* 2002, Rogalsky and Hickok 2009). There is also a robust two-way interaction between task-relevant (e.g., grammatically incorrect and correct sentences) and task-irrelevant (e.g., prosocial favourable and unsocial-negative) conditions, eliciting higher oscillation of beta-band frequencies for unsocial-incorrect sentences than unsocial-correct ones.

Unsocial words in English are processed quicker and much earlier than prosocial words. This rapid neurocognitive mechanism of unsocial terms is reflected in the early positive potential peak within 100 ms (P100). The early recognition is associated with unsocial words because they are always sensitive to life and threat. Many unsocial words such as threat, kill, warning, disharmony, etc, are used infrequently in our daily lives. Therefore, the processing of unsocial words demands rapid time with more considerable neural resources that can facilitate early recognition. When the main task is to attend to the syntactic structures of the sentences, the interference of unsocial words is inevitable within 100 ms. The early rapid and robust effect shows that the P1 cognitive component is underlying or attentive to unsocial terms. Like processing positive and negative emotional words that profoundly impact decision-making (Dillon *et al* 2006), prosocial and unsocial words have strongly been linked with human reproductive and preservation tactics.

Further, the positive modulation of delta-band frequencies is associated with unsocial negative words in the early stage of the time domain, while prosocial stimuli represent negative oscillation in the late stage of the time domain. Moreover, these two forms of delta-band frequency showed a significant difference in the neurocognitive mechanisms that can distinguish the processing of prosocial and unsocial words in the human brain. The prefrontal (PF) and frontal cortex of the brain always process the cognitive burdens or loads which are primarily affected and influenced by the perceptual mechanisms of anti- and prosocial stimuli, as many studies have highlighted the importance of PFCs for semantic retention, regulation, and interpretations (Demb *et al* 1995, Wagner *et al* 2001). Therefore, the impact of early and late delta activity in connection to these prosocial positive and unsocial negative stimuli involves a change in the neurocognitive shifts in the brain.

Literature on language processing suggests that the cognitive component of N400 within a time window from 380 to 500 ms is associated with the violation of meaning or semantic ambiguities at the sentential level (Friederici *et al* 2002, Tabullo *et al* 2011, van de Meerendonk *et al* 2013). However, the positive component of P600 within a time window from 500 to 700 ms indicates grammatically incorrect or syntactic violation (Kutas and Hillyard 1980, 1984). In this regard, our findings revealed a long sluggish wave of late positive peak (P500—600 ms) that is linked to grammatical violations in the context of prosocial positive and antisocial negative sentences. In addition, it has been shown that grammatically correct sentences are computed in the right-side, but incorrect ones are computed in the left side of the brain. The processing of incorrect and correct sentences is also reflected in the beta-band frequencies (13–40 Hz). Therefore, the inaccurate sentences demand a more significant cognitive effort on the right side, whereas the accurate sentences need a tremendous step on the left side of the prefrontal and occipital areas. This laterality division for incorrect and correct sentences with the presence of prosocial positive and unsocial negative words is consistent with the previous research on affective visuals, which establish that unpleasant images are computed in the right side of the brain, whereas positive images are interpreted in the left side of the brain (Aftanas *et al* 2001, Alves *et al* 2008, Wyczesany *et al* 2018).

Earlier studies have not analysed the different brain lobes engaged with the computation of prosocial and unsocial sentences. In this chapter, we have shown that the regions of the brain such as prefrontal (PF), temporal (T), and parietal (P) and occipital (O) areas are primarily involved in the computation of prosocial and unsocial words. Furthermore, a previous fMRI investigation explores that negative emotional comments have shown more prominent activation in the anterior and prefrontal cortex (PFC) than positive emotional words (Kensinger and Schacter 2006). Furthermore, it is observed that, during the comprehension of pro- and antisocial words, the prefrontal temporal, parietal and occipital lobes have been significantly involved in the process of computation. To summarise, our study contributes to the theory of neurocognitive and computational mechanisms of prosocial and unsocial language processing, supporting the earlier stand that the temporal cortex establishes a link to the limbic area through the insula, allowing it to encode prompt and rapid processing of unsocial negative words and to transmit the information to action or event network (Augustine 1996, Rizzolatti *et al* 2001). These resultant findings related to the rapid processing of unsocial words have linked with the pro-self or selfish words processed through the dorsolateral prefrontal cortex because of the high cognitive burden or load for analysing and evaluating the cost–benefit of selfish stimuli. However, the prosocial stimuli are processed through the anterior area of the superior temporal sulcus (STS) due to human harmony and communicative cooperation (Haruno and Frith 2010).

According to the findings of earlier studies, language provides or serves as a pragmatic context for processing non-verbal aspects or modals of emotion displaying face, image and pictures (Barrett and Kensinger 2010, Doyle *et al* 2021). In this chapter, the pragmatic and contextual statement is expanded and linked to the computational aspects of prosocial positive and unsocial negative words that facilitate sentence processing. Moreover, the emotional sentiment can be extended to understand the processing of pro- and antisocial linguistic behaviours that offer a background for sentence processing in the human brain. The neurocognitive mechanisms in allocating the neurocognitive resource for the computation of prosocial positive words broadly vary from unsocial negative words in sentences. This result implies that prosocial and antisocial words are used to create a positive impact on the human brain. Furthermore, neuro-genetic studies demonstrate that the additional hormones such as testosterone and oxytocin have a positive effect on the activation or presence of pro-self or unsocial behaviours and antisocial activities because these negative antisocial behaviours demand more considerable brain activity and a substantial neurocognitive load for executing or interpreting such events (Lambert *et al* 2017). Contrarily, prosocial behaviours are influenced by essential neuronal hormones, demanding a limited brain load to execute such events or actions.

9.5 Conclusion

This chapter describes the delta, theta and beta band frequencies of anti- or unsocial negative and prosocial positive words in the context of grammatically inaccurate and accurate sentences. It is observed that prosocial words used in either accurate or accurate sentences take a less cognitive load in late processing. However, unsocial words used in accurate or inaccurate sentences take a more extensive cognitive load in early processing. Unsocial negative words take more behavioural time and mental effort as compared to the cognitive resource of prosocial words in sentences. Similar to the processing of happy, pleasant and joyful events or actions, the sentences with prosocial words are computed more quickly than unsocial negative words. Our brain anticipates and recognises the unsocial negative words very early (P100), and such identification of unsocial words occur considerably sooner than semantic (N400) and grammatical (P600) violation.

To sum up, this chapter discloses that positive and prosocial languages have vast influence and significant control on the computation of grammar. The neurocognitive and behavioural mechanisms of prosocial and positive language may justify considering the findings as a diagnostic, clinical, pathological and behavioural tool for the intervention, prevention and treatment of negative moods and attitudes that always accelerate stress and depression. From the societal point of view, these findings help correct the behaviours and regulate adverse reactions by enhancing happiness and social stability. The findings offer additional avenues for further research into the function of expectation failure in the compatibility and incongruency of pro and antisocial words in various languages.

References

Adolphs R, Baron-Cohen S and Tranel D 2002 Impaired recognition of social emotions following amygdala damage *J. Cogn. Neurosci.* **14** 1264–74

Aftanas L, Varlamov A, Pavlov S, Makhnev V and Reva N 2001 Event-related synchronization and desynchronization during affective processing: emergence of valence-related time-dependent hemispheric asymmetries in theta and upper alpha band *Int. J. Neurosci.* **110** 197–219

Alves N T, Fukusima S S and Aznar-Casanova J A 2008 Models of brain asymmetry in emotional processing *Psychol. Neurosci.* **1** 63–66

Augustine J R 1996 Circuitry and functional aspects of the insular lobe in primates including humans *Brain Res. Rev.* **22** 229–44

Barrett L F and Kensinger E A 2010 Context is routinely encoded during emotion perception *Psychol. Sci.* **21** 595–9

Bieleke M, Gollwitzer P M, Oettingen G and Fischbacher U 2017 Social value orientation moderates the effects of intuition versus reflection on responses to unfair ultimatum offers *J. Behav. Decis. Mak.* **30** 569–81

Boyd R and Mathew S 2015 Third-party monitoring and sanctions aid the evolution of language *Evolut. Human Behav.* **36** 475–9

Carter C S and Van Veen V 2007 Anterior cingulate cortex and conflict detection: an update of theory and data *Cogn. Affect. Behav. Neurosci.* **7** 367–79

Christopoulos G I and King-Casas B 2015 With you or against you: social orientation dependent learning signals guide actions made for others *Neuroimage* **104** 326–35

Cohn M A, Mehl M R and Pennebaker J W 2004 Linguistic markers of psychological change surrounding September 11, 2001 *Psychol. Sci.* **15** 687–93

Collins A M and Loftus E F 1975 A spreading-activation theory of semantic processing *Psychol. Rev.* **82** 407

Cooper J C, Kreps T A, Wiebe T, Pirkl T and Knutson B 2010 When giving is good: ventromedial prefrontal cortex activation for others' intentions *Neuron* **67** 511–21

Cowell J M and Decety J 2015 The neuroscience of implicit moral evaluation and its relation to generosity in early childhood *Curr. Biol.* **25** 93–7

Crocker J 2008 From egosystem to ecosystem: implications for relationships, learning, and well-being *Transcending Self-Interest:Psychological Explorations of the Quiet Ego* (New York: American Psychological Association) pp 63–72

Crockett M J, Clark L, Hauser M D and Robbins T W 2010 Serotonin selectively influences moral judgment and behavior through effects on harm aversion *Proc. Natl Acad. Sci.* **107** 17433–8

Dale R, Marshall-Pescini S and Range F 2020 What matters for cooperation? The importance of social relationship over cognition *Sci. Rep.* **10** 1–14

De Cremer D and Tyler T R 2004 Managing group behavior: the interplay between procedural justice, sense of self, and cooperation *Adv. Exp. Soc. Psychol.* **37** 151–218

De Dreu C K and Kret M E 2016 Oxytocin conditions intergroup relations through upregulated in-group empathy, cooperation, conformity, and defense *Biol. Psychiatry* **79** 165–73

de Greck M *et al* 2012a Altered brain activity during emotional empathy in somatoform disorder *Human Brain Mapp.* **33** 2666–85

de Greck M, Shi Z, Wang G, Zuo X, Yang X, Wang X, Northoff G and Han S 2012b Culture modulates brain activity during empathy with anger *Neuroimage* **59** 2871–82

De Waal F B 2000 Primates–a natural heritage of conflict resolution *Science* **289** 586–90

Decety J and Cowell J M 2018 Interpersonal harm aversion as a necessary foundation for morality: a developmental neuroscience perspective *Develop. Psychopathol.* **30** 153–64

Decety J and Grèzes J 2006 The power of simulation: imagining one's own and other's behavior *Brain Res.* **1079** 4–14

Declerck C H, Boone C and Kiyonari T 2014 The effect of oxytocin on cooperation in a prisoner's dilemma depends on the social context and a person's social value orientation *Soc. Cogn. Affect. Neurosci.* **9** 802–9

Demb J B, Desmond J E, Wagner A D, Vaidya C J, Glover G H and Gabrieli J D 1995 Semantic encoding and retrieval in the left inferior prefrontal cortex: a functional MRI study of task difficulty and process specificity *J. Neurosci.* **15** 5870–8

Descorbeth O, Zhang X, Noah J A and Hirsch J 2020 Neural processes for live pro-social dialogue between dyads with socioeconomic disparity *Soc. Cogn. Affect. Neurosci.* **15** 875–87

Dillon D G, Cooper J J, Grent T, Woldorff M G and LaBar K S 2006 Dissociation of event-related potentials indexing arousal and semantic cohesion during emotional word encoding *Brain Cognit.* **62** 43–57

Dixon T 2013 *Altruism: morals from history Evolution, Games and God: The Principle of Cooperation* eds M Nowak and S Coakley (Cambridge, MA: Harvard University Press) pp 60–81

Doyle C M, Gendron M and Lindquist K A 2021 Language is a unique context for emotion perception *Affect. Sci.* **2** 171–7

Dvash J, Gilam G, Ben-Ze'ev A, Hendler T and Shamay-Tsoory S G 2010 The envious brain: the neural basis of social comparison *Human Brain Mapp.* **31** 1741–50

Eisenberg N, Hofer C, Sulik M J and Liew J 2014 The development of prosocial moral reasoning and a prosocial orientation in young adulthood: concurrent and longitudinal correlates *Dev. Psychol.* **50** 58

Eisenberg N, Lennon R and Roth K 1983 Prosocial development: a longitudinal study *Dev. Psychol.* **19** 846

Ensor R and Hughes C 2005 More than talk: relations between emotion understanding and positive behaviour in toddlers *Br. J. Dev. Psychol.* **23** 343–63

Estes Z and Verges M 2008 Freeze or flee? Negative stimuli elicit selective responding *Cognition* **108** 557–65

Fan M, Jie J, Luo P, Pang Y, Xu D, Yu G, Zhao S, Chen W and Zheng X 2021 Social exclusion down-regulates pain empathy at the late stage of empathic responses: electrophysiological evidence *Front. Human Neurosci.* **15** 88

Feng C, Li Z, Feng X, Wang L, Tian T and Luo Y J 2016 Social hierarchy modulates neural responses of empathy for pain *Soc. Cogn. Affect. Neurosci.* **11** 485–95

Fiske S T, Cuddy A J and Glick P 2007 universal dimensions of social cognition: warmth and competence *Trends Cogn. Sci.* **11** 77–83

Friederici A D, Hahne A and Saddy D 2002 Distinct neurophysiological patterns reflecting aspects of syntactic complexity and syntactic repair *J. Psycholinguist. Res.* **31** 45–63

Frimer J A, Aquino K, Gebauer J E, Zhu L L and Oakes H 2015 A decline in prosocial language helps explain public disapproval of the US Congress *Proc. Natl Acad. Sci.* **112** 6591–4

Gan T, Wang L, Zhang L, Fang W and Gu R 2016 The neural correlates of evaluating the outcome of prosocial-helping decisions *NeuroReport* **27** 1293–8

Gilbert P 2016 *Human Nature and Suffering* (London: Routledge) (https://doi.org/10.4324/9781315564258)

Girard L C, Pingault J B, Doyle O, Falissard B and Tremblay R E 2017 Expressive language and prosocial behaviour in early childhood: longitudinal associations in the UK Millennium Cohort Study *Eur. J. Dev. Psychol.* **14** 381–98

Greene J D, Nystrom L E, Engell A D, Darley J M and Cohen J D 2004 The neural bases of cognitive conflict and control in moral judgment *Neuron* **44** 389–400

Gross J T, Stern J A, Brett B E and Cassidy J 2017 The multifaceted nature of prosocial behavior in children: links with attachment theory and research *Soc. Develop.* **26** 661–78

Gui D Y, Gan T and Liu C 2016 Neural evidence for moral intuition and the temporal dynamics of interactions between emotional processes and moral cognition *Soc. Neurosci.* **11** 380–94

Gurven M 2004 Reciprocal altruism and food sharing decisions among Hiwi and Ache hunter–gatherers *Behav. Ecol. Sociobiol.* **56** 366–80

Hackel L M, Wills J A and Van Bavel J J 2020 Shifting prosocial intuitions: neurocognitive evidence for a value-based account of group-based cooperation *Soc. Cogn. Affect. Neurosci.* **15** 371–81

Haidt J 2001 The emotional dog and its rational tail: a social intuitionist approach to moral judgment *Psychol. Rev.* **108** 814

Hajcak G, MacNamara A and Olvet D M 2010 Event-related potentials, emotion, and emotion regulation: an integrative review *Deve. Neuropsychol.* **35** 129–55

Hare B 2017 Survival of the friendliest: homo sapiens evolved via selection for prosociality *Annu. Rev. Psychol.* **68** 155–86

Hare T A, Camerer C F and Rangel A 2009 Self-control in decision-making involves modulation of the vmPFC valuation system *Science* **324** 646–8

Haruno M and Frith C D 2010 Activity in the amygdala elicited by unfair divisions predicts social value orientation *Nat. Neurosci.* **13** 160–1

Heekeren H R, Wartenburger I, Schmidt H, Schwintowski H P and Villringer A 2003 An fMRI study of simple ethical decision-making *Neuroreport* **14** 1215–19

Heffner J, Vives M L and FeldmanHall O 2021 Emotional responses to prosocial messages increase willingness to self-isolate during the COVID-19 pandemic *Pers. Individ. Differ.* **170** 110420

Hein G, Silani G, Preuschoff K, Batson C D and Singer T 2010 Neural responses to ingroup and outgroup members' suffering predict individual differences in costly helping *Neuron* **68** 149–60

Henrich J and Muthukrishna M 2021 The origins and psychology of human cooperation *Annu. Rev. Psychol.* **72** 207–40

Henrich J P, Boyd R, Bowles S, Fehr E, Camerer C and Gintis H (ed) 2004 *Foundations of Human Sociality: Economic Experiments and Ethnographic Evidence from Fifteen Small-Scale Societies* (Oxford: Oxford University Press)

Hertrich I, Dietrich S and Ackermann H 2020 The margins of the language network in the brain *Front. Commun.* **5** 93

Hilbig B E, Glöckner A and Zettler I 2014 Personality and prosocial behavior: linking basic traits and social value orientations *J. Person. Soc. Psychol.* **107** 529

Hu X, Xu Z and Mai X 2017 Social value orientation modulates the processing of outcome evaluation involving others *Soc. Cogn. Affect. Neurosci.* **12** 1730–9

Hutcherson C A, Plassmann H, Gross J J and Rangel A 2012 Cognitive regulation during decision making shifts behavioral control between ventromedial and dorsolateral prefrontal value systems *J. Neurosci.* **32** 13543–54

Jansari A, Tranel D and Adolphs R 2000 A valence-specific lateral bias for discriminating emotional facial expressions in free field *Cogn. Emot.* **14** 341–53

Jie J, Fan M, Yang Y, Luo P, Wang Y, Li J, Chen W, Zhuang M and Zheng X 2021 Establishing a counter-empathy processing model: evidence from functional magnetic resonance imaging *Soc. Cogn. Affect. Neurosci.*

Jie J, Luo P, Zhuang M, Fan M, Wang Y, Yang Y and Zheng X 2019a Gender differences in empathic responses to others' economic payoffs: an event-related potentials study *Exp. Brain Res.* **237** 1347–59

Jie J, Luo P, Zhuang M, Li B, Pang Y, Li J and Zheng X 2019b Self-interest induces counter-empathy at the late stage of empathic responses to others' economic payoffs *Front. Psychol.* **10** 372

Joireman J and Duell B 2005 Mother Teresa versus Ebenezer Scrooge: mortality salience leads proselfs to endorse self-transcendent values (unless proselfs are reassured) *Person. Soc. Psychol. Bull.* **31** 307–20

Kacewicz E, Pennebaker J W, Davis M, Jeon M and Graesser A C 2014 Pronoun use reflects standings in social hierarchies *J. Lang. Soc. Psychol.* **33** 125–43

Kanske P and Kotz S A 2007 Concreteness in emotional words: ERP evidence from a hemifield study *Brain Res.* **1148** 138–48

Keltner D, Kogan A, Piff P K and Saturn S R 2014 The sociocultural appraisals, values, and emotions (SAVE) framework of prosociality: core processes from gene to meme *Ann. Rev. Psychol.* **65** 425–60

Kensinger E A and Schacter D L 2006 Amygdala activity is associated with the successful encoding of item, but not source, information for positive and negative stimuli *J. Neurosci.* **26** 2564–70

Kissler J, Herbert C, Winkler I and Junghofer M 2009 Emotion and attention in visual word processing—an ERP study *Biol. Psychol.* **80** 75–83

Kitts J A 2006 Collective action, rival incentives, and the emergence of antisocial norms *Am. Sociol. Rev.* **71** 235–59

Knoch D and Fehr E 2007 Resisting the power of temptations: the right prefrontal cortex and self-control *Ann. N.Y. Acad. Sci.* **1104** 123–34

Kogan A, Saslow L R, Impett E A, Oveis C, Keltner D and Saturn S R 2011 Thin-slicing study of the oxytocin receptor (OXTR) gene and the evaluation and expression of the prosocial disposition *Proc. Natl Acad. Sci.* **108** 19189–92

Krahé B 2020 *The Social Psychology of Aggression* (London: Routledge)

Kuepper Y, Alexander N, Osinsky R, Mueller E, Schmitz A, Netter P and Hennig J 2010 Aggression—interactions of serotonin and testosterone in healthy men and women *Behav. Brain Res.* **206** 93–100

Kutas M and Hillyard S A 1980 Reading senseless sentences: brain potentials reflect semantic incongruity *Science* **207** 203–5

Kutas M and Hillyard S A 1984 Brain potentials during reading reflect word expectancy and semantic association *Nature* **307** 161–3

Lambert B, Declerck C H, Emonds G and Boone C 2017 Trust as commodity: social value orientation affects the neural substrates of learning to cooperate *Soc. Cogn. Affect. Neurosci.* **12** 609–17

Lane J D, Wellman H M, Olson S L, Miller A L, Wang L and Tardif T 2013 Relations between temperament and theory of mind development in the United States and China: biological and behavioral correlates of preschoolers' false-belief understanding *Dev. Psychol.* **49** 825

Lapsley D K and Narvaez D 2004 A social–cognitive approach to the moral personality *Moral Development, Self, and Identity* (Hove: Psychology Press) pp 201–24

Lebreton M, Jorge S, Michel V, Thirion B and Pessiglione M 2009 An automatic valuation system in the human brain: evidence from functional neuroimaging *Neuron* **64** 431–9

Lee M 2013 Self-denial and its discontents *Evolution, Games, and God: The Principle of Cooperation* eds M Nowak and S Coakley (Cambridge, MA: Harvard University Press) pp 186–97

Leuthold H, Kunkel A, Mackenzie I G and Filik R 2015 Online processing of moral transgressions: ERP evidence for spontaneous evaluation *Social Cog. Affect. Neurosci.* **10** 1021–9

Levy D J and Glimcher P W 2012 The root of all value: a neural common currency for choice *Curr. Opin. Neurobiol.* **22** 1027–38

Li J, Zhu L, Gummerum M and Sun Y 2013 The development of social value orientation across different contexts *Int. J. Psychol.* **48** 469–80

Luo P, Pang Y, Li B, Jie J, Zhuang M, Yang S and Zheng X 2018 Competitive intensity modulates the pain empathy response: an event-related potentials study *Front. Psychol.* **9** 1854

McLeod J D and Owens T J 2004 Psychological well-being in the early life course: variations by socioeconomic status, gender, and race/ethnicity *Soc. Psychol. Q* **67** 257–78

McNally L and Jackson A L 2013 Cooperation creates selection for tactical deception *Proc. R. Soc. B: Biol. Sci.* **280** 20130699

McNally L, Brown S P and Jackson A L 2012 Cooperation and the evolution of intelligence *Proc. R. Soc. B: Biol. Sci.* **279** 3027–34

Mesulam M M 2000 *Principles of Behavioral and Cognitive Neurology* (Oxford: Oxford University Press)

Midlarsky E 1991 Helping as coping *Prosocial Behaviour* ed M S Clark (Thousand Oaks, CA: SAGE) pp 238–264

Miller E K and Cohen J D 2001 An integrative theory of prefrontal cortex function *Ann. Rev. Neurosci.* **24** 167–202

Mink D, Henning A and Aschersleben G 2014 Infant shy temperament predicts preschoolers theory of mind *Infant Behav. Develop.* **37** 66–75

Moll J, de Oliveira-Souza R, Bramati I E and Grafman J 2002 Functional networks in emotional moral and nonmoral social judgments *Neuroimage* **16** 696–703

Montoya E R, Terburg D, Bos P A and Van Honk J 2012 Testosterone, cortisol, and serotonin as key regulators of social aggression: a review and theoretical perspective *Motivat. Emot.* **36** 65–73

Murphy R O and Ackermann K A 2014 Social value orientation: theoretical and measurement issues in the study of social preferences *Person. Soc. Psychol. Rev.* **18** 13–41

Newman M L, Pennebaker J W, Berry D S and Richards J M 2003 Lying words: predicting deception from linguistic styles *Person. Soc. Psychol. Bull.* **29** 665–75

Nowak M A and Coakley S 2013 Introduction: why cooperation makes a difference *Evolution, Games, and God: The Principle of Cooperation* eds M Nowak and S Coakley (Cambridge, MA: Harvard University Press) pp 1–34

Obsuth I, Eisner M P, Malti T and Ribeaud D 2015 The developmental relation between aggressive behaviour and prosocial behaviour: a 5-year longitudinal study *BMC Psychol.* **3** 1–15

Oxford R L and Curtis A 2021 Exploring peace language: hope, help and harmony *Peacebuilding in Language Education* (Bristol: Multilingual Matters) pp 228–41

Pagel M 2012 *Wired for Culture: Origins of the Human Social Mind* (New York: WW Norton & Company)

Palazova M, Mantwill K, Sommer W and Schacht A 2009 Effects of emotion in words are localized in post-lexical processing stages *Psychophysiology* vol 46 (Malden, MA: Wiley-Blackwell Publishing, Inc.) p S160

Pärnamets P, Shuster A, Reinero D A and Van Bavel J J 2020 A value-based framework for understanding cooperation *Curr. Direct. Psychol. Sci.* **29** 227–34

Pennebaker J W and King L A 1999 Linguistic styles: language use as an individual difference *J. Person. Soc. Psychol.* **77** 1296

Pletti C, Decety J and Paulus M 2019 Moral identity relates to the neural processing of third-party moral behavior *Soc. Cogn. Affect. Neurosci.* **14** 435–45

Rand D G, Dreber A, Ellingsen T, Fudenberg D and Nowak M A 2009 Positive interactions promote public cooperation *Science* **325** 1272–5

Rangel A and Hare T 2010 Neural computations associated with goal-directed choice *Curr. Opin. Neurobiol.* **20** 262–70

Reuter M, Frenzel C, Walter N T, Markett S and Montag C 2011 Investigating the genetic basis of altruism: the role of the COMT Val158Met polymorphism *Soc. Cogn. Affect. Neurosci.* **6** 662–8

Rhee S H *et al* 2013 The role of language in concern and disregard for others in the first years of life *Dev. Psychol.* **49** 197

Ripley J S and Worthington E L Jr 2002 Hope-focused and forgiveness-based group interventions to promote marital enrichment *J. Counsel. Dev.* **80** 452–63

Rizzolatti G, Fogassi L and Gallese V 2001 Neurophysiological mechanisms underlying the understanding and imitation of action *Nat. Rev. Neurosci.* **2** 661–70

Roehm D, Schlesewsky M, Bornkessel I, Frisch S and Haider H 2004 Fractionating language comprehension via frequency characteristics of the human EEG *Neuroreport* **15** 409–12

Rogalsky C and Hickok G 2009 Selective attention to semantic and syntactic features modulates sentence processing networks in anterior temporal cortex *Cereb. Cortex* **19** 786–96

Sanfey A G, Rilling J K, Aronson J A, Nystrom L E and Cohen J D 2003 The neural basis of economic decision-making in the ultimatum game *Science* **300** 1755–8

Sapolsky R M 2005 The influence of social hierarchy on primate health *Science* **308** 648–52

Satpute A B and Lieberman M D 2006 Integrating automatic and controlled processes into neurocognitive models of social cognition *Brain Res.* **1079** 86–97

Schaich Borg J, Hynes C, Van Horn J, Grafton S and Sinnott-Armstrong W 2006 Consequences, action, and intention as factors in moral judgments: an fMRI investigation *J. Cogn. Neurosci.* **18** 803–17

Scheepers D and Derks B 2016 Revisiting social identity theory from a neuroscience perspective *Curr. Opin. Psychol.* **11** 74–8

Schupp H, Cuthbert B, Bradley M, Hillman C, Hamm A and Lang P 2004 Brain processes in emotional perception: motivated attention *Cogn. Emot.* **18** 593–611

Schupp H T, Junghöfer M, Weike A I and Hamm A O 2003 Attention and emotion: an ERP analysis of facilitated emotional stimulus processing *Neuroreport* **14** 1107–10

Singer T, Seymour B, O'Doherty J P, Stephan K E, Dolan R J and Frith C D 2006 Empathic neural responses are modulated by the perceived fairness of others *Nature* **439** 466–9

Somel M, Liu X and Khaitovich P 2013 Human brain evolution: transcripts, metabolites and their regulators *Nat. Rev. Neurosci.* **14** 112–27

Spinrad T L, Eisenberg N, Cumberland A, Fabes R A, Valiente C, Shepard S A, Reiser M, Losoya S H and Guthrie I K 2006 Relation of emotion-related regulation to children's social competence: a longitudinal study *Emotion* **6** 498

Stouten J, De Cremer D and Van Dijk E 2005 All is well that ends well, at least for proselfs: emotional reactions to equality violation as a function of social value orientation *Eur. J. Soc. Psychol.* **35** 767–83

Tabibnia G, Satpute A B and Lieberman M D 2008 The sunny side of fairness: preference for fairness activates reward circuitry (and disregarding unfairness activates self-control circuitry) *Psychol. Sci.* **19** 339–47

Tabullo Á, Sevilla Y, Pasqualetti G, Vernis S, Segura E, Yorio A, Zanutto S and Wainselboim A 2011 Expectancy modulates a late positive ERP in an artificial grammar task *Brain Res.* **1373** 131–43

Takahashi H, Kato M, Matsuura M, Mobbs D, Suhara T and Okubo Y 2009 When your gain is my pain and your pain is my gain: neural correlates of envy and schadenfreude *Science* **323** 937–9

Triandis H C 1978 Some universals of social behavior *Person. Soc. Psychol. Bull.* **4** 1–16

Tyler T R and Blader S L 2003 The group engagement model: procedural justice, social identity, and cooperative behavior *Person. Soc. Psychol. Rev.* **7** 349–61

van de Meerendonk N, Rueschemeyer S A and Kolk H H 2013 Language comprehension interrupted: both language errors and word degradation activate Broca's area *Brain Lang.* **126** 291–301

Van Lange P A 2000 Beyond self-interest: a set of propositions relevant to interpersonal orientations *Eur. Rev. Soc. Psychol.* **11** 297–331

Vandenberghe R, Nobre A C and Price C J 2002 The response of left temporal cortex to sentences *J. Cogn. Neurosci.* **14** 550–60

Von Hippel W and Trivers R 2011 Reflections on self-deception *Behav. Brain Sci.* **34** 41

Wagner A D, Paré-Blagoev E J, Clark J and Poldrack R A 2001 Recovering meaning: left prefrontal cortex guides controlled semantic retrieval *Neuron* **31** 329–38

Weinberg A and Hajcak G 2010 Beyond good and evil: the time-course of neural activity elicited by specific picture content *Emotion* **10** 767

Wellman H M, Lane J D, LaBounty J and Olson S L 2011 Observant, nonaggressive temperament predicts theory-of-mind development *Dev. Sci.* **14** 319–26

Williams P B, Poljacik G, Decety J and Nusbaum H C 2018 Loving-kindness language exposure leads to changes in sensitivity to imagined pain *J. Posit. Psychol.* **13** 429–33

Wispe L G 1972 Positive forms of social behavior: an overview *J. Soc. Issues* **28** 1–19

Wrangham R 2019 *The Goodness Paradox: How Evolution Made us Both More and Less Violent* (London: Profile Books)

Wyczesany M, Capotosto P, Zappasodi F and Prete G 2018 Hemispheric asymmetries and emotions: evidence from effective connectivity *Neuropsychologia* **121** 98–105

Yamada M, Lamm C and Decety J 2011 Pleasing frowns, disappointing smiles: an ERP investigation of counter empathy *Emotion* **11** 1336

Yang A, Hsee C and Urminsky O 2014 Eager to help yet reluctant to give: how pro-social effort and pro-social choices diverge *SSRN* (https://dx.doi.org/10.2139/ssrn.3448153)

Yang Q, Tang P, Gu R, Luo W and Luo Y J 2015 Implicit emotion regulation affects outcome evaluation *Soc. Cogn. Affect. Neurosci.* **10** 824–31

Yoder K J and Decety J 2014 Spatiotemporal neural dynamics of moral judgment: a high-density ERP study *Neuropsychologia* **60** 39–45

Yoder K J and Decety J 2014 The good, the bad, and the just: justice sensitivity predicts neural response during moral evaluation of actions performed by others *J. Neurosci.* **34** 4161–6

Zhu L, Jenkins A C, Set E, Scabini D, Knight R T, Chiu P H, King-Casas B and Hsu M 2014 Damage to dorsolateral prefrontal cortex affects tradeoffs between honesty and self-interest *Nat. Neurosci.* **17** 1319–21

IOP Publishing

Neurocognitive Perspectives of Prosocial and Positive Emotional Behaviours
Theory to application
Shashikanta Tarai and Arindam Bit

Chapter 10

Stress and mood disorder management using pharmacological and epigenetic factors

Arindam Bit, Pratistha Bhagat and Shashikanta Tarai

Mood disorientations are categorized by behavioural irregularities that include cognitive and mnemonic dysfunction and disturbances of emotional regulation. These effects represent a major cause of disability in psychiatric patients. Depression is a leading cause of disability globally and also a major contributor to the worldwide burden of disease. Integrating neurophysiological techniques of stress and affective disorders, topical findings are highlighted in this review, current problems, and ongoing challenges in efforts to combat these deficits and enhance pharmacological ramifications of antidepressant agents, mood stabilizers, and other psychiatric agents used to treat these symptoms. Although we have had effective treatments for depression for 50 years, these have always had major shortcomings, including the delayed onset of fast action antidepressant activity. In recent years, there has been a major advancement in identifying ketamine, as a glutamate N-methyl-D-aspartate receptor antagonist, as a fast-acting antidepressant.

In addition to this clinical advancement, our understanding of the mechanisms of depression and antidepressant responses have advanced at the neural and molecular levels, implicating alterations in brain plasticity in both the causes of depression and the mechanism underlying effective treatments. Synaptic plasticity is facilitated by an antidepressant-induced increased brain-derived neurotrophic factor (BDNF) in the central nervous system (CNS), reversing and ameliorating mood deficits and other symptoms of depressive illness associated with limbic circuitry. Epigenetic factors also influence the functional connectivity of these neural circuits to influence stress resilience and vulnerability and the development and course of depressive disorders. Altered function of the neuroendocrine and central nervous systems can influence behavioural resilience in which adaptive mechanisms promote recovery from stress. Stressors and the pro-inflammatory modules contribute to a distinctive

doi:10.1088/978-0-7503-3383-2ch10

moniker of cytokines and trophic factors in the CNS, enhancing neuronal survival and neurogenesis.

Conversely, maladaptive mechanisms can lead to the opposite effects in limbic brain regions. Furthermore, there is a substantial overlap between stress-induced adaptations that influence depressive illness and drug addiction vulnerability. Glucocorticoids, neurotrophic factors, inter-cellular signaling molecules, and endocannabinoids (eCB) dominate the behavioural and synaptic plasticity in addiction, as well as stress disorders. It is expected that the prospective research on neuronal dynamics and cellular revisions to stress that promotes resilience over vulnerability will aid the development of more effective behavioural and pharmaceutical therapies by addressing the etiology of stress-induced synaptic dysregulation in mood disorders.

10.1 Introduction

Major mood disorder (MMD) is one of the emerging causes of morbidity among the younger generation and adults worldwide, much of which is associated with traumatic lifetime events. In the United States, MDD has a lifetime incidence of 17% (Kessler *et al* 2005). The World Health Organization estimates that MMD will be the front runner for the cause of disability by 2020 (Reddy 2010). It has also created a large financial implication with an estimated cost of $210.5 billion annually for medicaments (Gerhard *et al* 2016). Furthermore, at the time of death, approximately 23% of suicide victims are currently on anti-depressant treatments (Karch *et al* 2012), reflecting the relationship between depression and suicide.

Moreover, depression, anxiety, and mood-related disorders are prevalent among the younger generation, potential sufferers of negligence, maltreatment, and trauma. During early life, stressful experiences have elongated repercussions on brain development, affecting the capacity to respond to various stressful challenges later in life, since the experience modulates neuroendocrine, autonomic, metabolic, and immune systems functions (Anda *et al* 2010). Moreover, depending on the severity and extent of stressful experiences, they can promote resilience to late-life stressors and the development of MDD or increase susceptibility to MDD. Therefore, understanding the processes that promote resilience or confer susceptibility will be important for developing better medications to treat MDD and related conditions.

Current antidepressant treatments have substantial shortcomings, including delayed onset and lack of efficacy or inadequate responses in some patients (Gerhard *et al* 2016). Moreover, not all symptoms show equal responses to treatment, and some symptoms can be exacerbated in the presence of other co-morbid conditions. Most patients with mood disorders exhibit cognitive dysfunction and memory impairments poorly treated by current antidepressant treatments. Work to improve antidepressant treatments currently focuses on two aspects of antidepressant therapy that are poorly treated, stress vulnerability and cognitive impairment. In regard to the role of stress in depressive illness, advancements have been made in recent years examining stress-induced epigenetic changes. Indeed, epigenetic regulation of DNA methylation is associated with the growth of vulnerability for developing depression resulting from early life trauma. Methylation in the serotonin transporter (*SLC6A4*), BDNF, glucocorticoid receptor (NR3C1), and FK506 binding protein (FKBP5) genes are well known to envisage the progression of anxiety and depression in clinical samples (Bagot *et al* 2014). Ina counter-response to the stress, these genes are modified in mood disorders, and one of the major consequences is alterations in synaptic plasticity (McEwen *et al* 2015). Currently, alterations in signalling in certain neural pathways associated with low-neurotrophic factor levels have been considered an underlying factor in the development of mood disorders (Autry *et al* 2011). Increased signalling of neurotrophins, including BDNF and nerve growth factor (NGF), is strongly linked with anti-depressant responses via TrkB receptors in limbic brain regions such as the hypothalamus, hippocampus and medial prefrontal cortex. In these regions, the treatment of chronic stress and depressive-like behaviour (Naert *et al* 2011, Calabrese *et al* 2012) with antidepressant drugs increases BDNF mRNA and protein levels (Calabrese *et al* 2011). Moreover, the fast-acting antidepressant ketamine also promotes the expression of proteins associated with neuronal plasticity, neurogenesis, synaptogenesis, neuronal survival and axonal elongation (Castrén 2013).

Broad changes in neural function are observed after stress. Stress-related brain atrophy is observed in limbic brain structures, as well as reductions in overall brain volume. On a cellular level, reductions in neuronal and glial cell numbers and disruptions of synaptic functions are detected in patients with mood disorders. Many different physiological and psychological stressors have been shown to influence these processes and contribute to the development of brain changes that could be termed 'pro-depressive'. High-fat-diets (HFD) that accelerate the growth of obesity and insulin resistance are associated with neuronal atrophy, including decreased numbers of progenitor cells, reduced glucocorticoid kinase-1 (GK1) expression, and reduced neurogenesis in cortical and limbic brain regions (Popelova 2015). Increased neurogenesis is associated with antidepressant treatment responses, while reduced neurogenesis has been associated with depression pathogenesis and the dysregulation of the hypothalamic-pituitary-adrenal (HPA) axis (David *et al* 2009, Zunszain *et al* 2012). In the prefrontal cortex (PFC) and hippocampus regions, it is observed that there is a decrease in synaptic number and functioning of neurons following increased activity of the HPA axis that includes changes in corticotrophin-releasing hormone receptor-1 (CRHR1) and adrenal glucocorticoids in patients with mood disorders (Liu *et al* 2008). Cell-surface expression of excitatory and inhibitor receptors, and proteins that are associated with the readily releasable pool (RRP) of synaptic vesicles (SVs), are involved in maintaining αamino3hydroxy5methyl4isoxazolepropionic acid (AMPA) glutamate receptor and γ-amino butyric acid receptor type-A ($GABA_A$) mediated changes in synaptic strength, interim plasticity and inter-synaptic crosstalk. These aspects of excitatory and inhibitory synaptic function are influenced by BDNF, vascular-endothelial growth (VEG), and insulin-like growth factor-1 (IGF1), which are predominantly needed for creating and maintaining the synaptic connections and neural plasticity in the CNS. In particular, BDNF and glucocorticoid changes facilitate synaptic plasticity and the accompanying morphological and molecular modifications by which depressive symptoms are ameliorated by antidepressants (Nestler *et al* 2002). Inhibition of nuclear factor-B (NFκB) resulting from IκB kinase (IKK) phosphorylation of IκB has a significant role in synaptic plasticity and the regulation of neuronal morphology (Gutierrez *et al* 2005). In particular, the IKK–NFκB beckoning pathway regulates hippocampal neuroplasticity and memory consolidation (Lubin and Sweatt 2007). Stress has been shown to affect long-term potentiation (LTP), assessed *in vitro*, and alters the stability of place cells and impedes the formation of spatial memories (Kim *et al* 2007). The BLA–ventral hippocampus (vHPC) circuit has also been recognized in terms of anxiety-related societal interactions, using optogenetic approaches (Allsop *et al* 2014).

There is also a relationship between stress, drugs of abuse, and synaptic plasticity (Grueter *et al* 2012, Koob *et al* 2014) that involves changes in synaptic plasticity and connectivity in the limbic brain regions. Moreover, genome-wide association studies for addiction liability have shown that genetic contributions to addiction primarily alter genes that might influence synaptic plasticity and connectivity through genetic variation in neural cell adhesion molecule genes (for a summary of these results, see Hall *et al* 2013). However, this recent work in the genetics of addiction in humans is founded on a long history of studies indicating that drugs of abuse produce profound changes in brain function. In brief, to understand this context, consider cocaine, which increases extracellular dopamine levels, activating post-synaptic dopamine receptors, but it is also associated with an elevation in synaptic glutamate levels (Smith *et al* 1995). These acute changes in dopaminergic and glutamatergic function promote longer-term changes in synaptic plasticity, including alterations in dendritic spine density (Robinson and Kolb 2004, Waselus *et al* 2013). These synaptic changes alter the intrinsic excitability of inputs to nucleus accumbens (NAc) medium spiny neurons (MSN) to affect cocaine-seeking behaviour but are also known to affect synaptic functions in other limbic brain regions as well. Many of these changes have been shown to occur after exposure to various drugs of abuse and after exposure to stressors, producing cross-sensitization with the reinforcing effects of drugs of abuse that have divergent mechanisms (Fitzgerald *et al* 1996). There is also a long history of the study of early life social isolation showing that it alters monoaminergic function, limbic reactivity and increases responses and self-administration of drugs of abuse (see Hall (1998), Hall and Perona (2012) for a review of this topic). Indeed, the social loss is a major contributing factor to the development of post-traumatic stress disorder (PTSD) (Charuvastra and Cloitre (2008)), which reflects several processes, including the protective effects of social buffering against the consequences of stress that are lost in individuals that become socially withdrawn or isolated. Moreover, social stressors such as social defeat are associated with alterations in these same structures, for instance, functional increases in post synaptic current (mEPSCs) in NAc-MSNs (Christoffel *et al* 2011). Further contributing to this picture, epigenomic analyses of these molecular and cellular circuits have identified plausible biomarkers for stress and mood-related disorientations that involve changes in neuroendocrine, immune and central nervous systems (LaSalle 2011).

The advancement of N-methyl-D-aspartate (NMDA) receptor antagonist ketamine is utilized to treat mood disorders, implying the role of stress in mood disorder resilience and vulnerability. Synaptic plasticity resulting from antidepressant treatments have long been thought to involve changes in mechanisms underlying synaptic plasticity. However, the more rapid actions of ketamine suggest that these processes can be accelerated in some way and provide a way to approach the identification of key common mechanisms. Introspecting these neurobiological and epigenetic mechanisms of stress and mood disorientations in the light of this recent advancement, the present review considers the new challenges and opportunities promoting synaptic plasticity and trophic factor signaling may afford for improved antidepressant treatments.

10.2 Developmental phases of stress and affective disorder

Stress disorders are characterized by the impairment of cognitive, emotional and motivational function. These occur in part through the instigation of the hypothalamic-pituitary-adrenal (HPA) axis but involve changes in the limbic system and the prefrontal cortex, amygdala, and hippocampus. Each has different roles in the cognitive and emotional symptoms of stress disorders. These regions of the brain are influenced differentially by acute and chronic stress. Acute stress results in modifications of morphology and chemistry which are strongly rescindable, but prolonged stress (for months or years) produces irreversible effects on brain function. Animal studies, in particular, have shown that brain plasticity associated with chronic stress involves a wide range of brain mechanisms. However, these include excitatory amino acids, glucocorticoids, BDNF, tissue plasminogen activator (tPA), and polysulfated neural cell adhesion molecule (PSA-NCAM), among others, which can be adaptive or maladaptive depending on the circumstances. Many of those studies are discussed in more detail in subsequent sections. Investigation of the mechanisms underlying the relationship between stress and consequent pathology necessitates, in many instances, animal models, but these studies have been supported in many ways by clinical studies. For example, early childhood maltreatment is associated with reduced hippocampal and prefrontocortical gray matter (Gorka *et al* 2014). Indeed, although many such effects of this type relate to the impact of chronic stress early in life, ongoing stress, perhaps associated with increased stress sensitivity in some individuals, may be an important aspect of continuing psychopathology.

Thus, differences in hippocampal volume are associated with sensitivity to daily stressors measured in terms of cortisol responses (Collip *et al* 2013). Indeed, many established genetic associations with MDD and other stress-related disorders have also been shown to interact with stressful experiences, particularly early in life, to promote the development of stress-related disorders. For example, a SERT polymorphism that affects levels of SERT expression interacts with early life stressors or trauma to predispose individuals to depressive and anxiety disorders (Karg *et al* 2011). In addition, the short allele (S) in the serotonin transporter-linked polymorphic region (5-HTTLPR) is associated with increased sensitivity with life stressors that increase the likelihood of developing depression. Moreover, using functional magnetic resonance imaging (fMRI), this polymorphism has been shown to increase acute sensitivity to stressors during threat anticipation in a network of connected brain regions that include the amygdala, hippocampus, medial prefrontal cortex, and a number of other limbic brain regions (Drabant *et al* 2012).

The factor associated with depression and upgrading and social and traumatic stress influences the white matter abnormalities, cortical or cerebellar atrophy, and basal ganglia wound as shown in magnetic resonance imaging (MRI) studies (Li *et al* 2017, Sacchet *et al* 2017, Shinoda *et al* 2017). These abnormalities are also related to obesity which is also responsible for glucocorticoids and inflammatory cytokines (Zass *et al* 2017). Metabolic disorders are consequently associated with disrupting the same neural, immune and endocrine circuits linked to stress- and illness-induced disruption that contributes to mood disorders. Aberrant motivation, affect, and anxiety is observed in depression as a result of the disruption of these mechanisms (Pasquali 2012). Stress, depression and anxiety are complicated conditions influenced by numerous peripheral physiological processes that regulate circulating factors related to stress. This includes cytokines and glucocorticoids, but it also performs transportation of leptin and adiponectin-associated peptides from stomach source to adipose tissue and ghrelin destination (Lago *et al* 2007). Many of these mechanisms are involved in feeding, energy homeostasis, and weight regulation and be disrupted in metabolic syndrome (Rosen *et al* 2006).

Moreover, emerging data also indicates that this gut microbiome influences the endocrine as well as neurocrine systems. This symbiotic interaction is just starting to be elaborated, but nonetheless, there is accumulating evidence that a psychiatric illness, including depression and anxiety, was somehow connected to the imbalanced microbiome–brain interaction (Mayer *et al* 2014, Petra *et al* 2015). These influences may work in various ways, but the reduction in synaptic plasticity has been shown to result from high-fat diet (HFD)-induced diabetes and insulin resistance; this effect will create neuronal atrophy in cortical and limbic formation animal model (Stranahan *et al* 2008). We can improve the insulin resistance in the cortical and limbic portion by utilizing HFD as well as step down the stimulation based on insulin-dependent of Akt, S6 kinase (S6K), glycogen synthase kinase (GSK)–3β and mTORC1 signalling (Arnold *et al* 2014). Furthermore, we can control the AMPK by Energy metabolism. This AMPK was the main regulator for mTORC1 signaling as well as synaptic protein synthesis. For energy metabolism and cellular respiration, BDNF was responsible for that (Markham *et al* 2012, Marosi and Mattson 2014), and as we will discuss, plays a critical role in synaptic plasticity as well as a consequence of stress on synaptic plasticity. As will be discussed throughout this review, the brain structures affected by HFD are critical structures involved in stress-related psychiatric disorders, and many of the same mediators of these changes are involved in the contributions of other stressors to the development of disease states.

10.3 Stress-induced alterations and affective disorder

Several animal models have been developed that demonstrate increased sensitivity to stressors resulting in behavioural changes similar to affective disorders. One example of this is serotonin transporter knockout (SERT KO) mice, in which the gene for the serotonin transporter (SERT; SLC6A4) is absent. Under at least some circumstances, these mice have been shown to exhibit behavioural traits reminiscent of anxiety and depression (Holmes *et al* 2003). This genetic model has parallels to the 5HTTLPR polymorphism in humans that was discussed above. Indeed, an orthologous polymorphism in the rhesus macaque (*Macaca mulatta*) SERT gene produces a similar gene × environment interaction potentiating stress responses in monkeys exposed to a stressful early-life environment (Barr *et al* 2004). Interestingly, this gene × environment interaction was observed in females, while elevated stress responses resulted solely from the genetic differences alone in males. This is particularly interesting given the well-known increase in the incidence of many stress-related disorders in females.

One recent study in the SERT KO mouse found that although SERT KO mice were impaired in learning the Morris Water Maze, they were not impaired in learning the Barnes maze (Karabeg *et al* 2013). The authors recommended that the difference between the two tests was the degree of stress evoked by the circumstance, which was supported by greater corticosterone responses in SERT KO mice. In addition, hippocampal immunohistochemistry revealed greater immediate early gene activation (cFos and Arc) associated with increased proliferation marker Ki67 and a marker for immature neurons (NeuroD) at baseline. However, SERT +/+ exposure to the water maze was associated with increases in Ki67 and NeuroD in several hippocampal subregions, while SERT −/− was not. Moreover, learning was correlated with neurogenesis in SERT KO mice, e.g., poor learning mice were slower learners.

Serotonin system genes besides SERT have also been repeatedly linked with MDD, other stress-related disorders and being involved in the actions of many treatments for those disorders. Consequently, many of these genes have been of interest in animal studies of stress and depression-related phenotypes. It has already been mentioned that the neurotrophic factor BDNF has been associated with stress-related disorders and antidepressant mechanisms that may involve the serotonin transporter (Murphy *et al* 2003). Studies of heterozygous BDNF knockout (BDNF +/−) mice have contributed to this understanding. Although not different at baseline, these mice have greater responses in behavioural despair tests after stress exposure (Advani *et al* 2009). Moreover, BDNF +/− mice, or mice with a forebrain specific reduction in BDNF, demonstrated a region-specific, stress-induced reduction in 5-HT1A receptor function in the hippocampus compared to control mice (Burke *et al* 2013). These effects could be reversed by chronic fluoxetine treatment. These chronic fluoxetine treatments were linked by the step-up activation of the high-affinity BDNF receptor, TrkB. Although not assessed in this study, other studies have associated 5-HT1A receptor activation with neurogenesis (Fricker *et al* 2005). The stress used here was a relatively mild stressor, which does not usually produce changes in 5-HT1A function, although more severe or chronic stressors have been shown to have these effects (McKittrick *et al* 1995, Lopez *et al* 1998).

Research has also investigated other more central genes to stress mechanisms, such as the receptor for corticotropin-releasing factor receptor 2 (CRFR-2).

CRFR-2 KO mice are hyperresponsive to stress as measured in cortisol activation, anxiety, and an inability to adopt active coping strategies (Bale *et al* 2000, Bale and Vale 2003, McEun *et al* 2008). Another factor associated with stress-related psychiatric dysfunction was found to be associated with the neural and behavioural disruptions observed in these mice—neuroinflammatory responses mediated by astrocytes (Gerber and Bale 2012). Treatment with anti-inflammatory drugs prevented both increased glial fibrillary acidic protein (GFAP) in the hippocampus, prefrontal cortex, and paraventricular nucleus of the hypothalamus and rescuing HPA-axis dysfunction in these mice. The authors described the effects of CRFR-2 KO as altered 'astrocyte-mediated plasticity'.

These context-dependent genetic features are transferred by amygdale PFC circuits (Tronson *et al* 2012). Injections of BDNF can reduce the progression of depressive behaviours in the hippocampus (Egan *et al* 2003, Taliaz *et al* 2011). Endocannabinoids which are key modulators of synaptic function are also induced by brain-derived neurotrophic factor. Endocannabinoid (eCB) signalling is affected by ageing, neuroinflammation, and neurodegenerative processes associated with various disease states (Marzo, Vincenzo Di 2015). Immune cells which interfere with the brain parenchyma also express eCB receptors (Hegde *et al* 2010). Deregulation of eCB signalling, therefore, affects the immune, endocrine and neuronal cell signalling (Russell and Kahn 2007). Two primary eCB receptors are CB1 and CB2. CBI receptors are linked throughout the brain, and these receptors are bounded to the Gi/o proteins (Howlett *et al* 2002). However, CB2 receptors mostly bounded to Gi proteins instead of the Go proteins (Glass and Northup 1999). In the mature brain, CB1 cannabinoid receptors are found in an abundant amount in a particular area, and these are used by the endocannabinoids, which act as retrograde messengers, which are used to regulate the brain-related and shut off the extra synaptic activity (Galve-Roperh *et al* 2009). CB2 receptor expression in neuronal cells is heavily restricted, and CB2 receptors were used to perform some brain population-related activity and NP/stem cells. The serine kinase mammalian target of rapamycin (mTOR) was used to regulate the CB1 receptor (Gomez *et al* 2011). Growth factors like EGF gets are modulated by mTOR signaling pathway. And this pathway is highly correlated with SPIED in an antagonistic manner in the case of mouse embryonic fibroblasts (Cunningham *et al* 2007) with $r = 0.55$ and 0.44 for EGFR and FGFR antagonist, respectively. Irrespective of animal model study related to oligodendrocyte precursor cell line and corresponding regulatory transcripts (Gobert *et al* 2009), mild scores of correlation of mTOR with CB antagonistic profile were obtained at $r < 0.25$. Endocannabinoids are anti-inflammatory (Klein 2005), this may relate to conditions that predispose individuals to neuroinflammation that exacerbates other conditions. eCB-related receptors and Cannabinoid in glial cells and neurons also change independently in neurological disease states (Stella 2010). eCB levels and signalling have been predicted for ABHD6MGL and FAAH. These enzymatic hubs regulate several distinct signalling lipids and target a wider panel of receptors within a signaling network, enhancing symptomatic relief (allcviation of spasticity) in chronic or rclapsing Enccphalomyclitis (EAE). BDNF shows a brain shield effect in myelin oligodendrocyte glycoprotein-induced EAE.

Different molecular components are involved in eCB signaling in the brain and peripheral tissues. ECB signalling is affected by age, but the bioactivity of cannabinoid-based therapeutics varies with age (Velayudhan *et al* 2014). Being a functionalized molecular integrator, mTOR facilitates sensing of nutrient transfer to cells which are bound to the energy homeostasis via/MAPK–Akt pathway. mTORC1 regulates cognitive functions and synaptic plasticity using the *de novo* protein synthesis routeway. This process provides nutrients under the situation of starvation. With the ageing of tissues, autophagy gets reduced (Kapahi *et al* 2010), and it is being induced in cancer cells by eCB signalling (Salazar *et al* 2009, Koay *et al* 2014).

10.4 Evidence for stress-induced changes in synaptic structure and function

The extracellular signal-regulated kinase-dependent pathway triggers excitatory neurotransmitter glutamate, and these are used to control the signaling of chain of intracellular. Neuronal depolarization has been done by glutamate by activating postsynaptic ionotropic receptors having to increase intercellular Na^+. In terms of brain regions involved in cognitive function, the hippocampus is most sensitive to stress. In response to sustained stress, the hippocampus transforms itself to adaptive modification. Cumulative stress has been changed by another part of the brain, such as the amygdala and prefrontal cortex and shortened dendrite in the medial prefrontal cortex. At the same time, it provides dendrite growth in the amygdala (Vyas *et al* 2002) and the orbitofrontal cortex (Liston *et al* 2006). The prefrontal cortex and amygdala also contain adrenal steroid receptors, which facilitates tissue plasminogen activator (tPA) to withstand stress by activating indices of structural plasticity and anxiety (Melchor *et al* 2003). The amygdala's medial and central region is involved in this phenomenon, releasing CRH through CRH1 receptors (Matys *et al* 2004). Prefrontal cortex remodelling (structural) leads to induction of behavioural correlation with attention set-shifting.

The hippocampus is vulnerable to stress-associated illness because this brain region contributes to the high density of corticoid receptors (Webster *et al* 2002). There are substantial bidirectional connections that exist between the prefrontal and amygdala. Early assessment of cellular mechanisms underlying cognitive deficits has oriented to primary memory (Martin *et al* 2000) and decreases dendritic spines' thickness (Chen *et al* 2010). These changes involve interactions between limbic regions as well as the effects of glucocorticoids and monoaminergic inputs. The electrical stimulus of BLA interrupts the induction of long-term potentiation (LTP) in the sub-region CA1 of primary memory (Vouimba and Richter-Levin 2005). p25 is a stress-regulated protein that promotes plasticity in the hippocampus after repeated stress in an amygdala-dependent manner. These changes contribute to stress associated learning and memory deficits. p25/Cdk5 dependent phosphorylation on Ser211 of GR was energizing by the above mechanism (Gräff *et al* 2012). These phenomena increase histone deacetylase 2 (HDAC2) (Gräff *et al* 2012). Continuous stress has been generated by the Cdk5 (cyclin-dependent kinase 5)-

activator p25, step-up controlling of glucocorticoid receptors (GR) as well as step up and step down the HDAC2 expression and memory-related genes expression in the hippocampus (Rei *et al* 2015). Molecular mechanisms of trans-repression between GR and NGFI-B, for the need to model Swi/Snf chromatin Brgl and ATPase activity, are important for forming stable complexes between GR and NGFI-B between GR and HDAC2. Acetylated histone H4 regulates the promotion based recruitment of both HDAC2 and GR throughout the gene. Collection of trans-repression machinery at the POMC promotes simultaneously interrupting initiation of transcription. Enrollment of GR lowers transcription by blocking NGFI-B-dependent activation. At the same time, modification of Brgl/NGFI-B/GR complex also recruits HDAC (Bilodeau *et al* 2006). Expression of the gene for learning and memory have been preventing by the HDAC2 (Gräff *et al* 2012). The hippocampal is protected from the detrimental effect of repulsive stress by the blockade of p25 generation (Rei *et al* 2015). N-methyl-D-aspartate (NMDA) receptors were energized by the above phenomenon and cause the accumulation of Ca^{2+} in huge amounts (Chetkovich *et al* 1991). The path in between the p25 generation and HDAC2 is responsible for reduced learning and memory genes. These phenomena boot up the memory loss shown by the previous studies (Guan *et al* 2009, Gräff *et al* 2012).

Some mediators of neural plasticity include inhibitory and excitatory neurotransmitters, gluco-corticoid, inter-cellular signaling molecules, NGF, and endocannabinoids. They conduct in a nonlinear network and execute reciprocal interactions and biphasic actions leading to pathophysiology and disruption (McEwen 2006). The longitudinal effect of stressful experiences in childhood results in attenuated development and capacity to respond to stressful propagative crises (Anda *et al* 2010). The mature brain can provide a stressful environment by executing functional and reversible structural plasticity, including dendritic remodelling, neuronal replacement, and synaptic turnover in the hippocampus region. Further, this region is influenced by environmental risk factors that regulate depression through the convergence of molecular and cellular interferences, disrupting neuronal execution and affecting cellular morphology. Molecular changes include synaptic deficits resulting in malfunction of circuitry related to the regulation of mood and cognitive function (Duman and Duman 2014). Continued stress result shows the body's decreasing weight and medium change in adrenal and thymus weights. This result produces the important saturation on the length and branch points of CA3 pyramidal neurons inside the elongated ridges on the floor of each lateral ventricle of the brain (Watanabe *et al* 1992). The impact of stress on the interneuron population estimates cell loss because of a dip in parvalbumin concentration in neurons. Anti-depression treatment safeguards from effective stress by modulating the hippocampal GABA-ergic system. Hippocampal function changes over age, so it would be expected to interact differently with age.

Ketamine and other nonselective NMDA antagonists treat stress and mood problems and other disorders that involve glutamatergic function. Interest in NMDA receptor antagonism in treating psychiatric disorders began with an interest in the cellular toxicity associated with several different neurological conditions. In some cases, these conditions involve particular NMDA receptor subunits. For example, GluN2B subunits, including extra-synaptic and synaptic NMDA receptors, have major significance in excitotoxicity while mediating the role of stroke-induced damage (Martin and Wang 2010). Ketamine and other rapid-acting compounds affect the fast-acting ionotropic glutamate receptors in the fast-acting phenomena. Actions at these targets tend to be 'all-or-nothing'; agonism producing excitotoxicity and seizures, and antagonism producing anaesthesia and impairing memory. It was found that the metabotropic glutamate receptors (G-protein) were important elements for the treatment of different neurological and psychiatric conditions, including emotional disorders, because of the poor dynamic range of action of antidepressants. Patients with stress and mood disorder have impairments in the neural modulation of perceptual input to primary cortices and amygdale (Shin and Liberzon 2010), influencing the activity of higher cortical regions mediating perception of emotional and affective behaviour. Perception of safe context can be more normalized by anxiety patients (Lissek *et al* 2014).

Altered neural representations influence instrumental cognitions that influence affective behaviour in particular regions within which neural pathways participate in affective modulation: the putamen for gain, the ACC for loss, and the amygdala for both gain and loss (Breiter *et al* 2001, Moustafa *et al* 2017). Amygdala activity correlates with a behavioural generalization about emotion following auditory cortex activation, differentiating between anxiety patients and controls (Laufer *et al* 2016). Because of fundamental changes in the case of patients how they perceive affective stimuli with anxiety and mood disorders and to what extent they discriminate affective content from other non-affective stimuli, differences between these groups emerge (Hartley *et al* 2012). To make the subjects more prone to exhibiting anxiety symptoms, changes are induced in the representation of conditioned stimuli in the amygdala and primary sensory regions by affective stimuli (Pattwell *et al* 2012).

The foregoing discussion involves studies that have used different approaches to induce stress. This raises the question of how stress is defined, operationalized, or measured. This is not a trivial question. Several different physiological indicators have been used as stress indicators (Romero 2004), including heart rate, plasma cortisol, behavioural indicators in animal studies, salivary or plasma cortisol, salivary α-amylase, and subjectively assessed negative affect in human studies. In different studies, different stressors are used. More research needs to consider the nature of the stressor and whether this impacts the outcome independently of the stressor's duration, frequency, and intensity. This is particularly true in the case of psychosocial stressors early in development, which also impacts other types of neuro-developmental mechanisms (see Hall and Perona (2012) for a discussion of this issue). In any case, studies have shown that there are genetic differences in acute and chronic stress responses using such measures in both humans and animal models. For example, acute stress responses are observed in individuals with a functional deletion α2b adrenoreceptor (due to a polymorphism in the *ADRA2B* gene), but not in non-deletion carriers, during exposure to psychosocial stress (violent movie scenes) (Cousijn *et al* 2010). Acute stress refers to a single and time-limited exposure to a physical, psychological, or social stressor, but it would not be surprising that there would be cumulative effects. They repeat acute stress effects. Such changes may influence the cognitive processing of emotionally relevant stimulants in other respects as well. Deletion carriers had blunted amygdala reactivity in response to neutral facial expressions (Li *et al* 2015), which suggests that there may also be a shift in responding towards greater responses to stimuli with strong emotional valence. Thus, increased right hippocampal activation is increased by *ADRA2B* functional deletion for fearful faces after stress (Cousijn *et al* 2010); for control conditions, to show responses with neutral faces, amygdala responses are increased in deletion carriers (Li *et al* 2015). Under stress, in response to neutral faces, the amygdala has been blunted by these deletion carriers, but they increase amygdala responses to neutral faces under control conditions.

In addition to changes in function responses to acute stressors in individuals with particular genetic differences, there is evidence for atrophy of limbic brain structures and reduced whole brain volume in patients with mood disorders. The ventromedial prefrontal (vmPFC) and the dorsolateral prefrontal cortex (DLPFC) are included in stress resilience/coping when these changes occur within a set of interconnected structures. However, other structures such as the amygdala, hippocampus, and hypothalamus are engaged in stress reactivity and distress-signalling. Chronic stress and stress-related illnesses are associated with changes in the structure of all of these brain regions. However, these gross anatomical changes are accompanied by changes in genes/proteins, which are known to regulate synaptic plasticity, so that these gross changes probably reflected changes occurring at a cellular level, particularly in terms of differences in cell morphology. Analysis of CREB and BDNF indicates that in patients with depression, the loss of neural plasticity results from CREB and BDNF function. Environmental challenges can prepare an organism for later stressors or impair the ability to deal with later stressors, fostering resilience or imbuing the organism with a vulnerability to stress, but which way this process goes may depend on genetic predisposition. BDNF is central to this mechanism that promotes adaptation to later environmental challenges, e.g., adaptive plasticity. Genetic epidemiological studies show that approximately 40%–50% of the risk for depression is genetically related (Fava and Kendler 2000), but this genetic risk may depend on stress exposure, as was discussed previously about SERT manipulations in animal models.

Resilient coping results from neural plasticity promoted during stress by certain types of neural activity (Sinha *et al* 2016). When subjects are exposed to highly stressful, threatening stimuli, a particular physiological and endocrine increase produces temporally distinct neural activation patterns in brain circuits. Positive responses to stressors appear to involve different neural patterns that allow adaptation to new conditions. Acute functional neuroplasticity at the time of stress comprising distinct and separable brain networks encompasses critical components of the stress response that are either positive or negative with respect to long-term coping and resilience. Changes within vmPFC circuitry promote stress-resilient coping (Fleshner *et al* 2011), as shown in figure 10.1. This occurs as limbic-striatal activation increases during stress and in the ventromedial prefrontal cortex (vmPFC) and dorsolateral prefrontal cortex (DLPFC). For neuroplasticity vmPFC is taken as one of the critical loci in a resilience-coping network where signals are increased in response to emotionally evocative stimuli, influencing behavioural control and the extent of active coping. At the time of exposure to emotionally significant or stressful stimuli, disrupted vmPFC connectivity with the amygdala, and poor adaptive coping, blunted vmPFC activation associated with childhood trauma, cumulative adversity, and a history of mood disorders or post-traumatic stress disorder (PTSD) (Gee *et al* 2013, Seo *et al* 2014). These cortical structures appear to act as breaks on limbic reactivity, and reduced functioning leads to increased stress reactivity and distress-signalling involving the amygdala, hippocampus, and hypothalamus.

Depression disrupts mood-related circuitries and is also associated with reductions in the prefrontal cortex (PFC) and hippocampus volumes. The extension of stress is connected with the duration of illness and the duration of treatment response for depression. The result of a cumulative loss of neurons and glia in the

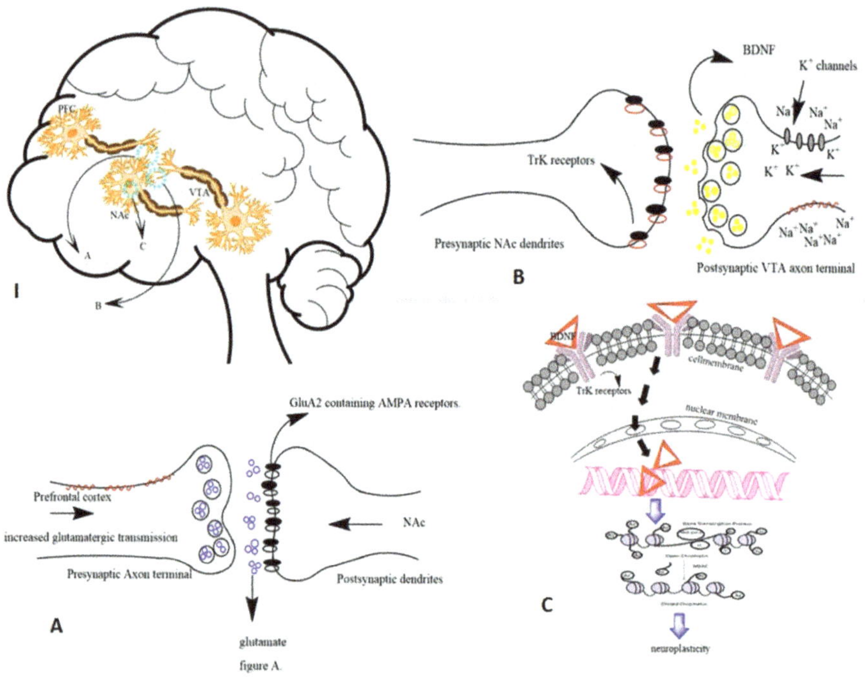

Figure 10.1. Stress influences neuroplasticity in a resilience-coping network that involves the prefrontal cortex, VTA and nucleus accumbens. Synaptic changes modify proteins crucial for cellular ion homeostasis, including Na^+, Ca^{2+} ATPases, and glucose and glutamate transport proteins, resulting in membrane-associated oxidative stress as shown in (A) and (B). Neuronal depolarization and increase in intracellular Na^+ signals is caused by the activation of the excitatory neurotransmitter glutamate. Prolonged bouts of stress via mechanisms that involve down-regulation of BDNF and BDNF-mediated neuroplasticity alters neural circuits, connecting PFC and VTA. BDNF increases the spine density in the NAc and strengthens excitatory synapses on VTA neurons, as represented in (B). Neuronal dysfunction results in anatomical changes accompanied by genes/protein expression changes, including CREB and BDNF function reductions, as shown in (C).

PFC and hippocampus is due to tissue atrophy caused by exposure to stress. Studies with a comparison of hippocampal volumes in patients with schizophrenia and patients with major depressive disorder (MDD), and healthy controls, suggest that volume differences in hippocampal regions may provide important information regarding the pathophysiology of schizophrenia and MDD (Savitz and Drevets 2009, Ota *et al* 2016) as the reduction of PFC and hippocampal volumes are associated with the length of illness and the time of treatment response.

In part because of observations of decreased volumes in limbic brain regions, neurotrophic hypotheses of depression and antidepressant response, and in particular BDNF, have been widely proposed (Castrén and Rantamäki 2010). Indeed, clinical studies illustrate that a BDNF polymorphism is connected with decreased hippocampal volumes in normal subjects and patients with depression (Hajek *et al* 2012) and is associated with impaired executive function and cognition (Soliman *et al* 2010). Given the known roles of BDNF in the formation and maintenance of synapses, it is not surprising that the amount and function of synapses are disrupted in depression, consistent with the model shown in figure 10.1. Synaptic plasticity in the somatosensory and visual cortex that influences the ability to perceive and access information and make appropriate, adaptive responses to subsequent related stimuli is also disrupted in depression and mood disorders (Holtmaat *et al* 2009). Other regulators of synaptic plasticity are also certainly involved. Glycogen synthase kinase-3 and upstream wingless (Wnt)–frizzled (Fz) regulates signalling pathways in mood disorders through multiple physiological processes, which include neuroplasticity, neuroprotection and neurogenesis (Krishnan and Nestler 2008). Interactions between signalling pathways regulate synaptogenesis, and disruption of these key neural pathways is involved in depression, including reductions in neurotrophic factors, interruption of estradiol cycling, and elevation of inflammatory cytokines. GSK3 regulates cAMP response element-binding (CREB), influencing hippocampal neurogenesis and neuroprotection that has been implicated in the action of antidepressant treatments (Li *et al* 2010). In addition, GSK3 increases the production of amyloid β-peptides (Phiel *et al* 2003), contributing to inflammatory responses in monocytes, microglia, and astrocytes. This could contribute to increases in inflammatory cytokines observed in patients with depression (Raison and Miller 2003).

Although some responses, such as neuroinflammation and immune activation, may be largely systemic, a complex repertoire of neuroplastic mechanisms in distinct brain regions is elicited by acute and chronic exposure to stress, including subregions of the hippocampus, which depend on the level of hormone release. These effects influence various aspects of hippocampal function. Stress and elevated glucocorticoids (Pavlides *et al* 1996) affect primed-burst stimulation and long-term potentiation (LTP) (Felix-Ortiz *et al* 2013). The dentate gyrus-CA3 system within the hippocampus shows adaptations in structural plasticity in response to stress that affects episodic memory (Lisman and Otmakhova 2001). CA3 pyramidal neurons, in response to restraint stress, undergo a reversible remodelling of their dendrites in the CA3 region (McEwen 2010), as do dentate granule neuron dendrites (Gould *et al* 1990). Many actions of glucocorticoids may contribute to these effects. The calcium ion conductances are regulated by the primary effect of corticosteroids in the hippocampal region, which affects neural excitability and plasticity, influences stress responses, and changes in hippocampal function with ageing (Kerr *et al* 1989). Hippocampal neurons undergo re-modelling during stress in the presence of vital mediators that include steroid hormones (Sousa *et al* 2000). Excitatory amino acid release synergizes with glucocorticoids, promoting excitotoxic damage under some conditions. However, these effects are highly concentration-dependent, with lower concentrations reducing excitotoxic effects through actions on mitochondrial metabolism but higher concentrations promoting excitotoxic effects (Du *et al* 2008). Several other factors influence cell excitability and plasticity, such as tumour necrosis factor-α (TNF), which is synthesized in response to cellular activity in neuronal circuits. TNF triggers neural receptors associated with the regulation of transcription factor NF-kB, thereby modulating neuronal vulnerability and excitability during excitotoxicity of neurons (Albensi and Mattson 2000).

Many of the studies discussed above focused on neural plasticity in the hippocampus related to certain aspects of learning and memory. Stress works through similar mechanisms in many other brain regions to influence other functions associated with long-term changes in response to stress, including circuits involved in motivation and the predisposition to drug addiction. Dysfunction in the mesolimbic dopaminergic pathway, in the ventral tegmental area (VTA) dopaminergic cells and other portions of the related circuitry, is linked with many neuropsychiatric disorders, including those that are well-known to be stress-related (Krishnan *et al* 2007). Enhanced release of BDNF in the nucleus accumbens (NAc) accompanies enhanced firing rates of VTA dopaminergic neurons that are enhanced by social defeat, expands post-synaptic densities, and increases miniature excitatory postsynaptic currents (mEPSCs) in NAc medium spiny neurons (Moron *et al* 2013). These functional changes in response to stress are accompanied by structural changes within mesocorticolimbic brain systems that regulate motivation and mood (Christoffel *et al* 2011). Chronic stress and mood disorders associated with chronic stress affect structural and neurochemical plasticity in many different regions of the brain that include the ventromedial prefrontal cortex (vmPFC), hippocampus and amygdala (Liston *et al* 2006, Liston *et al* 2006, Bruce 2007). Allostatic load refers to the cumulated physiological consequences of chronic stress. The cumulative effects of allostatic load are produced as the body attempts to maintain homeostasis leading to neural and physiological vulnerability to later stressors, combining with other risk factors leading to greater and greater maladaptive responses. Mal adaptations to stressors are observed specifically in parts of the limbic system, including the amygdala, hippocampus, and associated circuitry. Changes in brain activation observed with fMRI techniques indicate that neural adaptations associated with allostasis result in a loss of resilience to future stressors, which is a key feature of disorders of stress adaptation, including some types of anxiety and depression as PTSD. Increases in stress symptoms in soldiers are associated with greater amygdala and hippocampus responsiveness to stress-related stimuli (Admon *et al* 2009), although the changes in these regions exhibit different temporal relationships.

Amygdala reactivity before stress predicts later stress symptoms, while changes in hippocampal responsiveness are associated with later stress responses. These systems have substantial distinct stress susceptibility/resistance, and genetic differences contribute to these differences. The adrenergic receptor alpha 2B (ADRA2B) gene affects the phasic amygdala, including ventro-visual regions covering the primary visual cortex to the fusiform gyrus (Murty 2012). appears to influence Mnemonic function in part by distorting the stability of place cell firing rates is influenced (Sandi and Pinelo-Nava 2007) by the appearance of the vulnerability to stress associated with amygdala activity and hippocampal plasticity (Admon *et al* 2009). Behaviour impairment is due to memory deficits captured through probe trial performance tasks (Eichenbaum 1992, Damien *et al* 2015).

Epigenomic analyses define epigenetic modifications of DNA methylation (and other epigenetic mechanisms) acting at the interface of genetic and environmental factors. Increased understanding of the causes of neuropsychiatric diseases must consider the interaction of genetic, epigenetic, and the development of circuit-level mechanisms that underlie disease pathogenesis. This work will require technological innovation allowing the functional dissection of the molecular mechanisms underlying changes in distinct brain circuits and circuit connectivity discussed in previous sections. The new improvement of procedures for epigenetic/epigenomic examinations (LaSalle 2011) and optogenetic neural actuation or silencing (Manuscript and Tools 2013) will assist with clarifying the sub-atomic instruments and cell circuits adding to pressure-related problems (Pfau and Russo 2015). Neuroendocrine, insusceptible, and sensory systems add to this strength (Ménard *et al* 2016). Versatility is a coordinated cycle by which versatile instruments in different frameworks elevate and foster reactions to stressors that standardize work; the disappointment of strength prompts changes pertinent to numerous sickness states. Understanding versatility is consequently a basic piece of treating pressure related issues. Comprehension of this interaction will give expected focuses to foster biomarkers explicit to sorts of pressure (formative setting, nature, chronicity, and so on), and for different components that might impact pressure and flexibility, like gender, age, hereditary foundation, provocative state, etc. For example, distinguishing proof of gender-subordinate favourable to flexibility markers will empower the improvement of more viable medicines for problems with considerable gender reliance or may have a fairly unique hidden premise in people, just like the case for temperament. In the previous conversations, the sub-atomic instruments assumed significant parts in atypical reactions to stretch, adding to mindset problems and push flexibility.

Hippocampus has long been known to have roles in memory function, and important aspects include morphological re-arrangements in responses to various experiences, including stressful experiences (McEwen 2001). As discussed above, plasticity in hippocampal and other circuits involved in memory and emotional responses has an important roles in stress-related disorders, as discussed in a previous section. In many pieces of this circuitry, intense pliancy related to aversive learning and variations to upsetting upgrades brings about the initiation of the excitatory synapse glutamate, which causes neuronal depolarization (Tsai and Coyle 1998). The ensuing actuation of N-methyl-D-aspartate (NMDA) receptors and the convergence of Ca^{2+} particles is a significant starting advance prompting long term potentiation (see figure 10.1). However, numerous other signaling molecules are contributions that regulate the release of glutamate, the consequences of glutamate release, or other aspects of downstream signaling that ultimately determine the extine of structural and functional plasticity (Northoff and Panksepp 2008). In addition, these processes are affected by antidepressant treatments (Christoffel *et al* 2011, Duman and Duman 2014), which will be discussed in more detail in a subsequent section. Plasticity in several brain regions is associated with neuro-psychiatric diseases, including depression, anxiety, and drug addiction (Holtmaat *et al* 2009, Russo *et al* 2011).

As is clear from some of the preceding discussion, many mechanisms have been found to contribute to neural plasticity in circuitry relevant to mood disorders. In part, this results from strong neural activation occurring during exposure to stressors that results in neuroplasticity. Strong neural inputs producing plasticity often involved combinations of mechanisms that influence downstream signal trans-duction. Several such molecular mechanisms have been linked to depressive behaviours, and manipulations of these mechanisms have been suggested as potential novel therapeutic approaches (Sharif *et al* 2007). Mitogen-activated protein kinase phosphatase-1 (MKP-1), from the tyrosine and serine/threonine phosphatase family, is upregulated in the hippocampal area of individuals deter-mined to have misery. Phosphorylation of serine or threonine deposits of proteins containing carboxy-terminal proline at one side adds to the serious level of proline-coordinated phosphorylation (Huttlin *et al* 2010, Lundby *et al* 2012). N-terminal/stress-actuated kinases (JNKs) and extracellular sign controlled kinases (ERKs) seem to assume a significant part in these pathways (Beręsewicz *et al* 2008), including both JNK (p-JNK/NJNK) and dynamic ERK1/2 (p-RK1/2/ERK1/2), in the hippocampus. JNKs govern brain morphogenesis and the plasticity of developmental and adult axodendritic morphology, consequently regulating many important neuron-specific functions involving NMDA glutamate receptors (NMDAR) (Lissin *et al* 1998). NMDAR actuation delivers calcium influx and enrollment of AMPARs that lead to dependable synaptic transmission and memory arrangement changes. These cycles are modulated by an assortment of components, incorporating pathophysiological measures found in intense mind wounds (Ziebell *et al* 2015), for example, peril related sub-atomic examples (DAMPs), a bunch of sub-atomic determinants got from cell flotsam, and jetsam, intracellular proteins, or atomic DNA/RNA delivered from harmed cells following calamitous occasions (Seong and Matzinger 2004), and perhaps during other types of cellular stress. As noted above, these signalling pathways also interact with immune and neuro-endocrine signals stimulated by stressful states. Cytokines are stunningly touchy particles created and delivered by microglial cells in a unique situation and cell-dependent fashion. Numerous cytokines influence the Janus kinase (JAK)/signal transducer and activator of transcription (STAT) pathways by means of silencer of cytokine signalling (SOCS) group of proteins that are significant negative controllers of the JAK/STAT pathway (Moniaga *et al* 2015). Ultimately, MAPK signalling is a critical mediator of glutamatergic signalling involved in BDNF-regulated neural plasticity underlying learning and memory. Consequently, approaches have been developed to modulate these processes. For example, GLYX-13 (rapastinel), acting at the glycine site of glutamate NMDA receptors, has been developed as a potential antidepressant drug, but also improves performance in hippocampal-dependent learning tasks (Zhang *et al* 2008). The is just one of many mechanisms that overlap between learning and stress-related neuroplasticity. Postsynaptic endocytosis in glutamatergic neurons is controlled by mGluR5 and α1-adrenergic receptor (AR)-subordinate LTDs, where α1-AR-started LTD intervenes regulation of motioning through calcium-penetrable AMPA receptors (Sachser *et al* 2017). This ionotropic glutamate receptor (IGluR)-subordinate signalling supporting post-synaptic versatility initiating the drawn-out potentiation (LTP) and driving the cell premise of long-term memory (LTM) (Sachser *et al* 2017), and seems to be modulated by stress and stress-related disorders.

Another important signalling pathway regulating glutamatergic synaptic plasticity involves IκB kinase (IKK), which phosphorylates IκB, thereby increasing the function of NFκB (Mercurio *et al* 1999), which regulates synaptic plasticity and neuronal morphology (Gutierrez *et al* 2005). This pathway has a role in memory consolidation (O'Mahony *et al* 2006, Lubin and Sweatt 2007). Other parts of signalling pathways influencing synaptic plasticity have also been identified. Stress affects Gq-receptor-subordinate pliancy, including glutamatergic transmission in the bed nucleus of the stria terminalis (BNST) and glutamate-enacted Gq-connected signalling pathways. Tension is constrained by various neuronal circuits that share strong and equal associations with the BNST, a key design controlling negative enthusiastic states (Ressler 2010). The BNST incorporates different contributions from mind locales engaged with pressure reactions and stress-related pathology above to tweak nervousness. Contributions to the BNST from the infralimbic cortex (ILCx) and ventral subiculum/CA1 (SUV/CA1) manage BNST movement at the single-cell level (Glangetas *et al* 2017). vSUB/CA1 incitement can advance various types of *in vivo* pliancy at the single-cell level in the anteromedial part of the BNST (among). vSUB/CA1-driven LTP in the among gets fitting reactions to anxiogenic setting, instead of overstated reactions, and brokenness of this component might underlie pathologic nervousness states (Glangetas *et al* 2017).

Given the implications of these mechanisms for the structural plasticity of synapses, and other cellular structures, they may involve other mechanisms that regulate cellular structure. Actin dynamics and structural plasticity have been shown to affect Cannabinoid Receptor CB1 signalling by regulating the WAVE1 protein complex (Njoo *et al* 2015). Cannabinoids, of course, influence synaptic plasticity, memory, and motivational states (Zhu 2006, Akirav 2011), and some cannabinoids have been suggested to have antidepressant effects (de Mello *et al* 2014). WAVE macromolecules act as nucleation-promoting factors linking upstream signals to the activated actin-related protein 2/3 (ARP2/3) moving CB1 receptor assembles during a multiprotein platform. Studies on useful malleability in pain circuits have provided mechanistic insights linking numerous modulatory factors to changes in perception and behaviour. This plasticity occurs in the context of structural remodelling and reorganisation of synapses, cells and circuits, potentially contributing to the long-term nature of chronic pain (Kuner and Flor 2016), including pathological pain states that may share some similar mechanisms to other types of stress-induced neural dysfunctions. That changes in CB1 signalling relevant to these states may involve lipid rafts, it is perhaps not surprising that synaptic neurotransmission and plasticity are also affected by membrane-derived bioactive phospholipids triggered to different degrees, at different loci, and by different mechanisms of action (Garcia *et al* 2015). Finally, across a few synapse frameworks associated with neuroplasticity, including glutamatergic, GABAergic, and endocannabinoid signalling, receptors present in the outer layer of the film and the size of the readily releasable pool (RRP) of synaptic vesicles (SVs) are the significant determinants for keeping up with synaptic strength, momentary pliancy, and intersynaptic crosstalk (Millar *et al* 2002, Vithlani *et al* 2011). Phospholipids go about as nearby couriers in action subordinate GABAergic STD in a Ca^{2+}-subordinate, spike-free way (Garcia *et al* 2015).

Many things manipulate chemokine release that affects those cells signalling pathways, which include harm and cell pressure in CNS cells, and macrophage inflammatory protein-1a (MIP-1a or CCL3), monocyte chemotactic protein-1 (MCP-1 or CCL2) (Losy and Zaremba 2001), and CCL5 (or RANTES) (Zaremba *et al* 2006). These signals stimulate peripheral immune cells, producing protective effects that have been suggested to have a potential for cell-based therapies. Not all of these mechanisms involve the plasticity of synapses and may affect other neural processes through actions. When the adaptive immune system is uncovered to myelin antigens (McMahon *et al* 2006, Mecha *et al* 2013), provided via way of means of dendritic cells (DCs) to antigen-unique T cells, this results in demyelination of the CNS (Dittel *et al* 1999). It is also becoming clear that phospholipids are also involved in regulating synaptic plasticity and glutamatergic signalling. Table 10.1 specifies the summary of the literature related to molecular mechanisms of depression and mood disorder, following the receptors of these disorders.

As discussed in this review, central factors contributing to stress-related illness interact substantially with various peripheral factors, including immune factors related to illness, stress, and other factors contributing to a general inflammatory state in the body, like metabolic syndrome. Circulating inflammatory cytokines increase in case psychological and social stressors increase in humans (Steptoe *et al* 2007). Immune signaling has also been shown to influence synaptic plasticity, in part by acting through some of the signaling pathways discussed above. These immune influences occur through microglia as well as more classic immune mechanisms. Among other effects discussed below, antidepressant treatments also normalize cytokine function (Dowlati *et al* 2010). Resident innate immune cells of the brain, microglia, have the property to secrete inflammatory cytokines that influence neuroplasticity (Jensen *et al* 2013). Low levels of TNF-α and IL-1β are responsible for synaptic plasticity caused by PI3K-Akt signaling. Mitogen-activated protein kinase (MAPK) phosphatase-1 (MKP-1) are present in greater amounts in the hippocampal region of the post-mortem brain from an individual having a history of depression. Targeting the MKP-1 protein may be the new approach to develop new efficacious antidepressants (Akbarian and Davis 2010) in the amygdala and other structures (Moussavi and Chatterji 2007, Price *et al* 2009) through the enzyme and cytokine receptors that also influence this pathway. Stress and mood disorders also change the function of neurotrophins, in particular BDNF and

Table 10.1. Classification of molecular mechanisms and receptors involved in depression and mood disorders.

Authors	Molecular and genetic mechanisms	Molecular receptors	Brain regions for stress and mood disorder
Price *et al* (2010)	Phosphotransferases	Enzyme	Hippocampus, amygdala
	Mitogen-activated protein kinases (MAPK)	Eukaryote	Ventral-dorsal midline
Morrison *et al* (2003)	MAPK1 RNA	Cytokines, cellular stressors	Hippocampus
McEwen *et al* (1999)	BDNF	Glucocorticoid	ADC, PFC, hippocampus
Shirayama *et al* (2002), Saarelainen *et al* (2003)	BDNF and CREB	TrkB	Hippocampus
Zhang *et al* (2008), Burgdorf *et al* (2011), Burgdorf *et al* (2013)	Cytoplasmic membrane	Glycine-site modulator NMDARs	Hippocampus, PFC
	BSTc/BNSTs	Gq-linked receptors	Dorsolateral and ventrolateral bed nucleus
Majewska *et al* (2006), Holtmaat *et al* (2009)	Cytoplasm, chemokines	Cytoskeleton receptor, eukaryotic	Hippocampus, PFC
Carboni *et al* (1998), Kennedy *et al* (2007), Lein *et al* (2007)	*JNKs* mRNA	NMDAR or NMDA	Neocortex, hippocampus, hypothalamus
Kim *et al* (2007), Yang *et al* (2011)	JNK1	AMPAR	Hippocampus
Chengrui *et al* (2013)	Neuromuscular junction	ACh	Cerebellum, cerebrum
Hanisch *et al* (2007) Lalancette-Hébert *et al* (2007)	Cytokines, chemokines and adhesion molecules	Purinergic receptors—P2 receptors, ATP	Hippocampus, visual cortex
de Vos *et al* (2002), Mecha *et al* (2013)	Myelin antigens	T-cells receptors	Hippocampus
Jauch *et al* (2006)	Endothelial cells	BBB	CVOs
Walz *et al* (1993)	Microglia or gelial cell	Cytokine	Brain and spinal cord; CNS
Pertwee *et al* (2010), Njoo *et al* (2015)	WAVE1	Cannabinoid receptor CB1; Gq/11 or G12/13	DRG

Pierce *et al* (2001), Troy-Fioramonti *et al* (2015)	GPCRs; WAVE proteins; plasma membrane	Endocytosis of CB1; action related protein 2/3	CNS
García-Morales *et al* (2015)	Membrane-derived bioactive phospholipids	LPA; LPA1/Gαi/o-protein/phospholipase	Embryonic cerebral cortex; CNS; motor neurons area
Moreno-López *et al* (2011), Vithlani *et al* (2011)	Postsynaptic membrane; GABA	$GABA_A$Rs; AMPARs	Brainstem; neocortex; hypothalamus

NT-3, following stimulation of glucocorticoid receptors in the hippocampus and prefrontal cortex (McEwen 1999, Shirayama *et al* 2002). For instance, chronic electroconvulsive seizures increase BDNF and its receptor, trkB, in the brain's frontal regions (Saarelainen *et al* 2003).

The mechanisms of antidepressant effects are discussed in more detail below. A summary of the molecular mechanisms involved in stress-related disorders is found in table 10.1. In response to stress, these collective mechanisms or pre-existing differences that influence subsequent responses to stress are undoubtedly mediated by epigenetic changes mediated by the changes in gene transcription discussed here. Adaptations to particular environments resulting from experience are thought to increase survival and reproductive success and thus are genetically programmed to produce epigenetic modifications. Although such benefits may be highly short-term in nature in the case of stress, longer-term consequences of the same changes may be deleterious. Thus, the same adaptations could produce maladaptation later or for other environments, resulting in allostatic overload (Juster *et al* 2010).

10.5 Antidepressant drugs and synaptic plasticity

Changes in neuroplasticity are thought to underlie the development of mood disorders and stress-related contributions to mood disorders in particular and underlie antidepressant responses. In a general way, these antidepressant responses are opposite to those that promote the development of stress-related psychiatric disorders. Several trophic factors, including VEGF, BDNF, and IGF1, play significant roles in depression and stress-related illness, as well as antidepressant responses. As discussed in detail below, findings unite several pro-depressive factors, including stress, to reductions in BDNF function, while therapeutic responses to antidepressants, and other experiences promoting resilience to depression, are associated with increases in BDNF function (Schmidt and Duman 2010). In general, reductions in BDNF and other factors promote aberrant stress responses and depression, while increases produce the opposite effects, stress resilience and alleviation of depressive symptomatology. Although the role of several growth factors in antidepressant effects has already been established, these effects are most well-elaborated and strongest for BDNF. The secretion and functionality of BDNF in the blood and the brain depend heavily on the level of stress and depression, in particular the PFC and hippocampus (Numakawa *et al* 2013). BDNF is essential for synaptic connections, survival and maintenance in these brain regions, with reductions being associated with reduced neuroplasticity and increases associated with increased neuroplasticity (Holtmaat and Svoboda 2009). The strong genetic contribution to depression may act in part by influencing this process. Individuals with a BDNFVal66Met allelic polymorphism reduced hippocampal volumes associated with impaired executive function and episodic memory (Smith *et al* 2011). Such changes may require certain types of experience to occur. Modification of neural circuits occurs due to constant depression and stress via mechanisms that involve down-regulation of BDNF and BDNF-mediated neuroplasticity (Bahi *et al* 2014). However, the presence of the BDNFVal66Met allele alone is enough to result in neuron atrophy in medial PFC (mPFC) and hippocampus (Liu *et al* 2012), so that even ordinary stressors may be sufficient to produce these effects. In other words, this could be described as a reduction in resilience to mild stressors of everyday life, resulting in more extreme responses characteristic of more extreme stress. Hippocampal volume reduction was seen in met carriers (Bueller *et al* 2006), and the amygdala and ventromedial prefrontal cortex show reduction in neural activity (Soliman *et al* 2010). That such effects are characteristic of more severe stressors, animal studies using chronic stress models of depression have shown reductions inBDNF mRNA and protein levels in brain regions associated with depression and stress responses (Nair *et al* 2007). This is consistent with the rather broad finding that glucocorticoid signaling influences neuronal plasticity in response to stress, as well as antidepressant treatments (Arango-Lievano *et al* 2015). It appears neural plasticity and structural remodelling of several brain structures are increased by antidepressants via effects mediated by neurotrophins. Moreover, those factors also influence the impact of stress upon neuroplasticity, perhaps in both directions. Thus, BDNF increases glucocorticoid receptor (GR) expression, increasing hippocampally-mediated HPA feedback and reducing subsequent stressor effects. Reduction in BDNF produces the opposite effects. The other factors that have been discussed here that contribute to the integrated signalling of stress responses, including via the TrkB-MAPK pathway, result in sustained GR phosphorylation and changes in GR function. By contrast, cognition, perception, and mood are affected by continuous stimulation of glucocorticoid receptors, resulting in structure and function changes of brain circuits due to remodelling of dendritic spines in brain regions underlying those functions (Liston *et al* 2013). Remodelling neurons increases stress-mediated glucocorticoids and hinders cognitive ability, which are common features of major depression (Pariante 2006). GR function is influenced by stress-sensitive pathways (Jeanneteau and Chao 2013); further GR activity during stress is modulated through the cellular pathway. Fluoxetine prevents neuroplastic changes induced by priming GR phosphorylation, during chronic stress, at sites that are BDNF-sensitive (Lievano *et al* 2015). Although most antidepressants have acute actions on the re-uptake or breakdown of monoamines, they ultimately appear to produce their actions by enhancing synaptic plasticity, including neurogenesis and synaptogenesis in the adult hippocampus, via enhanced neurotrophic factor expression; in CNS, neural plasticity is associated broadly with BDNF, including changes in plasticity involved with affective disorders.

10.5.1 Working phenomena of antidepressant drugs

Synaptic plasticity changes response to stress and antidepressants may reverse or prevent those changes; the mechanisms underlying synaptic plasticity to antidepressants share many common mechanisms with which stress influences the same outcomes (Nestler *et al* 2002). For example, glucocorticoids (GCs) act to influence cAMP response element-binding protein (CREB) and, TrkB signaling to influence synaptic plasticity (Gray *et al* 2013). On the other hand, BDNF mainly does synaptic plasticity regulation with rapid response, which influences memory and learning functions following stressful events and the development of depression and anxiety and the reversal of those deficits by treatments. In part, these responses may reflect a failure of resilience that is BDNF mediated. Thus, in CA3 increased BDNF levels goes back to the baseline levels sometime after exposure to chronic stress (Lakshminarasimhan and Chattarji 2012). Furthermore, changes in the BDNF level initiates stress-induced remodelling of the prefrontal cortex, hippocampus, and amygdala, which has been displayed as an important factor that promotes growth in newly born neurons (Gray *et al* 2013). This may reflect a normal and adaptive (e.g., resilient) response. However, when these responses are weak or short-lasting, maladaptations may result, reflecting in neurogenesis and synaptogenesis changes.

Neuronal plasticity associated with antidepressants involves gene and protein expression changes in hippocampal pyramidal neurons (GABAergic interneurons of the cerebral cortex, hippocampal pyramidal CA1 neurons) and neurons in the temporal and frontal cortex (Calabrese *et al* 2010). Some of these have been related to resiliency. Chronic treatment with agomelatine affects the fibroblast growth factor (FGF-2), brain-derived neurotrophic factor (BDNF), and activity-regulated cytoskeleton-associated protein (Arc) (Calabrese *et al* 2011). Along with gene expression, increases in BDNF also modulate fibroblast growth factor (FGF-2) (Turner *et al* 2006) and are associated with antidepressant effects (Bachis *et al* 2008). Significant changes are found in the hippocampus, where agomelatine produces a steady increment of the neurotrophin mRNA (BDNF) after treatment. Stress influence reduced hippocampal neurogenesis, hippocampal volume, and hippocampal pyramidal cell dendritic branching and spine density (Hu and Wang 2010). Similar stress-induced alternation may result from the severe application of Glucocorticoids (GCs) and following the elevated cortisol activation resulting from the amygdala regions and hippocampus stress (Mitra and Sapolsky 2008). Stress-alleviating and antidepressant effects have the opposite effects in the hippocampus and related structures such as the amygdala (Mitra *et al* 2005). Remodeling of the amygdala, prefrontal cortex and hippocampus is similar to stress-induced differences that involve BDNF expression and function alterations. Hippocampal atrophy resulting from chronic stress is related to reduced BDNF function. NT-3 and NGF are coupled with the same signal transduction pathways through their respective receptors. And they attenuate self-expression, resulting in structural and functional modification of subpopulations of hippocampal neurons in connection to complementary receptors expressed within corresponding cells (Duman and Monteggia 2006). Attenuated expression of NGF (other types) also regulates the destructive influence of stress. Long-term immobilized stress also influences attenuating NGF and NT-3 region of the hippocampus (Ueyama *et al* 1997).

In neurogenesis, glucocorticoid stimulation affects downstream mechanisms causing oligodendrocyte (mRNA) abnormalities like amyotrophic lateral sclerosis via up-regulation of SGK1. Diminishing the multiplication of human hippocampal progenitor cells includes SGK1 as a key catalyst that lessens neurogenesis. Glucocorticoid removal leads to maintenance of serine residues phosphorylation at S203 and S211 of GR. For antidepressant outcomes mediated by manipulation of SGK1, neurogenesis is important (David *et al* 2009), critically involved in depression pathogenesis, and influenced by regulation of the HPA axis (Anacker *et al* 2013). Utilizing optogenetic manipulation, the BLA–ventral hippocampus (vHPC) circuit has found a significant role in anxiety-related social interaction, optogenetic excitation and precisely behaviours (Allsop *et al* 2014). BLA and hippocampus association and interaction is regulated by stress (Allsop *et al* 2014). Essentially, BLA shows unmistakable neural capacity in anxiety and reward conditioning. Further, BLA neurons can encode encounters with both negative and positive emotions (Namburi *et al* 2015) along with addiction conditions and reward learning (Koob 2009). Effects of BLA in the presence of stress lead to specific synaptic mechanisms and micro-circuits (Anisman and Matheson 2005). It is evidenced by electrical stimulation that dynamic hippocampal synaptic plasticity is established by time-dependent cholinergic. Different types of hippocampal schaeffer collateral (SC) results from stimulation septal cholinergic inputs with an optogenetic approach (Gu *et al* 2012) that adds up to CA1 synaptic plasticity. At different synapses, cholinergic input manages various types of plasticity (Stephan *et al* 2006, Martin *et al* 2000), subject to local glutamatergic activity regarding time and context. Different types of cholinergic influence as mediated by nicotinic acetylcholine receptors (nAChR) or metabotropic receptors (mAChR) (Opendak and Gould 2015). Nicotine affects memory and learning mechanisms under the influence of nAChRs receptors. However, differences in their functional properties revealed diversified effects on these cognitive properties (Kenney and Gould 2008). Contextual stimuli based on ethanol exposure when subjected to rabbits having trained to self-administered ethanol (Dayas *et al* 2007), enhances hippocampal e-fos expression and drug-seeking behaviour (Due *et al* 2002).

Mechanisms for neuronal degeneration and dysfunction involve lipid peroxidation, which produces 4-hydroxynonenal, which covalently alters proteins critical for cellular ions homeostasis, including Na^+, ATPases, Ca^{2+}, glucose, and glutamate transport proteins, bringing about membrane-induced oxidative pressure (Mattson 2009). The risk for uncontrolled excitation of neuronal activity and stroke increases due to the intake of excess calories, which principally occur because of the blood–brain barrier (Kanoski *et al* 2010). Molecular mechanisms synaptic plasticity and control behavioural in addiction and stress disorders. NAC shell is a limbic–motor interface that leads to integrating salience reward and adversive stimuli through its target regions in the brain (Chen *et al* 2010). Newborn cells are migrated into the granule cell layer with their morphological and physiological characteristics (van Praag *et al* 2002).

Further, these newborn cells transform from immature to activated mature cells enlarging the soma, reducing cell surface up-regulation of myeloid markers. Ketamine, despite these limitations, increases the action of an antidepressant with potentially fewer side effects (Iadarola *et al* 2015), which has contributed to the interest in this approach. Ketamine was originally developed as a dissociative anaesthetic (Curran and Morgan 2000), although it is now primarily used in veterinary medicine. Acute ketamine therapy triggers a quick course of cellular and molecular events which underlie the ever-steady behaviour and synaptic reaction (Gureviciene 2008) associated with chronic stress and depression (Gerhard *et al* 2016). Psychotomimetic effects of Ketamine may lower its role as an antidepressant (Berman *et al* 2000). The NMDA, NR2B subunits, found in the neocortex and hippocampus (Monyer *et al* 1994), are linked to synaptic plasticity, which influences cognitive functions (von Engelhardt *et al* 2008).

These mechanisms underlying the effects of classical antidepressants, including selective serotonin reuptake inhibitors (SSRIs), is known to have an important role in the effects of so-called 'rapid-acting' antidepressants (Duman *et al* 2000). Scopolamine and Ketamine have emerged as fast-acting antidepressant drugs that act through NMDA receptors increment mTORC1 signalling through Akt and ERK activation, leading to a functional synaptic increase in the PFC52. The dis-inhibition of glutamate neurons is made by ketamine via blockade of NMDA mTORC1 signaling pathway regulating protein translation alternating the neuronal activity for developing synaptic plasticity (Dwyer *et al* 2015). Molecular signalling changes PFC pyramidal neurons and improves the function and number of dendritic spines after the ketamine treatment (Li and Jope 2010, Voleti *et al* 2013). Moreover, the treatments enhance synaptic plasticity and combat the cellular effects of depression and stress through glutamatergic agents. Glycine-binding sites containing GluN1 are present in almost all neurons throughout development. However, four different genes (GluN2A, B, C, and D) generate the GluN2 and produce several physiological, biochemical, pathophysiological properties (Wyllie *et al* 2013) throughout the forebrain. The regulation of several HDACs are influenced by chronic stress and can get dysregulated (Cousijn *et al* 2010), resulting in silencing or repression of various critical genes regulating synaptic plasticity related to several correlated psychiatric conditions associated with depression. Thus, it might be suggested that reversing these changes might have therapeutic effects or be involved in the outcomes of treatments. Cdk5 promoter modification can be done using recombinant transcription factors like zinc finger protein (ZFP).

Reactive oxygen species (ROS) induce oxidative stress-sensitive genes that have a sensitizing effect on neurodegeneration, thus affecting the viability and regeneration process of certain specific regions in the brain's hippocampus: the apical dendrites of pyramidal neurons (CA3). Research explains that intrinsic factors like cocaine concentrations (high/low) being located in axon, soma and dendrites can modulate excitability by directly blocking Na^+ and K^+ channels at high cocaine concentration, whereas low cocaine concentration (transposed via standard chronic regimens (i.e., <3 μM)), can indirectly change the functions of these channels. So, conclusively, this constant cocaine interference ultimately altering the intrinsic neuronal excitability can be explained by a mechanism where it can be observed that: extracellular dopamine activates dopamine receptors (DAR) in response to a high level of increasing cocaine concentration in specific hippocampal regions, as mentioned earlier. Thus, precisely, dual effects are experienced by cocaine, including both intrinsic and synaptic effects of nucleus accumbens (NAc) MSN excitability. Eventually, this drug-driven neuronal excitability transiently induces an alteration in the synaptic and intrinsic excitability to shape final NAc MSN, which results in cocaine-seeking behaviour or addiction to that specific drug (where the brain wants to experience that same feeling over and over again) by activation of the neural circuit and driven by a specific cocaine-associated behaviour.

10.6 Alternative treatment to current therapeutic approaches

Recent statistical data suggests that almost one in every five people are troubled by major depression, making it a severe and debilitating illness. The current treatments have various limitations like therapeutic time lag, low efficacy rates, and undesirable side effects, thus limiting the overall efficiency of available treatments. Apart from that, study shows that physical activity like running can enhance neurogenesis in the brain's hippocampal region. Also, exercise can be beneficial in a genetic animal model of depression and depressed humans as an antidepressant. So, a goal of treatment must be to restore neural plasticity and reverse the shortfalls as identified: to be evidenced for atrophy of neurons in limbic and cortical regions of the brain associated with depression which modulates mood and emotion.

Moreover, the rapid-acting antidepressants and classical ones have a treatment effect on brain neural plasticity, possibly by adapting to multiple intracellular signaling pathways. Also, antagonists of the NMDA receptor (ketamine) that show rapid improvement in depressive symptoms, and similar actions on neural plasticity might mediate these actions better than classically acting antidepressant drugs. This antagonist opposes the damage caused by chronic stress by increasing the synaptic connections in the PFC. While on the other hand, indirect blocking of the GABA-A receptor increases glutamate transmission, thus facilitating AMPA receptor activity, which might also treat cognitive impairment, as cell adhesion molecules and growth factor signaling are stimulated, which would also affect synaptic plasticity. The muscarinic cholinergic system also regulates the pathophysiological parameters of MDD. Moreover, scopolamine may have fast-acting antidepressant effects.

Other drugs, not specifically intended to affect any of these mechanisms, may provide additional insight nonetheless. Additionally, it was observed that even when some of the symptoms respond to treatment provided, a significant proportion of patients with major depressive disorder (MDD) continue to experience cognitive impairment. Several novel approaches may help improve these aspects of treatment. Clinically, it has been observed that several drugs (antidiabetic agents, galantamine, modafinil, N-acetylcysteine, melatonin, omega-3 fatty acids, scopolamine, statins, curcumin, minocycline, erythropoietin, insulin) might improve cognitive function in MDD. For example, cardiovascular illness-related patients with lower blood cholesterol are often prescribed 'Statins' as they have anti-atherosclerotic effects, thus positively correlating with the percent decrease in LDL cholesterol. Other examples: in rodents, the hippocampal BDNF levels are enhanced by the effects of atorvastatin, and in stress-related murine models, Simvastatin might have anxiolytic and antidepressant-like effects. It is interesting to note that these drugs also affect inflammatory signalling, which may indicate a mechanism for influencing CNS functions in this way. For example, a tetracycline antibiotic, minocycline generally used in the treatment of infections in the respiratory tract, acne, and mild rheumatoid arthritis, is also shown to enhance the hippocampal neurogenesis and triggers anti-apoptotic and anti-inflammatory activities, thereby the down-regulating expression of pro-inflammatory cytokines (IL-2, TNF-α, IL-6, IL-1β, INF-γ) and up-regulating anti-inflammatory cytokines (IL-10). Yet another substance identified as Acetyl-L-carnitine (ALC) was found to enhance mitochondrial neuronal metabolism and prevent cells from various toxicity like glutamate-mediated neurotoxicity and hypothalamic-adrenocortical hyperactivity. It also improves the insulin-resistant state by producing both lipid and carbohydrate metabolism. Melatonin is a pineal gland hormone, regulates the maintenance of circadian rhythms and modulates energy metabolism.

The general inflammatory state associated with metabolic syndrome may also contribute to the pathogenesis of depression. Impaired insulin resistance and signalling play a significant role in the pathogenesis of MDD via effects on synaptic plasticity and cell survival in the hippocampus and medial temporal cortex. Angiotensin-converting enzyme (ACE) inhibitors modulate immune features and attenuate cytokine production (e.g., IL-1, TNF-α) by interfering with NF-κB activation. Erythropoietin (EPO) alleviates symptoms of MDD, including impairment of verbal memory and attention. EPO is produced by the kidney and acts as a hormone for the regulation of erythropoiesis. It has also been shown to cross the blood–brain barrier and exert neuroprotective and antidepressant effects while enhancing hippocampus-dependent memory and neuroplasticity. EPO is predominantly produced in the fetal liver and adult kidney. That EPO and its receptor (EPOR) are expressed in the brain led to EPO regulating hematopoiesis-independent effects on the nervous system. The effects of EPO on memory may involve effects on neuroplasticity.

Other approaches may be particularly useful for treating cognitive impairments in depression, including many that do not respond well to current treatments. For example, adult patients with attention deficit hyperactivity disorder (ADHD), when exposed to a pro-drug for D-amphetamine, i.e., Lisdexamfetamine dimesylate (LDX), improved executive dysfunction and cognitive function, as did adults in post-remission of MDD. Patients with mild MDD, when augmented with DX, significantly improve executive function. Additionally, for the treatment of narcolepsy, a stimulant-like agent called Modafinil is used. It directly affects dopamine and norepinephrine but indirectly affects several neurotransmitters, including

GABA, serotonin, orexin, glutamate, and histamine. A cholinergic agent like modafinil, named galantamine, is a potent modulator of nicotinic receptors and other neurotransmitter systems like GABA, glutamate, monoamines. Also, N-acetylcysteine (NAC) is generally used in treating psychiatric disorders. NAC has many additional roles like improving mitochondrial function and neurogenesis, inhibiting pro-inflammatory cytokines and modulation of apoptosis. It also acts as a regulator of synaptic glutamate using cysteine-glutamate exchanger while increasing glutathione and oxidative defences.

Beyond pharmacological treatments, consideration of cellular treatments might also be considered in depressive disorders. Human pluripotent stem cells produce neural cells that can be transplanted to protect against neural toxicity. This is done using embryonic stem (ES) cells fabricated on a specialized hydrogel matrix called polyethene glycol to mimic the modelling of cellular interactions within the brain by using a serum-free culture medium. The CNS receptors blind matrix molecules present in the extracellular space during the developmental stage. By the force of binding and contraction, the developing neurons either push or pull the neurite forward. Neural precursor cells of the developing brain are multipotent to self-renew or differentiate from neurons or glia (Leipzig and Shoichet 2009). distinct cell types like glial cells, neuronal cells, endothelial cells, and microglial cells, along with the secreted cellular signals, involve themselves in different cellular interactions in between themselves thus having a greater relevance to the developing brain than genotoxicity (Lidsky and Schneider 2003, Bystron *et al* 2008, Kettenmann *et al* 2011, Arnold and Betsholtz 2013). The miscellaneous cell populace of neuronal and glial cells tend to interconnect with branches of vascular networks to form branched microglial structures. While the developing brain is less sensitive to many types of toxic insults, the consequences of toxic insults are greater during early childhood because of the developmental consequences (Rice and Barone 2000). Thus, early developmental effects, whether resulting from toxins or experiences influencing neurodevelopment in other respects, are important determinants of the incidence of neurodevelopmental disorders worldwide (Grandjean and Landrigan 2014).

To set up a lab-based *in vitro* human cellular-based modelling of neurotoxicity screening, a fused collaborative strategy of diverse field areas is needed to be implemented such as: bioinformatics; stem cell biology; tissue engineering; and machine learning. The administration of various application-based strategies explains the importance and vitality of this human cell-based model in predicting toxicology to provide a safety assessment for drug and chemical use beforehand (Schwartz *et al* 2015). It is important to study the adverse effects of chemical substances and physical agents on the developing nervous system focus to provide a relevant understanding of the etiopathogenesis of complex brain disorders. Stress and mood disorders have a disadvantageous outcome for neurodevelopment. Alternations in the developmental neurogeneration can have unwanted effects on the developing nervous system and the adult brain, where neurogenesis is believed to play a vital role in learning, memory, and even depression. Having a sound knowledge of the complex process of nervous system development and its understanding to the core can be coupled with the field of neurotoxicology using cultured neural stem or progenitor cells to inspect the influences of neurotoxic stimuli on cell survival, proliferation and differentiation, with directional focus on heritable effects in the adult brain. Moreover, implementations of developmental neurotoxicity layout are vital together with relevant data for the apprehension of the etiopathogenesis of complex brain disorders of the adult brain (Tamm and Ceccatelli 2017).

10.7 Conclusion

Neuronal plasticity, which contributes to resilience to stress and mood disorders, is observed in adulthood far greater than previously appreciated following therapeutic responses to treatment. The mechanisms involved in maintaining brain function and emotional system, referred to as the allostatic control systems can negatively affect homeostasis in exposure to persistent stressful conditions. Moreover, neuroplasticity in limbic, prefrontal and hippocampus regions is associated with the development of these conditions and treatment. Clinical diagnosis of stress and mood disorder has shown the reduced volume of hippocampal and prefrontal grey matter. Blunted vmPFC activation is a result of exposure to cumulative stress. Depression and mood disorders disrupt synaptic plasticity in the somatosensory and visual cortex. Inflammatory mechanisms that disrupt neural, immune and endocrine circuits due to stress and mood disorder bring morphological and metabolic changes in humans.

MRI studies also capture the effect of MDD, which produces the white matter (made of myelinated axons) anomalies, cortical or cerebral shrinkage and abrasion of the group of subcortical nuclei responsible for motor control (i.e., basal ganglia). Mood disorders are associated with alterations in cellular resilience and structural plasticity, either as a predisposing or precipitating factor in developing those conditions. Pre-clinical and clinical investigations reveal the significance of signaling pathways influencing cell survival and death, as well as neurogenesis and synaptogenesis. Thus, the prospect of improved treatments for stress-related conditions and mood disorders focuses on critical CNS mechanisms underlying these pathways. Further, serotonin and SERT have also been linked with MDD.

BDNF induces endocannabinoids, modulating synaptic function, which changes the disease state. These modulators can help with stressful environments by executing functional and reversible structural plasticity. In this context, ketamine and NMDA antagonists are potential agents for its treatment. Stress associated neuropsychiatric disorders also affect the mesolimbic dopaminergic pathway in VTA. The lowering of BDNF promotes aberrant stress responses and depression in the presence of primary stress and mood disorder. Ketamine treatment leads to modulation in molecular signaling in PFC pyramidal neurons and dendritic spines. Optogenetic neural activation and epigenomic analyses elucidate the molecular mechanisms contributing to stress-related disorders. JNKs govern brain morphogenesis, including adult axodendritic morphology that regulate NMDA glutamate receptors. Several neurotransmitter systems, including glutamatergic, GABAergic, and endocannabinoid signaling, are involved in neuroplasticity, and they are vital determinants for maintaining the toughness of synapse, transient plasticity, and interactions between them inter-synapses. Major depression alters the neuronal structure, interrupting cognitive performance and amplifying stress-driven escalation in hormone levels, glucocorticoids. Neuronal dysfunction also involves lipid peroxidation, which adjusts the protein conformation covalently, which are vital for ion homeostasis in the cellular microenvironment and membrane-linked oxidative stress. Moreover, excessive caloric intake has unfavourable outcomes reflected in integrity of the blood–brain barrier, which increases excitation of neuronal activity and stroke. In animal studies, heart rate, plasma cortisol, and behavioural markers are considered for stress indication.

Neuronal plasticity is observed in adulthood to a far greater degree than previously appreciated, which contributes to resilience to stress and mood disorders, and is critically involved in therapeutic responses to treatments for that specific disorganization. Earlier, it was observed that allostatic directed arrangements could irreversibly influence homeostasis in unabated stress. Neuroplasticity in limbic regions is associated with both the development of these conditions and their treatment. Mood disorders are associated with alterations in cellular resilience and structural plasticity, either as a predisposing or precipitating factor in developing those conditions. The prospect of improved treatments for stress-related conditions and mood disorders focuses on critical CNS mechanisms underlying these pathways (Calabrese *et al* 2009).

References

Admon R, Lubin G, Stern O, Rosenberg K, Sela L, Ben-Ami H and Hendler T 2009 Human vulnerability to stress depends on amygdala's predisposition and hippocampal plasticity *Proc. Natl Acad. Sci.* **106** 14120–5

Advani T, Koek W and Hensler J G 2009 Gender differences in the enhanced vulnerability of BDNF+/− mice to mild stress *Int. J. Neuropsychopharmacol.* **12** 583–8

Ahn H J, Hernandez C M, Levenson J M, Lubin F D, Liou H C and Sweatt J D 2008 c-Rel, an NF-κB family transcription factor, is required for hippocampal long-term synaptic plasticity and memory formation *Learning Mem.* **15** 539–49

Akbarian S and Davis R J 2010 Keep the 'phospho' on MAPK, be happy *Nat. Med.* **16** 1187–8

Akirav I 2011 The role of cannabinoids in modulating emotional and non-emotional memory processes in the hippocampus *Front. Behavioral Neurosci.* **5** 34

Albensi B C and Mattson M P 2000 Evidence for the involvement of TNF and NF-κB in hippocampal synaptic plasticity *Synapse* **35** 151–9

Allsop S A, V Weele C M, Wichmann R and Tye K M 2014 Optogenetic insights on the relationship between anxiety-related behaviours and social deficits *Front. Behav. Neurosci.* **8** 241

Anacker C *et al* 2013 Role for the kinase SGK1 in stress, depression, and glucocorticoid effects on hippocampal neurogenesis *Proc. Natl Acad. Sci.* **110** 8708–13

Anda R F, Butchart A, Felitti V J and Brown D W 2010 Building a framework for global surveillance of the public health implications of adverse childhood experiences *A. J. Prevent. Med.* **39** 93–8

Anisman H and Matheson K 2005 Stress, depression, and anhedonia: caveats concerning animal models *Neurosci. Biobehav. Rev.* **29** 525–46

Arango-Lievano M, Lambert W M, Bath K G, Garabedian M J, Chao M V and Jeanneteau F 2015 Neurotrophic-priming of glucocorticoid receptor signaling is essential for neuronal plasticity to stress and antidepressant treatment *Proc. Natl Acad. Sci.* **112** 15737–42

Arnold T and Betsholtz C 2013 Erratum to: the importance of microglia in the development of the vasculature in the central nervous system *Vasc. Cell* **5** 1–7

Arnold S E *et al* 2014 High fat diet produces brain insulin resistance, synaptodendritic abnormalities and altered behavior in mice *Neurobiol. Dis.* **67** 79–87

Autry A E, Adachi M, Nosyreva E, Na E S, Los M F, Cheng P F, Kavalali E T and Monteggia L M 2011 NMDA receptor blockade at rest triggers rapid behavioural antidepressant responses *Nature* **475** 91–5

Bachis A, Mallei A, Cruz M I, Wellstein A and Mocchetti I 2008 Chronic antidepressant treatments increase basic fibroblast growth factor and fibroblast growth factor-binding protein in neurons *Neuropharmacol.* **55** 1114–20

Bagot R C, Labonté B, Peña C J and Nestler E J 2014 Epigenetic signaling in psychiatric disorders: stress and depression *Dialogues Clin. Neurosci.* **16** 281

Bahi A, Chandrasekar V and Dreyer J L 2014 Selective lentiviral-mediated suppression of microRNA124a in the hippocampus evokes antidepressants-like effects in rats *Psychoneuroendocrinol.* **46** 78–87

Bailey S L, Carpentier P A, McMahon E J, Begolka W S and Miller S D 2006 Innate and adaptive immune responses of the central nervous system *Critical Rev. Immun.* **26** 945–55

Bale T L, Contarino A, Smith G W, Chan R, Gold L H, Sawchenko P E, Koob G F, Vale W W and Lee K F 2000 Mice deficient for corticotropin-releasing hormone receptor-2 display anxiety-like behaviour and are hypersensitive to stress *Nat. Gen.* **24** 410–4

Bale T L and Vale W W 2003 Increased depression-like behaviors in corticotropin-releasing factor receptor-2-deficient mice: sexually dichotomous responses *J. Neurosci.* **23** 5295–301

Barr C S, Newman T K, Lindell S, Shannon C, Champoux M, Lesch K P, Suomi S J, Goldman D and Higley J D 2004 Interaction between serotonin transporter gene variation and rearing condition in alcohol preference and consumption in female primates *Arch. Gen. Psych* **61** 1146–52

Beręsewicz M, Kowalczyk J E and Zabłocka B 2008 Kalirin-7, a protein enriched in postsynaptic density, is involved in ischemic signal transduction *Neurochem. Res.* **33** 1789–94

Berman R M, Cappiello A, Anand A, Oren D A, Heninger G R, Charney D S and Krystal J H 2000 Antidepressant effects of ketamine in depressed patients *Biol. Psychiatry* **47** 351–4

Bilodeau S *et al* 2006 Role of Brg1 and HDAC2 in GR trans-repression of the pituitary POMC gene and misexpression in Cushing disease *Genes Dev.* **20** 2871–86

Breiter H C, Aharon I, Kahneman D, Dale A and Shizgal P 2001 Functional imaging of neural responses to expectancy and experience of monetary gains and losses *Neuron* **30** 619–39

Brown E S, Rush A J and McEwen B S 1999 Hippocampal remodeling and damage by corticosteroids: implications for mood disorders *Neuropsychopharmacol.* **21** 474–84

Bueller J A, Aftab M, Sen S, Gomez-Hassan D, Burmeister M and Zubieta J K 2006 BDNF Val66Met allele is associated with reduced hippocampal volume in healthy subjects *Biol. Psychiatry* **59** 812–15

Burgdorf J, Zhang X L, Weiss C, Matthews E, Disterhoft J F, Stanton P K and Moskal J R 2011 The N-methyl-D-aspartate receptor modulator GLYX-13 enhances learning and memory, in young adult and learning impaired aging rats *Neurobiol. Aging* **32** 698–706

Burgdorf J, Zhang X L, Nicholson K L, Balster R L, Leander J D, Stanton P K, Gross A L, Kroes R A and Moskal J R 2013 GLYX-13, a NMDA receptor glycine-site functional partial agonist, induces antidepressant-like effects without ketamine-like side effects *Neuropsychopharmacol.* **38** 729–42

Burke T F, Advani T, Adachi M, Monteggia L M and Hensler J G 2013 Sensitivity of hippocampal 5-HT1A receptors to mild stress in BDNF-deficient mice *Int. J. Neuropsychopharmacol.* **16** 631–45

Bystron I, Blakemore C and Rakic P 2008 Development of the human cerebral cortex: Boulder Committee revisited *Nat. Rev. Neurosci.* **9** 110–22

Calabrese F, Molteni R, Racagni G and Riva M A 2009 Neuronal plasticity: a link between stress and mood disorders *Psychoneuroendocrinol.* **34** S208–16

Calabrese P, Le Doussal P and Rosso A 2010 Free-energy distribution of the directed polymer at high temperature *EPL Europhys. Lett.* **90** 20002

Calabrese F, Molteni R, Gabriel C, Mocaer E, Racagni G and Riva M A 2011 Modulation of neuroplastic molecules in selected brain regions after chronic administration of the novel antidepressant agomelatine *Psychopharmacology* **215** 267–75

Calabrese V, Cornelius C, Mancuso C, Lentile R, Stella A G and Butterfield D A 2010 Redox homeostasis and cellular stress response in aging and neurodegeneration *Free Radicals and Antioxidant Protocols* (Totowa, NJ: Humana Press) pp 285–308

Carboni L, Carletti R, Tacconi S, Corti C and Ferraguti F 1998 Differential expression of SAPK isoforms in the rat brain: an in situ hybridisation study in the adult rat brain and during post-natal development *Mol. Brain Res.* **60** 57–68

Castrén E and Rantamäki T 2010 The role of BDNF and its receptors in depression and antidepressant drug action: reactivation of developmental plasticity *Developmental Neurobiol.* **70** 289–97

Castrén E 2013 Neuronal network plasticity and recovery from depression *JAMA Psychiatry* **70** 983–9

Charuvastra A and Cloitre M 2008 Social bonds and posttraumatic stress disorder *Annu. Rev. Psychol.* **59** 301–28

Chen Y, Rex C S, Rice C J, Dubé C M, Gall C M, Lynch G and Baram T Z 2010 Correlated memory defects and hippocampal dendritic spine loss after acute stress involve corticotropin-releasing hormone signaling *Proc. Natl Acad. Sci.* **107** 13123–8

Chetkovich D M, Gray R, Johnston D and Sweatt J D 1991 N-methyl-D-aspartate receptor activation increases cAMP levels and voltage-gated Ca2+ channel activity in area CA1 of hippocampus *Proc. Natl Acad. Sci.* **88** 6467–71

Christoffel D J, Golden S A and Russo S J 2011 Structural and synaptic plasticity in stress-related disorders *Rev. Neurosci.* **22** 535–49

Collip D, Habets P, Marcelis M, Gronenschild E, Lataster T, Lardinois M, Nicolson N A and Myin-Germeys I 2013 Hippocampal volume as marker of daily life stress sensitivity in psychosis *Psychol. Med.* **43** 1377–87

Cousijn H, Rijpkema M, Qin S, Van Marle H J, Franke B, Hermans E J, van Wingen G and Fernández G 2010 Acute stress modulates genotype effects on amygdala processing in humans *Proc. Natl Acad. Sci.* **107** 9867–72

Covington H E III *et al* 2011 A role for repressive histone methylation in cocaine-induced vulnerability to stress *Neuron* **71** 656–70

Cunningham J T, Rodgers J T, Arlow D H, Vazquez F, Mootha V K and Puigserver P 2007 mTOR controls mitochondrial oxidative function through a YY1–PGC-1α transcriptional complex *Nature* **450** 736–40

Curran H V and Morgan C 2000 Cognitive, dissociative and psychotogenic effects of ketamine in recreational users on the night of drug use and 3 days later *Addiction* **95** 575–90

David D J *et al* 2009 Neurogenesis-dependent and-independent effects of fluoxetine in an animal model of anxiety/depression *Neuron* **62** 479–93

Dayas C V, Liu X, Simms J A and Weiss F 2007 Distinct patterns of neural activation associated with ethanol seeking: effects of naltrexone *Bio. Psych.* **61** 979–89

Dehay C and Kennedy H 2007 Cell-cycle control and cortical development *Nat. Rev. Neurosci.* **8** 438–50

de Mello Schier A R, de Oliveira Ribeiro N P, Coutinho D S, Machado S, Arias-Carrión O, Crippa J A, Zuardi A W, Nardi A E and Silva A C 2014 Antidepressant-like and anxiolytic-like effects of cannabidiol: a chemical compound of Cannabis sativa *CNS & Neurol. Disorders-Drug Targets* **13** 953–60

Di Marzo V, Stella N and Zimmer A 2015 Endocannabinoid signalling and the deteriorating brain *Nat. Rev. Neurosci.* **16** 30–42

Dittel B N, Visintin I, Merchant R M and Janeway C A 1999 Presentation of the self antigen myelin basic protein by dendritic cells leads to experimental autoimmune encephalomyelitis *J. Immunol.* **163** 32–9

Dowlati Y, Herrmann N, Swardfager W, Liu H, Sham L, Reim E K and Lanctôt K L 2010 A meta-analysis of cytokines in major depression *Bio. Psych.* **67** 446–57

Drabant E M, Ramel W, Edge M D, Hyde L W, Kuo J R, Goldin P R, Hariri A R and Gross J J 2012 Neural mechanisms underlying 5-HTTLPR-related sensitivity to acute stress *Am. J. Psych.* **169** 397–405

Du L *et al* 2003 Intra-mitochondrial poly(ADP-ribosylation) contributes to NAD+ depletion and cell death induced by oxidative stress *J. Bio. Chem.* **278** 18426–33

Due D L, Huettel S A, Hall W G and Rubin D C 2002 Activation in mesolimbic and visuospatial neural circuits elicited by smoking cues: evidence from functional magnetic resonance imaging *Am. J. Psych.* **159** 954–60

Duman R S, Nakagawa S and Malberg J 2001 Regulation of adult neurogenesis by antidepressant treatment *Neuropsychopharmacol.* **25** 836–44

Duman R S and Monteggia L M 2006 A neurotrophic model for stress-related mood disorders *Bio. Psych.* **59** 1116–27

Duman R S 2014 Pathophysiology of depression and innovative treatments: remodeling glutamatergic synaptic connections *Dialogues Clin. Neurosci.* **16** 11

Duric V, Banasr M, Licznerski P, Schmidt H D, Stockmeier C A, Simen A A, Newton S S and Duman R S 2010 A negative regulator of MAP kinase causes depressive behavior *Nat. Med.* **16** 1328–32

Egan M F *et al* 2003 The BDNF val66met polymorphism affects activity-dependent secretion of BDNF and human memory and hippocampal function *Cell* **112** 257–69

Eichenbaum H 1992 The hippocampal system and declarative memory in animals *J. Cogn. Neurosci.* **4** 217–31

Fava M and Kendler K S 2000 Major depressive disorder *Neuron* **28** 335–41

Felix-Ortiz A C, Beyeler A, Seo C, Leppla C A, Wildes C P and Tye K M 2013 BLA to vHPC inputs modulate anxiety-related behaviors *Neuron* **79** 658–64

Fitzgerald L W, Ortiz J, Hamedani A G and Nestler E J 1996 Drugs of abuse and stress increase the expression of GluR1 and NMDAR1 glutamate receptor subunits in the rat ventral tegmental area: common adaptations among cross-sensitizing agents *J. Neurosci.* **16** 274–82

Fleshner M, Maier S F, Lyons D M and Raskind M A 2011 The neurobiology of the stress-resistant brain *Stress* **14** 498–502

Fricker A D, Rios C, Devi L A and Gomes I 2005 Serotonin receptor activation leads to neurite outgrowth and neuronal survival *Mol. Brain Res.* **138** 228–35

Fuchs E, Flugge G and Czeh B 2006 Remodeling of neuronal networks by stress *Front. Biosci.* **11** 2746–58

Galve-Roperh I, Palazuelos J, Aguado T and Guzmán M 2009 The endocannabinoid system and the regulation of neural development: potential implications in psychiatric disorders *Eur. Arch. Psych. Clin. Neurosci.* **259** 371–82

García-Morales V, Montero F, González-Forero D, Rodríguez-Bey G, Gómez-Pérez L, Medialdea-Wandossell M J, Domínguez-Vías G, García-Verdugo J M and Moreno-López B 2015 Membrane-derived phospholipids control synaptic neurotransmission and plasticity *PLoS Biol.* **13** e1002153

Gee D G, Gabard-Durnam L J, Flannery J, Goff B, Humphreys K L, Telzer E H, Hare T A, Bookheimer S Y and Tottenham N 2013 Early developmental emergence of human amygdala–prefrontal connectivity after maternal deprivation *Proc. Natl Acad. Sci.* **110** 15638–43

Gerber A R and Bale T L 2012 Antiinflammatory treatment ameliorates HPA stress axis dysfunction in a mouse model of stress sensitivity *Endocrinology* **153** 4830–7

Gerhard D M, Wohleb E S and Duman R S 2016 Emerging treatment mechanisms for depression: focus on glutamate and synaptic plasticity *Drug Discovery Today* **21** 454–64

Gewies A *et al* 2014 Uncoupling Malt1 threshold function from paracaspase activity results in destructive autoimmune inflammation *Cell Rep.* **9** 1292–305

Glangetas C *et al* 2017 NMDA-receptor-dependent plasticity in the bed nucleus of the stria terminalis triggers long-term anxiolysis *Nat. Commun.* **8** 1–7

Glasper E R, LaMarca E A, Bocarsly M E, Fasolino M, Opendak M and Gould E 2015 Sexual experience enhances cognitive flexibility and dendritic spine density in the medial prefrontal cortex *Neurobiol. Learn. Mem.* **125** 73–9

Glass M and Northup J K 1999 Agonist selective regulation of G proteins by cannabinoid CB1 and CB2 receptors *Mol. Pharmacol.* **56** 1362–9

Gomez O, Sanchez-Rodriguez A, Le M Q U, Sanchez-Caro C, Molina-Holgado F and Molina-Holgado E 2011 Cannabinoid receptor agonists modulate oligodendrocyte differentiation by activating PI3K/Akt and the mammalian target of rapamycin (mTOR) pathways *British J. Pharmacol* **163** 1520–32

Gould E, Woolley C S and McEwen B S 1990 Short-term glucocorticoid manipulations affect neuronal morphology and survival in the adult dentate gyrus *Neuroscience* **37** 367–75

Gräff J *et al* 2012 An epigenetic blockade of cognitive functions in the neurodegenerating brain *Nature* **483** 222–6

Grandjean P and Landrigan P J 2014 Neurobehavioural effects of developmental toxicity *Lancet Neurol.* **13** 330–8

Gray J D, Milner T A and McEwen B S 2013 Dynamic plasticity: the role of glucocorticoids, brain-derived neurotrophic factor and other trophic factors *Neuroscience* **239** 214–27

Grueter B A, Rothwell P E and Malenka R C 2012 Integrating synaptic plasticity and striatal circuit function in addiction *Curr. Opinion Neurobiol.* **22** 545–51

Gu Z, Lamb P W and Yakel J L 2012 Cholinergic coordination of presynaptic and postsynaptic activity induces timing-dependent hippocampal synaptic plasticity *J. Neurosci.* **32** 12337–48

Guan J S *et al* 2009 HDAC2 negatively regulates memory formation and synaptic plasticity *Nature* **459** 55–60

Gureviciene I 2008 Changes in hippocampal synaptic plasticity in animal models of age-related memory *Doctoral Dissertation* Kuopion Yliopisto

Guidotti G, Calabrese F, Auletta F, Olivier J, Racagni G, Homberg J and Riva M A 2012 Developmental influence of the serotonin transporter on the expression of npas4 and GABAergic markers: modulation by antidepressant treatment *Neuropsychopharmacol.* **37** 746–58

Gutierrez H, Hale V A, Dolcet X and Davies A 2005 NF-κB signalling regulates the growth of neural processes in the developing PNS and CNS *Development* **132** 1713–26

Hajek T, Kopecek M and Höschl C 2012 Reduced hippocampal volumes in healthy carriers of brain-derived neurotrophic factor Val66Met polymorphism: meta-analysis *World J. Biol. Psych.* **13** 178–87

Hall F S, Drgonova J, Jain S and Uhl G R 2013 Implications of genome wide association studies for addiction: are our a priori assumptions all wrong? *Pharmacol. Therapeut.* **140** 267–79

Hall F S, Wilkinson L S, Humby T, Inglis W, Kendall D A, Marsden C A and Robbins T W 1998 Isolation rearing in rats: pre-and postsynaptic changes in striatal dopaminergic systems *Pharmacol. Biochem. Behav.* **59** 859–72

Hall F S and Perona M T 2012 Have studies of the developmental regulation of behavioral phenotypes revealed the mechanisms of gene–environment interactions? *Physiol. Behav.* **107** 623–40

Hanisch U K and Kettenmann H 2007 Microglia: active sensor and versatile effector cells in the normal and pathologic brain *Nat. Neurosci.* **10** 1387–94

Hartley C A and Phelps E A 2012 Anxiety and decision-making *Biol. Psych.* **72** 113–8

Hegde V L, Nagarkatti M and Nagarkatti P S 2010 Cannabinoid receptor activation leads to massive mobilization of myeloid-derived suppressor cells with potent immunosuppressive properties *Eur. J. Immunol.* **40** 3358–71

Holmes A, Murphy D L and Crawley J N 2003 Abnormal behavioral phenotypes of serotonin transporter knockout mice: parallels with human anxiety and depression *Biol. Psych.* **54** 953–9

Holtmaat A and Svoboda K 2009 Experience-dependent structural synaptic plasticity in the mammalian brain *Nat. Rev. Neurosci.* **10** 647–58

Holtmaat A *et al* 2009 Long-term, high-resolution imaging in the mouse neocortex through a chronic cranial window *Nat. Protoc.* **4** 1128–44

Huttlin E L, Jedrychowski M P, Elias J E, Goswami T, Rad R, Beausoleil S A, Villén J, Haas W, Sowa M E and Gygi S P 2010 A tissue-specific atlas of mouse protein phosphorylation and expression *Cell* **143** 1174–89

Jauch R, Cho M K, Jäkel S, Netter C, Schreiter K, Aicher B, Zweckstetter M, Jäckle H and Wahl M C 2006 Mitogen-activated protein kinases interacting kinases are autoinhibited by a reprogrammed activation segment *EMBO J.* **25** 4020–32

Jeanneteau F and Chao M V 2013 Are BDNF and glucocorticoid activities calibrated? *Neuroscience* **239** 173–195

Jego S, Glasgow S D, Herrera C G, Ekstrand M, Reed S J, Boyce R, Friedman J, Burdakov D and Adamantidis A R 2013 Optogenetic identification of a rapid eye movement sleep modulatory circuit in the hypothalamus *Nat. Neurosci.* **16** 1637–43

Jensen C J, Massie A and De Keyser J 2013 Immune players in the CNS: the astrocyte *J. Neuroimmune Pharmacol.* **8** 824–39

Ji H J, Hu J F, Wang Y H, Chen X Y, Zhou R and Chen N H 2010 Osthole improves chronic cerebral hypoperfusion induced cognitive deficits and neuronal damage in hippocampus *Eur. J. Pharmacol.* **636** 96–101

Juster R P, McEwen B S and Lupien S J 2010 Allostatic load biomarkers of chronic stress and impact on health and cognition *Neurosci. Biobehav. Rev.* **35** 2–16

Kanoski S E, Zhang Y, Zheng W and Davidson T L 2010 The effects of a high-energy diet on hippocampal function and blood-brain barrier integrity in the rat *J. Alzheimer's Dis.* **21** 207–19

Kapahi P, Chen D, Rogers A N, Katewa S D, Li P W L, Thomas E L and Kockel L 2010 With TOR, less is more: a key role for the conserved nutrient-sensing TOR pathway in aging *Cell Metabol.* **11** 453–65

Karabeg M M *et al* 2013 5-HTT deficiency affects neuroplasticity and increases stress sensitivity resulting in altered spatial learning performance in the Morris water maze but not in the Barnes maze *PloS One* **8** e78238

Karg K, Burmeister M, Shedden K and Sen S 2011 The serotonin transporter promoter variant (5-HTTLPR), stress, and depression meta-analysis revisited: evidence of genetic moderation *Arch. General Psych.* **68** 444–54

Katewa S D and Kapahi P 2011 Role of TOR signaling in aging and related biological processes in Drosophila melanogaster *Exp. Gerontol.* **46** 382–90

Kenney J W and Gould T J 2008 Modulation of hippocampus-dependent learning and synaptic plasticity by nicotine *Mol. Neurobiol.* **38** 101–21

Kerr D S, Campbell L W, Hao S Y and Landfield P W 1989 Corticosteroid modulation of hippocampal potentials: increased effect with aging *Science* **245** 1505–9

Kessler R C, Berglund P, Demler O, Jin R, Merikangas K R and Walters E E 2005 Lifetime prevalence and age-of-onset distributions of DSM-IV disorders in the National Comorbidity Survey Replication *Arch. Gen. Psychiatry* **62** 593–602

Kettenmann H, Hanisch U K, Noda M and Verkhratsky A 2011 Physiology of microglia *Physiol. Rev.* **91** 461–553

Kim J J, Lee H J, Welday A C, Song E, Cho J, Sharp P E, Jung M W and Blair H T 2007 Stress-induced alterations in hippocampal plasticity, place cells, and spatial memory *Proc. Natl Acad. Sci.* **104** 18297–302

Klein T W 2005 Cannabinoid-based drugs as anti-inflammatory therapeutics *Nat. Rev. Immunol.* **5** 400–11

Koay L C, Rigby R J and Wright K L 2014 Cannabinoid-induced autophagy regulates suppressor of cytokine signaling-3 in intestinal epithelium *Am. J. Physiol.-Gastrointest. Liver Physiol.* **307** G140–8

Kokaia Z, Zhao Q, Kokaia M, Elmér E, Metsis M, Smith M L, Siesjö B K and Lindvall O 1995 Regulation of brain-derived neurotrophic factor gene expression after transient middle cerebral artery occlusion with and without brain damage *Exp. Neurol.* **136** 73–88

Koob G F 2009 Brain stress systems in the amygdala and addiction *Brain Res.* **1293** 61–75

Koob G F *et al* 2014 Addiction as a stress surfeit disorder *Neuropharmacol.* **76** 370–82

Krishnan V and Nestler E J 2008 The molecular neurobiology of depression *Nature* **455** 894–902

Krishnan V *et al* 2007 Molecular adaptations underlying susceptibility and resistance to social defeat in brain reward regions *Cell* **131** 391–404

Kuner R and Flor H 2017 Structural plasticity and reorganisation in chronic pain *Nat. Rev. Neurosci.* **18** 20–30

Iadarola N D, Niciu M J, Richards E M, Vande Voort J L, Ballard E D, Lundin N B, Nugent A C, Machado-Vieira R and Zarate C A Jr 2015 Ketamine and other N-methyl-D-aspartate receptor antagonists in the treatment of depression: a perspective review *Therap. Adv. Chronic Dis.* **6** 97–114

Lago F, Dieguez C, Gómez-Reino J and Gualillo O 2007 The emerging role of adipokines as mediators of inflammation and immune responses *Cytokine Growth Factor Rev.* **18** 313–25

Lakshminarasimhan H and Chattarji S 2012 Stress leads to contrasting effects on the levels of brain derived neurotrophic factor in the hippocampus and amygdala *PLoS One* **7** e30481

LaSalle J M 2011 A genomic point-of-view on environmental factors influencing the human brain methylome *Epigenetics* **6** 862–9

Laufer O, Israeli D and Paz R 2016 Behavioral and neural mechanisms of overgeneralization in anxiety *Curr. Biol.* **26** 713–22

Lein E S *et al* 2007 Genome-wide atlas of gene expression in the adult mouse brain *Nature* **445** 168–76

Leipzig N D and Shoichet M S 2009 The effect of substrate stiffness on adult neural stem cell behavior *Biomater.* **30** 6867–78

Lepack A E, Fuchikami M, Dwyer J M, Banasr M and Duman R S 2015 BDNF release is required for the behavioral actions of ketamine *Int. J. Neuropsychopharmacol.* **18** 033

Li N, Lee B, Liu R J, Banasr M, Dwyer J M, Iwata M, Li X Y, Aghajanian G and Duman R S 2010 mTOR-dependent synapse formation underlies the rapid antidepressant effects of NMDA antagonists *Science* **329** 959–64

Li X and Jope R S 2010 Is glycogen synthase kinase-3 a central modulator in mood regulation? *Neuropsychopharmacol.* **35** 2143–54

Lidsky T I and Schneider J S 2003 Lead neurotoxicity in children: basic mechanisms and clinical correlates *Brain* **126** 5–19

Lisman J E and Otmakhova N A 2001 Storage, recall, and novelty detection of sequences by the hippocampus: elaborating on the SOCRATIC model to account for normal and aberrant effects of dopamine *Hippocampus* **11** 551–68

Lissek S, Kaczkurkin A N, Rabin S, Geraci M, Pine D S and Grillon C 2014 Generalized anxiety disorder is associated with overgeneralization of classically conditioned fear *Bio. Psych.* **75** 909–15

Lissin D V, Gomperts S N, Carroll R C, Christine C W, Kalman D, Kitamura M, Hardy S, Nicoll R A, Malenka R C and Von Zastrow M 1998 Activity differentially regulates the surface expression of synaptic AMPA and NMDA glutamate receptors *Proc. Natl Acad. Sci.* **95** 7097–102

Liston C, Cichon J M, Jeanneteau F, Jia Z, Chao M V and Gan W B 2013 Circadian glucocorticoid oscillations promote learning-dependent synapse formation and maintenance *Nat. Neurosci.* **16** 698–705

Liston C, Miller M M, Goldwater D S, Radley J J, Rocher A B, Hof P R, Morrison J H and McEwen B S 2006 Stress-induced alterations in prefrontal cortical dendritic morphology predict selective impairments in perceptual attentional set-shifting *J. Neurosci.* **26** 7870–4

Logan J, Skopp N A, Karch D, Reger M A and Gahm G A 2012 Characteristics of suicides among US army active duty personnel in 17 US states from 2005 to 2007 *Am. J. Pub. Health* **102** S40–4

López J F, Chalmers D T, Little K Y and Watson S J 1998 Regulation of serotonin1A, glucocorticoid, and mineralocorticoid receptor in rat and human hippocampus: implications for the neurobiology of depression *Bio. Psych.* **43** 547–73

Losy J and Zaremba J 2001 Monocyte chemoattractant protein-1 is increased in the cerebrospinal fluid of patients with ischemic stroke *Stroke* **32** 2695–6

Liu R J, Lee F S, Li X Y, Bambico F, Duman R S and Aghajanian G K 2012 Brain-derived neurotrophic factor Val66Met allele impairs basal and ketamine-stimulated synaptogenesis in prefrontal cortex *Bio. Psych.* **71** 996–1005

Lu S, Gao W, Wei Z, Wang D, Hu S, Huang M, Xu Y and Li L 2017 Intrinsic brain abnormalities in young healthy adults with childhood trauma: a resting-state functional magnetic resonance imaging study of regional homogeneity and functional connectivity *Aus. New Zealand J. Psych* **51** 614–23

Lubin F D and Sweatt J D 2007 The IκB kinase regulates chromatin structure during reconsolidation of conditioned fear memories *Neuron* **55** 942–57

Lundby A, Secher A, Lage K, Nordsborg N B, Dmytriyev A, Lundby C and Olsen J V 2012 Quantitative maps of protein phosphorylation sites across 14 different rat organs and tissues *Nat. Commun.* **3** 1–10

Luppino F S, de Wit L M, Bouvy P F, Stijnen T, Cuijpers P, Penninx B W and Zitman F G 2010 Overweight, obesity, and depression: a systematic review and meta-analysis of longitudinal studies *Arch. Gen. Psych.* **67** 220–9

Magarin A M and McEwen B S 1995 Stress-induced atrophy of apical dendrites of hippocampal CA3c neurons: involvement of glucocorticoid secretion and excitatory amino acid receptors *Neuroscience* **69** 89–98

Maier S F 2003 Bi-directional immune–brain communication: implications for understanding stress, pain, and cognition *Brain, Behav. Immun.* **17** 69–85

Majewska A K, Newton J R and Sur M 2006 Remodeling of synaptic structure in sensory cortical areas in vivo *J. Neurosci.* **26** 3021–9

Markham A, Cameron I, Bains R, Franklin P, Kiss J P, Schwendimann L, Gressens P and Spedding M 2012 Brain-derived neurotrophic factor-mediated effects on mitochondrial respiratory coupling and neuroprotection share the same molecular signalling pathways *Eur. J. Neurosci.* **35** 366–74

Marosi K and Mattson M P 2014 BDNF mediates adaptive brain and body responses to energetic challenges *Trends Endocrinol. Metabol.* **25** 89–98

Martin H G and Wang Y T 2010 Blocking the deadly effects of the NMDA receptor in stroke *Cell* **140** 174–6

Martin S J, Grimwood P D and Morris R G 2000 Synaptic plasticity and memory: an evaluation of the hypothesis *Annu. Rev. Neurosci.* **23** 649–711

Mattson M P 2009 Roles of the lipid peroxidation product 4-hydroxynonenal in obesity, the metabolic syndrome, and associated vascular and neurodegenerative disorders *Exp. Gerontol.* **44** 625–33

Matys T, Pawlak R, Matys E, Pavlides C, McEwen B S and Strickland S 2004 Tissue plasminogen activator promotes the effects of corticotropin-releasing factor on the amygdala and anxiety-like behavior *Proc. Natl Acad. Sci.* **101** 16345–50

Mayer E A, Knight R, Mazmanian S K, Cryan J F and Tillisch K 2014 Gut microbes and the brain: paradigm shift in neuroscience *J. Neurosci.* **34** 15490–6

McElligott Z A, Klug J R, Nobis W P, Patel S, Grueter B A, Kash T L and Winder D G 2010 Distinct forms of Gq-receptor-dependent plasticity of excitatory transmission in the BNST are differentially affected by stress *Proc. Natl Acad. Sci.* **107** 2271–6

McEwen B S 1999 Stress and hippocampal plasticity *Annu. Rev. Neurosci.* **22** 105–22

McEwen B S 2001 Plasticity of the hippocampus: adaptation to chronic stress and allostatic load *Annal. NY Acad. Sci.* **933** 265–77

McEwen B S 2006 Protective and damaging effects of stress mediators: central role of the brain *Dialogues Clin. Neurosci.* **8** 367

McEwen B S and Milner T A 2007 Hippocampal formation: shedding light on the influence of sex and stress on the brain *Brain Res. Rev.* **55** 343–55

McEwen B S 2010 Stress, sex and neural adaptation to a changing environment: mechanisms of neuronal remodeling *Ann. NY Acad. Sci.* **1204** E38

McEwen B S 2008 Central effects of stress hormones in health and disease: understanding the protective and damaging effects of stress and stress mediators *Eur. J. Pharmacol.* **583** 174–85

McKittrick C R, Blanchard D C, Blanchard R J, McEwen B S and Sakai R R 1995 Serotonin receptor binding in a colony model of chronic social stress *Biol. Psych.* **37** 383–93

Mecha M, Feliú A, Carrillo-Salinas F J, Mestre L and Guaza C 2013 Mobilization of progenitors in the subventricular zone to undergo oligodendrogenesis in the Theiler's virus model of multiple sclerosis: implications for remyelination at lesions sites *Exp. Neurol.* **250** 348–52

Ménard C, Hodes G E and Russo S J 2016 Pathogenesis of depression: insights from human and rodent studies *Neurosci.* **321** 138–62

Mercurio F and Manning A M 1999 NF-κB as a primary regulator of the stress response *Oncogene* **18** 6163–71

Millar A G, Bradacs H, Charlton M P and Atwood H L 2002 Inverse relationship between release probability and readily releasable vesicles in depressing and facilitating synapses *J. Neurosci.* **22** 9661–7

Mitra R and Sapolsky R M 2008 Acute corticosterone treatment is sufficient to induce anxiety and amygdaloid dendritic hypertrophy *Proc. Natl Acad. Sci.* **105** 5573–8

Mitra R, Jadhav S, McEwen B S, Vyas A and Chattarji S 2005 Stress duration modulates the spatiotemporal patterns of spine formation in the basolateral amygdala *Proc. Natl Acad. Sci.* **102** 9371–6

Moniaga C S, Watanabe S, Honda T, Nielsen S and Hara-Chikuma M 2015 Aquaporin-9-expressing neutrophils are required for the establishment of contact hypersensitivity *Sci. Rep.* **5** 1–13

Monyer H, Burnashev N, Laurie D J, Sakmann B and Seeburg P H 1994 Developmental and regional expression in the rat brain and functional properties of four NMDA receptors *Neuron* **12** 529–40

Moreno-López C *et al* 2011 Excessive daytime sleepiness in multiple system atrophy (SLEEMSA study) *Arch. Neurol.* **68** 223–30

Moron-Concepcion J and Hipolito-Cubedo L 2013 T2. Effects of CFA-induced chronic inflammatory pain on opioid self-administration and accumbal dopamine release in heroin dependent rats *Neuropsychopharmacol.* **38** S273–434

Morrison D K and Davis R J 2003 Regulation of MAP kinase signaling modules by scaffold proteins in mammals *Annu. Rev. Cell Development. Biol* **19** 91–118

Moussavi S, Chatterji S, Verdes E, Tandon A, Patel V and Ustun B 2007 Depression, chronic diseases, and decrements in health: results from the World Health Surveys *Lancet* **370** 851–8

Mukhopadhyay S, Chapnick B M and Howlett A C 2002 Anandamide-induced vasorelaxation in rabbit aortic rings has two components: G protein dependent and independent *Am. J. Physiol. Heart Circul. Physiol.* **282** H2046–54

Murty V P, LaBar K S and Adcock R A 2012 Threat of punishment motivates memory encoding via amygdala, not midbrain, interactions with the medial temporal lobe *J. Neurosci.* **32** 8969–76

Naert G, Ixart G, Maurice T, Tapia-Arancibia L and Givalois L 2011 Brain-derived neurotrophic factor and hypothalamic-pituitary-adrenal axis adaptation processes in a depressive-like state induced by chronic restraint stress *Mol. Cell. Neurosci.* **46** 55–66

Nair A, Vadodaria K C, Banerjee S B, Benekareddy M, Dias B G, Duman R S and Vaidya V A 2007 Stressor-specific regulation of distinct brain-derived neurotrophic factor transcripts and cyclic AMP response element-binding protein expression in the postnatal and adult rat hippocampus *Neuropsychopharmacol.* **32** 1504–19

Namburi P *et al* 2015 A circuit mechanism for differentiating positive and negative associations *Nature* **520** 675–78

Nestler E J 2008 Transcriptional mechanisms of addiction: role of ΔFosB *Phil. Trans. R. Soc. Lond.* B **363** 3245–55

Nestler E J, Barrot M, DiLeone R J, Eisch A J, Gold S J and Monteggia L M 2002 Neurobiology of depression *Neuron* **34** 13–25

Njoo C, Agarwal N, Lutz B and Kuner R 2015 The cannabinoid receptor CB1 interacts with the WAVE1 complex and plays a role in actin dynamics and structural plasticity in neurons *PLoS Biol.* **13** e1002286

Northoff G and Panksepp J 2008 The trans-species concept of self and the subcortical–cortical midline system *Trends Cogn. Sci.* **12** 259–64

Numakawa T, Adachi N, Richards M, Chiba S and Kunugi H 2013 Brain-derived neurotrophic factor and glucocorticoids: reciprocal influence on the central nervous system *Neuroscience* **239** 157–72

O'Mahony A *et al* 2006 NF-κB/Rel regulates inhibitory and excitatory neuronal function and synaptic plasticity *Mol. Cell. Biol.* **26** 7283–98

Ota M, Sato N, Hidese S, Teraishi T, Maikusa N, Matsuda H, Hattori K and Kunugi H 2017 Structural differences in hippocampal subfields among schizophrenia patients, major depressive disorder patients, and healthy subjects *Psych. Res.: Neuroimag.* **259** 54–9

Pariante C M 2006 The glucocorticoid receptor: part of the solution or part of the problem? *J. Psychopharmacol.* **20** 79–84

Pasquali R 2012 The hypothalamic–pituitary–adrenal axis and sex hormones in chronic stress and obesity: pathophysiological and clinical aspects *Ann. NY Acad. Sci.* **1264** 20

Pattwell S S *et al* 2012 Altered fear learning across development in both mouse and human *Proc. Natl Acad. Sci.* **109** 16318–23

Pawlak R, Magarinos A M, Melchor J, McEwen B and Strickland S 2003 Tissue plasminogen activator in the amygdala is critical for stress-induced anxiety-like behavior *Nat. Neurosci.* **6** 168–74

Pavlides C, Ogawa S, Kimura A and McEwen B S 1996 Role of adrenal steroid mineralocorticoid and glucocorticoid receptors in long-term potentiation in the CA1 field of hippocampal slices *Brain Res.* **738** 229–35

Pertwee R G *et al* 2010 International Union of Basic and Clinical Pharmacology. LXXIX. Cannabinoid receptors and their ligands: beyond CB1 and CB2 *Pharmacol. Rev.* **62** 588–631

Pescini Gobert R *et al* 2009 Convergent functional genomics of oligodendrocyte differentiation identifies multiple autoinhibitory signaling circuits *Mol. Cell. Biol.* **29** 1538–53

Petra A I, Panagiotidou S, Hatziagelaki E, Stewart J M, Conti P and Theoharides T C 2015 Gut-microbiota-brain axis and its effect on neuropsychiatric disorders with suspected immune dysregulation *Clin. Therap.* **37** 984–95

Phiel C J, Wilson C A, Lee V M Y and Klein P S 2003 GSK-3α regulates production of Alzheimer's disease amyloid-β peptides *Nature* **423** 435–9

Pfau M L and Russo S J 2015 Peripheral and central mechanisms of stress resilience *Neurobiol. Stress* **1** 66–79

Pierce K L and Lefkowitz R J 2001 Classical and new roles of β-arrestins in the regulation of G-protein-coupled receptors *Nat. Rev. Neurosci.* **2** 727–33

Popelová A 2015 Impact of different types of antidiabetic interventions on the development of neurodegenerative changes in brains of diabetic mice and rats (https://dspace.cuni.cz/handle/20.500.11956/81341)

Price J L and Drevets W C 2010 Neurocircuitry of mood disorders *Neuropsychopharmacol.* **35** 192–216

Radell M L, Myers C E, Sheynin J and Moustafa A A 2017 Computational models of posttraumatic stress disorder (PTSD) *Comput. Models Brain Behav.* **43** 43–55

Raison C L and Miller A H 2003 Depression in cancer: new developments regarding diagnosis and treatment *Biol. Psych.* **54** 283–94

Reddy M S 2010 Depression: the disorder and the burden *Ind. J. Psychol. Med.* **32** 1–2

Rei D *et al* 2015 Basolateral amygdala bidirectionally modulates stress-induced hippocampal learning and memory deficits through a p25/Cdk5-dependent pathway *Proc. Natl Acad. Sci.* **112** 7291–6

Rennie G, Chen A C, Dhillon H, Vardy J and Damian D L 2015 Nicotinamide and neurocognitive function *Nutritional Neurosci.* **18** 193–200

Ressler K J 2010 Amygdala activity, fear, and anxiety: modulation by stress *Bio. Psych.* **67** 1117–9

Rice D and Barone S Jr 2000 Critical periods of vulnerability for the developing nervous system: evidence from humans and animal models *Environ. Health Persp.* **108** 511–33

Robinson T E and Kolb B 2004 Structural plasticity associated with exposure to drugs of abuse *Neuropharmacol.* **47** 33–46

Romero L M 2004 Physiological stress in ecology: lessons from biomedical research *Trends Ecol. Evol.* **19** 249–55

Rosen E D and Spiegelman B M 2006 Adipocytes as regulators of energy balance and glucose homeostasis *Nature* **444** 847–53

Russell S J and Kahn C R 2007 Endocrine regulation of ageing *Nat. Rev. Mol. Cell Biol.* **8** 681–91

Saarelainen T *et al* 2003 Activation of the TrkB neurotrophin receptor is induced by antidepressant drugs and is required for antidepressant-induced behavioral effects *J. Neurosci.* **23** 349–57

Sacchet M D and Gotlib I H 2017 Myelination of the brain in major depressive disorder: an in vivo quantitative magnetic resonance imaging study *Sci. Rep.* **7** 1–14

Sachser R M, Haubrich J, Lunardi P S and de Oliveira Alvares L 2017 Forgetting of what was once learned: exploring the role of postsynaptic ionotropic glutamate receptors on memory formation, maintenance, and decay *Neuropharmacol.* **112** 94–103

Salazar M *et al* 2009 TRB3 links ER stress to autophagy in cannabinoid antitumoral action *Autophagy* **5** 1048–9

Sandi C and Pinelo-Nava M T 2007 Stress and memory: behavioral effects and neurobiological mechanisms *Neural Plast.* 2007

Savitz J and Drevets W C 2009 Bipolar and major depressive disorder: neuroimaging the developmental-degenerative divide *Neurosci. Biobehav. Rev.* **33** 699–771

Schmidt H D and Duman R S 2010 Peripheral BDNF produces antidepressant-like effects in cellular and behavioral models *Neuropsychopharmacol.* **35** 2378–91

Seo D, Tsou K A, Ansell E B, Potenza M N and Sinha R 2014 Cumulative adversity sensitizes neural response to acute stress: association with health symptoms *Neuropsychopharmacol.* **39** 670–80

Seong S Y and Matzinger P 2004 Hydrophobicity: an ancient damage-associated molecular pattern that initiates innate immune responses *Nat Rev. Immunol.* **4** 469–78

Sharif O and Knapp S 2008 From expression to signaling: roles of TREM-1 and TREM-2 in innate immunity and bacterial infection *Immunobiol.* **213** 701–13

Shi J, Wittke-Thompson J K, Badner J A, Hattori E, Potash J B, Willour V L, McMahon F J, Gershon E S and Liu C 2008 Clock genes may influence bipolar disorder susceptibility and dysfunctional circadian rhythm Am. J. Med. Genetics *B* **147** 1047–55

Shin L M and Liberzon I 2010 The neurocircuitry of fear, stress, and anxiety disorders *Neuropsychopharmacol.* **35** 169–91

Shirayama Y, Chen A C H, Nakagawa S, Russell D S and Duman R S 2002 Brain-derived neurotrophic factor produces antidepressant effects in behavioral models of depression *J. Neurosci.* **22** 3251–61

Shors T J 2006 Stressful experience and learning across the lifespan *Annu. Rev. Psychol.* **57** 55–85

Sinha R, Lacadie C M, Constable R T and Seo D 2016 Dynamic neural activity during stress signals resilient coping *Proc. Natl Acad. Sci.* **113** 8837–42

Smith E E *et al* 2011 Correlations between MRI white matter lesion location and executive function and episodic memory *Neurology* **76** 1492–9

Soliman F *et al* 2010 A genetic variant BDNF polymorphism alters extinction learning in both mouse and human *Science* **327** 863–6

Sousa N, Lukoyanov N V, Madeira M D, Almeida O F X and Paula-Barbosa M M 2000 Reorganization of the morphology of hippocampal neurites and synapses after stress-induced damage correlates with behavioral improvement *Neuroscience* **97** 253–66

Stephan K E, Baldeweg T and Friston K J 2006 Synaptic plasticity and dysconnection in schizophrenia *Bio. Psych.* **59** 929–39

Steptoe A, Hamer M and Chida Y 2007 The effects of acute psychological stress on circulating inflammatory factors in humans: a review and meta-analysis *Brain Behavior Immun.* **21** 901–12

Stranahan A M, Norman E D, Lee K, Cutler R G, Telljohann R S, Egan J M and Mattson M P 2008 Diet-induced insulin resistance impairs hippocampal synaptic plasticity and cognition in middle-aged rats *Hippocampus* **18** 1085–8

Subhani A R, Kamel N, Saad M N M, Nandagopal N, Kang K and Malik A S 2018 Mitigation of stress: new treatment alternatives *Cogn. Neurodynam.* **12** 1–20

Taliaz D, Loya A, Gersner R, Haramati S, Chen A and Zangen A 2011 Resilience to chronic stress is mediated by hippocampal brain-derived neurotrophic factor *J. Neurosci.* **31** 4475–83

Tamm C and Ceccatelli S 2017 Mechanistic insight into neurotoxicity induced by developmental insults *Biochem. Biophys. Res. Commun.* **482** 408–18

Tenk C M, Wilson H, Zhang Q, Pitchers K K and Coolen L M 2009 Sexual reward in male rats: effects of sexual experience on conditioned place preferences associated with ejaculation and intromissions *Horm. Behav.* **55** 93–7

Thamhesl M, Apfelthaler E, Schwartz-Zimmermann H E, Kunz-Vekiru E, Krska R, Kneifel W, Schatzmayr G and Moll W D 2015 Rhodococcus erythropolis MTHt3 biotransforms ergopeptines to lysergic acid *BMC Microbiol.* **15** 1–13

Tronson N C, Corcoran K A, Jovasevic V and Radulovic J 2012 Fear conditioning and extinction: emotional states encoded by distinct signaling pathways *Trend. Neurosci.* **35** 145–55

Troy-Fioramonti S, Demizieux L, Gresti J, Muller T, Vergès B and Degrace P 2015 Acute activation of cannabinoid receptors by anandamide reduces gastrointestinal motility and improves postprandial glycemia in mice *Diabetes* **64** 808–18

Tsai G and Coyle J T 1998 The role of glutamatergic neurotransmission in the pathophysiology of alcoholism *Ann. Rev. Med.* **49** 173–84

Turner C A, Akil H, Watson S J and Evans S J 2006 The fibroblast growth factor system and mood disorders *Biol. Psychiatry* **59** 1128–35

Ueyama T, Kawai Y, Nemoto K, Sekimoto M, Toné S and Senba E 1997 Immobilization stress reduced the expression of neurotrophins and their receptors in the rat brain *Neurosci. Res.* **28** 103–110

Van Praag H, Schinder A F, Christie B R, Toni N, Palmer T D and Gage F H 2002 Functional neurogenesis in the adult hippocampus *Nature* **415** 1030–4

Velayudhan L, V Diepen E, Marudkar M, Hands O, Suribhatla S, Prettyman R, Murray J, Baillon S and Bhattacharyya S 2014 Therapeutic potential of cannabinoids in neurodegenerative disorders: a selective review *Curr. Pharm. Design* **20** 2218–30

Vithlani M, Terunuma M and Moss S J 2011 The dynamic modulation of GABAA receptor trafficking and its role in regulating the plasticity of inhibitory synapses *Physiol. Rev.* **91** 1009–22

Voleti B *et al* 2013 Scopolamine rapidly increases mammalian target of rapamycin complex 1 signaling, synaptogenesis, and antidepressant behavioral responses *Bio. Psych.* **74** 742–9

von Engelhardt J *et al* 2008 Contribution of hippocampal and extra-hippocampal NR2B-containing NMDA receptors to performance on spatial learning tasks *Neuron* **60** 846–60

Vos P E *et al* 2002 EFNS guideline on mild traumatic brain injury: report of an EFNS task force *Eur. J. Neurol.* **9** 207–19

Vouimba R M and Richter-Levin G 2005 Physiological dissociation in hippocampal subregions in response to amygdala stimulation *Cereb. Cortex* **15** 1815–21

Vyas A, Mitra R, Rao B S and Chattarji S 2002 Chronic stress induces contrasting patterns of dendritic remodeling in hippocampal and amygdaloid neurons *J. Neurosci.* **22** 6810–8

Walz W, Ilschner S, Ohlemeyer C, Banati R and Kettenmann H 1993 Extracellular ATP activates a cation conductance and a K+ conductance in cultured microglial cells from mouse brain *J. Neurosci.* **13** 4403–11

Waselus M, Flagel S B, Jedynak J P, Akil H, Robinson T E and Watson S J Jr 2013 Long-term effects of cocaine experience on neuroplasticity in the nucleus accumbens core of addiction-prone rats *Neurosci.* **248** 571–84

Watanabe Y, Gould E, Cameron H A, Daniels D C and McEwen B S 1992 Phenytoin prevents stress-and corticosterone-induced atrophy of CA3 pyramidal neurons *Hippocampus* **2** 431–5

Waters E M *et al* 2015 G-protein-coupled estrogen receptor 1 is anatomically positioned to modulate synaptic plasticity in the mouse hippocampus *J. Neurosci.* **35** 2384–97

Webster M J, Knable M B, O'Grady J, Orthmann J and Weickert C S 2002 Regional specificity of brain glucocorticoid receptor mRNA alterations in subjects with schizophrenia and mood disorders *Mol. Psych.* **7** 985–94

Wyllie D J A, Livesey M R and Hardingham G E 2013 Influence of GluN2 subunit identity on NMDA receptor function *Neuropharmacol.* **74** 4–17

Yang H C, Yuan C M, Liu T B, Li L J, Peng H J, Liao C P, Rong H, Fang Y R and Angst J 2011 Validity of the 32-item Hypomania Checklist (HCL-32) in a clinical sample with mood disorders in China *BMC Psych.* **11** 1–7

Yasokawa Y T, Shinoda J, Okumura A, Nakayama N, Miwa K and Iwama T 2007 Correlation between diffusion-tensor magnetic resonance imaging and motor-evoked potential in chronic severe diffuse axonal injury *J. Neurotrauma* **24** 163–73

Zaremba P D, Bialek M, Blaszczyk B, Cioczek P and Czuczwar S J 2006 Non-epilepsy uses of antiepileptic drugs *Pharmacol. Rep.* **58** 1

Zass L J, Hart S A, Seedat S, Hemmings S M and Malan-Müller S 2017 Neuroinflammatory genes associated with post-traumatic stress disorder: implications for comorbidity *Psych. Genetics* **27** 1–16

Zhang Y *et al* 2008 Model-based analysis of ChIP-Seq (MACS) *Genome Biol.* **9** 1–9

Zhou Z, Cao S, Li H and Li Y 2015 Treatment with escitalopram improves the attentional bias toward negative facial expressions in patients with major depressive disorders *J. Clin. Neurosci.* **22** 1609–13

Zhu H J, Wang J S, Markowitz J S, Donovan J L, Gibson B B, Gefroh H A and DeVane C L 2006 Characterization of P-glycoprotein inhibition by major cannabinoids from marijuana *J. Pharmacol. Exp. Therapeut.* **317** 850–7

Ziebell J M, Adelson P D and Lifshitz J 2015 Microglia: dismantling and rebuilding circuits after acute neurological injury *Metabol. Brain Dis.* **30** 393–400

Zunszain P A, Anacker C, Cattaneo A, Choudhury S, Musaelyan K, Myint A M, Thuret S, Price J and Pariante C M 2012 Interleukin-1 β: a new regulator of the kynurenine pathway affecting human hippocampal neurogenesis *Neuropsychopharmacol.* **37** 939–49

IOP Publishing

Neurocognitive Perspectives of Prosocial and Positive Emotional Behaviours
Theory to application
Shashikanta Tarai and Arindam Bit

Chapter 11

Adopting positive emotion and prosocial language in a classroom context: neurocognitive and behavioural well-being of learners

Shashikanta Tarai, Anbu Savekar and Arindam Bit

This chapter describes and explains the efficacy of the instructor's prosocial and positive communicative language in altering learning habits and behavioural changes in learners. The underpinnings of the socio-cognitive theory of behaviour, cognitive neuroscience, social and emotional learning and positive psychology are interpreted in the light of current observations and findings. We adapted Covey's (2013) nine habits to our study for learning English in a classroom context. The evaluation and comparative analysis of control and experimental groups ($N = 14$ each) based on self-rating response scores (prior and post-instruction) yielded positive results. We found awareness about the learner's habits, which changed when they were exposed to positive emotion and prosocial language. Findings validate the effect of social and emotional learning in creating favourable scenarios and bringing a positive transformation in the habits of learners. Thus, the efficacy of positive emotion and prosocial communication reinforces self-efficacy and establishes well-being and constructive behaviours in learners' minds.

11.1 Introduction

Social and emotional learning (SEL) from the point of view of neuroscience and neurobiology have vast implications in the efficacy of integrating behaviour, emotions and cognition leading towards learning, which is underpinned by skill development, emotional self-regulation, self-and social-awareness, social communication, well-being and prosocial behaviours (Brackett *et al* 2019, Immordino-Yang *et al* 2019, Jones *et al* 2019, Schonert-Reichl 2019, Wentzel 2019). The bi-directional link and reciprocal relation between emotion and social intelligence (EI and SI)

doi:10.1088/978-0-7503-3383-2ch11

enhance emotional and social competence. EI and SI are determined by learners' perception and information processing, which are correlated to the structural neural changes catalysed by the stimuli (Immordino-Yang *et al* 2019). Past literature has ample established evidence to suggest the interaction between the instructor and learner, which is symbiotic as their emotional and cognitive engagement factors influence the instructional-learning process (Brackett *et al* 2019, Jagers *et al* 2019). Emotions influence learning, which is consequently impacted by emotional conditions (Green and Batool 2017), modulating the emotive content of the lectures and learners' understanding (Meirovich 2012, Mercer *et al* 2016), as the modular system of emotions and its impact are illustrated in figure 11.1.

Studies ascertain the significance of interpersonal communication, rapport and empathy and based on the instructors' and learners' belief and motivation in the learning process (Aragão 2011, Barcelos 2015, Barcelos and Aragão 2018, Gläser-Zikuda *et al* 2018). Numerous scholars are inclined towards socio-cultural aspects that impact learning, where cooperative participation plays a vital role in stimulating interaction within the learning context (Avila 2019, Jagers *et al* 2019). When learners are exposed to emotive learning practices, improvements and changes are observable in learners' interaction skills, attitude, beliefs, perceptions and knowledge (Boyd and Pennebaker 2015, King 2016, Sauter 2017). Literature confirms that

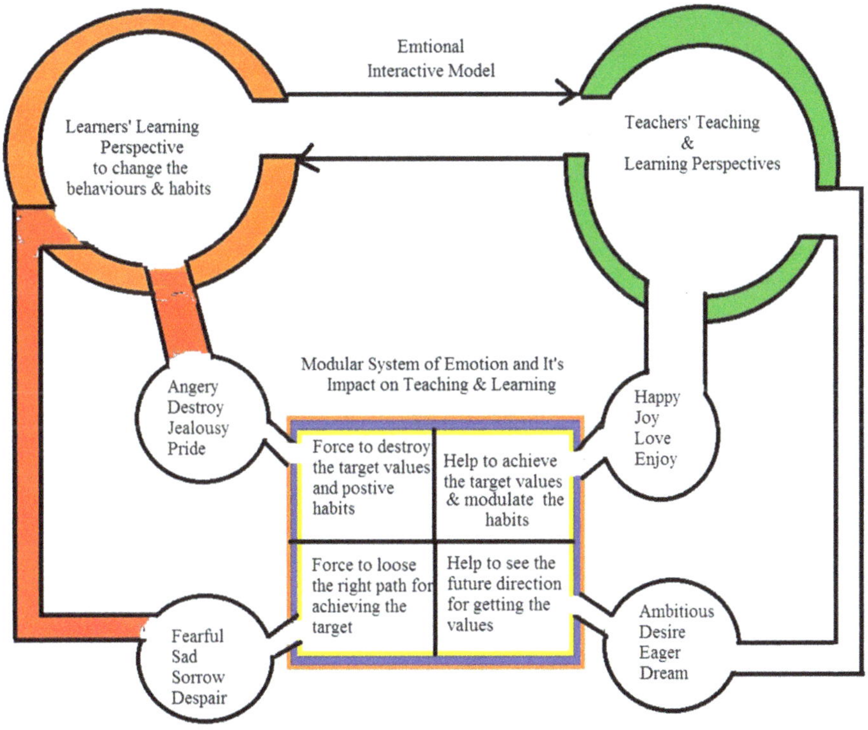

Figure 11.1. The modular system of emotion influences the behaviours and habits of learners in an interactive and parallel context.

emotions significantly influence teaching (Jennings and Greenberg 2009, Méndez López and Peña Aguilar 2013, MacIntyre and Vincze 2017) as well as learning (Hagenauer *et al* 2015, Barcelos and Aragão 2018, Henry and Thorsen 2018, Henry and Thorson 2019), yet none of the studies has examined the efficacy of prosocial and positive emotional communication in establishing an interactive, positive-prosocial learning condition, as the proposed interactive or parallel emotional model shows in figure 11.1. No research has attempted to quantitatively study the transformation of learners' pre-existing habits and behavioural attributes using prosocial and positive emotive communication strategies. Supporting this construct and further verifying the usage of prosocial and positive communication within the chosen curriculum of language learning, thus, hitherto remains unexplored.

We anticipate that learning a language like English for non-native speakers can improve significantly, incorporating prosocial and positive and emotional communicative language directed towards learners. Past research has evidence to substantiate the positive influence of prosocial vocabulary used towards enhancing learning (Kuykendall 1993). Furthermore, studies corroborate the significance of prosocial and positive language on establishing support of the masses (Frimer *et al* 2015) and strengthening study findings in cognitive neuroscience (Tarai *et al* 2019), which illustrated the effect of prosocial words on language processing. Would prosocial and positive emotion language be used judiciously with a pre-planned strategy to communicate with learners, transforming learners' learning inclination in terms of habit and behaviour? This study examines whether language with prosocial words and positive effect modulate learning behaviour (English language learning by non-native learners). Covey's (2013) effective habits are underpinned by behaviours that identify three essential domains of learning (cognitive, psychomotor and emotional skills): the first being knowledge, which relates to what to do; the second pertains to the skills which imply how to do; and the final one relates to the desire—why to do. Studies on cognitive, social neuroscience and behavioural theory have established a correlation between learner's emotional and socio-cultural contexts through imitative and observational learning (Atkinson 2014, 2018, Blake *et al* 2007, Brackett *et al* 2019, King and Chen 2019, Liand Jeong 2020, Thierry and Rebuschat 2020). Would the learning behaviour and habit be transformed and altered by the prosocial and positive language interaction due to the enhancement of positive and emotional aspects of learners?

11.1.1 Role of emotional instruction and learning

Coordination and purposeful planning of interaction is directed towards alignment. Thus, enhancing inter-and intra-group connections require a socio-emotional method (Atkinson *et al* 2018). Changes in behaviour are observable when learners are exposed to social and emotional connect through language (Atkinson 2014), as the social environment propels learners' inclination towards learning. This study validates the significance of pre-designed strategic use of prosocial language and positive emotion to engage instructions to generate productive knowledge effectively.

Learning about the functionality of language and contextual adaptations of culture within the social environment is largely influenced by emotions (Sieberer-Nagler 2016, Liand Jeong 2020). Emotion substantially influences learning, as it alters and transforms perception, evaluation, judgement and action (Frijda 2016, MacIntyre and Vincze 2017), in addition to amplifying attentional engagement and memory allotment (Green and Batool 2017). Learning through emotional experiences induces a positive attitude, empathy, self-confidence, motivation besides fostering self-growth (Jennings and Greenberg 2009). Consequently, the instructor's positive emotions generate a conducive learning environment, the ability to withstand stress, and an interactive social connection for the learner (Méndez López and Peña Aguilar 2013, Zinsser *et al* 2016, Oxford 2020). On the other hand, negative emotion and feeling amplifies learning anxiety and impedes the learning process in the absence of social support (Jin and Dewaele 2018). The emotional well-being of learners is considerably influenced by the instructors' skills and socio-emotional state (Srinivasan 2015, Mercer *et al* 2016, Chen 2019). The paradigm of well-being for both the instructors as well as learners lies within the constructs of positive psychology, which resolves several substantial concerns related to instructors' challenges, stress and strain during the interactions (MacIntyre and Mercer 2014, Oxford 2015, Dewaele *et al* 2019, Klimova and Pikhart 2020). For instance, language teaching-learning is likely to be significantly influenced by emotions, since emotions stimulate thinking (Constantinou *et al* 2014, Rodrigo-Ruiz 2016, Oxford 2020). A study has established that instructors are capable of managing and controlling the emotional reactions, besides influencing the behaviours and habits of their learners (Jennings and Greenberg 2009). The negative emotion of learners is reduced in the presence of positive interpersonal attitude based interactions, which is created by the instructor, reinforced by practical instructional skills, engaging interactions and creative activities (Méndez López and Peña Aguilar 2013, Gkonou and Mercer 2017, Oxford 2020).

The instructors' challenge of executing the tasks and activities are feasible through interpersonal communication. Therefore, Goetz *et al* (2013) support instructional practices and methods that employ an empathetic interaction style correlating substantially to learners' understanding, enthusiasm, attention, enjoyment, and pride. Furthermore, the nurturing instructional practice significantly reduces learning barriers ranging from boredom to anger and anxiety to helplessness in learners. This practice modulates instructors' resilience to withstand emotional labour, regulation and burnout (Green and Batool 2017, Gkonou *et al* 2020). Additionally, the negative emotions in the instructor, such as irritation, anger or frustration, are likely to be triggered by the adverse emotional reactions of the learners (King 2016, King *et al* 2020). Therefore, the retention of learning, starting off the learning process, and stimulation of attention in learners are underpinned by emotions, wherein instructors' emotions have considerable implications in the quality of the teaching–learning (King and Chen 2019). Thus, it can be said that emotional (positive and negative) instruction has a considerable role in impacting not only learning activities but also instructors' practices and overall outcomes

(Baudoin and Galand 2017, Dewaele *et al* 2019, Gkonou *et al* 2020, King *et al* 2020).

Generalisation occurs at one end of the spectrum when an emotional being is stereotyped as irrational, childish, out of control and destructive, rather than being considered a well-balanced, empathetic and mature individual (Sutton and Wheatley 2003). The attributes of emotion and cognition are divergent and opposing. Nonetheless, researchers are examining the effect of emotions on understanding in the context of learning (King and Chen 2019, Gkonou *et al* 2020). Tarai *et al* (2019) study in neurocognitive and behaviour domains ascertained that language processing involves less cognitive and neural resources when prosocial and positive emotion-based words are used. In the context of learning, the psychological theories of stimulus appraisal, emotional memory and value are reinforced by neurological perspectives.

Similarly, the neurobiological mechanisms of emotional stimulus appraisal support instructor–learner interaction (Schumann 1997). Thus, the innate foraging skills are behavioural attributes just as learning is, although learning involves acquiring information, knowledge or skill (Schumann 2001). Parallel to this construct, the early socialisation that processes the forms of joint attention influences the socio-emotional learning when learner experiences support the various conditions of self-esteem due to the positive instruction expressions and self-regulation (Zinsser *et al* 2016, Li and Jeong 2020).

11.1.2 Effect of positive language on learning

The framework of positive psychology posits that positive emotions generate a positive mindset that stimulates and sustains positive emotion, attention, relationship, and accomplishment (Seligman 2011), promoting social interaction and developing inclination towards learning and communication (MacIntyre and Vincze 2017). The instruction-based learning process is supported by the functional aspect of language usage (Ellis 2019). The impact is more significant when instructors focus upon ‘how they relate to the learners’ than just the ‘how’ and ‘what’ they impart to learners (Jennings and Greenberg 2009). The instructors’ effective instructional strategy of reframing, rephrasing and restating can counter harmful content, specifically in a non-responsive and non-productive session, thereby promoting behavioural change resulting in prosocial and positive emotional quotient (Aknin *et al* 2018).

The deliberate use of positive linguistic tools: inclusive (we) and exclusive (you) pronouns, unobtrusively engage or disengage instructor with learners; in addition to promoting interaction, as well as underpinning empathy, support, respect, dignity and trust in the learner (Pennebaker 2017). The pronoun ‘we’ reinforces the power of inclusiveness between both instructor and learner within the context of learning. Language wields substantial influence towards shaping thoughts. The efficacy of using grammatical or function words (*pronouns*: I, we, you, them; *prepositions*: of, for, to; *auxiliary verbs*: was, have, is; *adverbs*: very, really, so; *conjunctions*: or, since, and; *negations*: no, never, not; and *articles*: a, an, the); and lexical or content words (nouns, adjectives, regular verbs and adverbs), is substantial in communication. Function words promote social interaction and establish the interpersonal speaker–listener connection (Kuykendall 1993, Pennebaker 2017).

11.1.3 Augmenting learning through prosocial behaviour and language

A favourable learning environment is created by instructors' understanding, connection, and positive interactive communication, strengthening the interpersonal connection with learners (Hagenauer *et al* 2015). The emotional (EI) and social intelligence (SI) of the instructor co-create the connection between instructor and learner besides enhancing the socio-emotional skills of learners (Cain and Carnellor 2008, Garner 2010, Jin and Dewaele 2018). Instructors' socio-emotional patterns induce empathy and generate enthusiasm for learning (Henry and Thorsen 2019), wherein the EI and SI are mirrored in interactive discourse in communication (Pennebaker 2017, Sauter 2017, Gholamrezaee and Ghanizadeh 2018).

Prosocial vocabulary mirrors prosociality and distinctly offers help and social support through words conveying warmth, loving-kindness, cooperation and empathy; furthermore, prosocial language is processed quicker than unsocial and negative language (Kuykndall 1993, Frimer *et al* 2015, King and Chen 2019, Tarai *et al* 2019). Encouraging emotion is the catalysing agent that induces prosocial action resulting in prosocial behaviour (Aknin *et al* 2018). The altruistic behaviours of prosociality are characterised by generosity, kindness, caring, and helpful behaviour whilst serving society through conservation of the environment, making donations and reaching out to offer assistance, all of which is free from selfish financial profits (Kuykendall 1993, Padilla-Walker and Carlo 2015). Past evidence maintains that prosocial language and behaviour significantly elicit public support, drawing masses towards positive crowdfunding and generating speeches during public addresses (Decter-Frain and Frimer 2016). Interestingly, even exposure to prosocial-positive lyrics in musical compositions elicits greater empathy, prosocial thinking and behaviour attributes than listening to music with a highly emotional predisposition (Greitemeyer 2009, Ruth 2019).

11.1.4 Prosocial-positive language modulates neurocognitive aspects of learners

Multidisciplinary research in recent times has begun to approach learning from the point of view of neuro-education through the lens of neuroscience and neurobiological mechanisms. The literature from these multidisciplinary domains contributes towards enhancing learning orientation and identifying better instructional interaction strategies. The implication of neurobiology and neurocognition in learning pertains to the socio-emotional and cognitive stimuli that underpin the neural structural changes for developing neuroplasticity (Kweldju 2019, Zhang *et al* 2019, Thierry and Rebuschat 2020, Zhang *et al* 2020). The impact of learning or instructional engagement is observable in neuronal connections and neuronal structures in the brain, which identifies the presence of additional synaptic links due to the neuronal changes resulting in neuroplasticity. The synaptic neuronal connections increase or decrease, corresponding to the frequency of the links occurring and the manner of stimulation (Kweldju 2019). For instance, the instructors' instructional approach to ensure the efficacy of learning is associated with activation of the neuronal region responsible for creativity and skills. The learning process involves creating new memory and its storage which is recalled subsequently, thereby repeatedly activating and establishing the learners' synaptic connections. Structural and functional neuroimaging evidence corroborates the brain stimulation of memory and neural regions associated with the learning process triggered by the learners' extrinsic and intrinsic factors (Li and Jeong 2020, Thierry and Rebuschat 2020, Jeong *et al* 2021). Social factors such as social communication and behaviours are significant components of social neuroscience. These socio-cultural contexts of interactions influence the brain responses that are evident in the learner's processing of stimuli and subsequent reaction since encoding (learning) and information retrieval (memory) are co-dependent (Jeong *et al* 2010, Li and Jeong 2020). The behavioural response, social connections and well-being emerge as the outcome of cognitive, social, and emotional development associated with the learners (Immordino-Yang *et al* 2019, Jones *et al* 2019). Neuroscience literature suggests that brain neural development and neuroplasticity engage social-emotional experience (Schonert-Reichl 2019). Learning a second language is said to change neuronal network connectivity and improve cognitive neuronal plasticity since it involves the functioning of neural networks and activates various cognitive abilities such as reasoning, working memory, speech segmentation, sound discernment, task switching, syntax and semantic memory (Bubbico *et al* 2019).

11.1.5 Prosocial-positive instruction facilitates language learning

The shared positive-prosocial experiences of instructor and learner are considered as empathy, emotional expressions and emotional regulations, which are also the key to effective EI; and it provides positive associations vital for learning, positive behaviour, healthy interactional engagement and achieving the desired goals in language learning (Brackett *et al* 2019). The development of social skills is essential and occurs through the experiential learning of engaging in interpersonal connections with peers (Blake *et al* 2007). The positive and proactive engagement towards satisfying the emotional and social needs or deficits results in learners' emotional well-being, resilience, and emotional health as in emotional regulation. The frame of RULER is significant to incorporate social and emotional competence (RULER—recognising emotion, understanding emotion, labelling motion, expressing emotion and regulating emotion). The first three skills: 'recognising, understanding, and labelling' emotions-facilitate the instructor to identify and interpret others' feelings. The two remaining skills, expressing and regulating emotion, indicate how to manage the emotions to accomplish the predefined learning outcomes. Literature suggests that the impact of the RULER approach has an encouraging result for instructors. The instructors were found to experience lower levels of stress and burnout, and the learners' efficacy improved not only for learning but also for social skills and behavioural habits (Castillo *et al* 2013, Castillo-Gualda *et al* 2017, Brackett *et al* 2019).

Furthermore, the preventive science framework supports the negative consequences and offers positive outcomes to facilitate competencies and skills across social connections, emotional regulation and cognition (Jones *et al* 2019). The resilience and well-being in instructors, developed through positive emotional engagement (SEL—social and emotional learning or RULER approach), have seen a positive change leading to improved instructional (cognitive) engagement experiences with learners (Brackett *et al* 2019, King and Chen 2019). In addition, positive emotions have numerous benefits to the personal-self and social-self: building greater resilience and productive action and improving the cardiovascular functions by reducing stress, creating social connections and personal well-being (Dewaele *et al* 2019).

11.1.6 Prosocial language develops behavioural habits and the well-being of learners

The social and the psychological concurrence associate mainly with the social brain, wherein cognition integrates with language to establish a functional change in the social interactional connection (Mercer 2013). Language is transformational, and the positive-prosocial language influences the thinking and emotions to generate behavioural responses. The instructors' greater socio-emotional competence can be developed through training towards reducing emotional distress, better awareness, well-being and self-efficacy (Immordino-Yang *et al* 2019). Positive psychology is associated with positive subjective experience and positive personality attributes, which primarily associates with altruism, prosociality and positive interpersonal relationships (Seligman 2018). The positive and prosocial language of the instructor is instrumental in reducing the negative effect of the learners' anxiety and stress, as the instructor's relaxed and empathetic response pushes the learner to go past their fears (Dewaele *et al* 2019). The framework of positive psychology explicates the enjoyment during the instructional interaction, and the learning engagement leads to the transformation of behaviour, personal growth and identity (self-worth, self-image) and language competency (Dewaele *et al* 2019, Klimova and Pikhart 2020). Thus, learners' prosocial behaviours in a social context demonstrate healthy and positive engagement with instructors (McKeown and Taylor 2018, Schonert-Reichl 2019, Wentzel 2019).

11.1.7 Addressing the hypothesis and research questions

Language significantly influences emotional and social learning, wherein the learning process transforms and sustains positive behaviour besides generating social support during interactions (Sieberer-Nagler 2016, MacIntyre and Vincze 2017). Therefore, our study aims to examine the scope of using prosocial and positive emotion language to increase learning efficacy. Prosocial and positive language sustains prosocial behaviour, which fosters a positive attitude, emotion of empathy, support and help (Greitemeyer 2009, Decter-Frain and Frimer 2016, Tarai *et al* 2019). The robust evidence of prosocial-positive linguistic features is found in US Congressmen's discourses across political discussions in garnering community support and endorsement, which is established by Frimer (2015). In addition, an earlier study by Kuykendall (1993) maintains the relevance of planned and judicious use of polite language to elicit and augment prosocial skills in learners. The outcome of these studies presents us with the first premise for our research: language with prosocial words and positive emotion alters and transforms the habits and behaviour attributes of learners engaged in learning.

Learners' motivation is attributable to the significant role of emotion (Goetz *et al* 2013, Méndez López and Peña Aguilar 2013, King 2016, Baudoin and Galand 2017, Teimouri 2017). Moreover, emotional language can influence thinking and generate an interactive connection between speakers and listeners (Boyd and Pennebaker 2015). This construct presents us with the second premise for our study: to test whether positive emotional language does generate positive engagement aptitude in learners' habits and behaviour. Our study intends to ascertain the following enquiries and hypotheses (H1 and H2), using language infused with prosocial words and positive emotion in instructing the learners who are situationally challenged being non-native speakers of English.

H1

Instructors' prosocial language is likely to augment learners' empathy and build interpersonal connections.

H2

The learners' exposure to prosocial language may generate more significant levels of prosocial behaviour characteristics such as consideration, respect, mindful deliberation and commitment sustained by increased emotional regulation.

These hypotheses were verified using a quantitative technique and statistical approach for the selected protocol for performance and valuations, wherein the self-rating scores were gathered from prior- and post-interview engagements for analysis.

11.2 Methodological techniques

11.2.1 Participants

This study used the purposive sampling technique to identify the participants randomly for the study. This sampling approach was chosen to fulfil this study's objectives, as it achieves the specificity of testing the hypothesis in which the value judgment of selected participants can be generalised and considered to represent the population. The participants ($N = 30$, $M = 20$) were learners of the English language and essentially non-native speakers. These participants had a background knowledge of English as a subject which they studied during their school level. The socio-economic profile of participants indicated either rural or semi-urban populations. However, most of the bi-lingual speakers were inclined more towards Hindi (mother-tongue) due to the exposure to the language. The participants conceded their willingness to participate in the study through written consent forms. All of the personal demographic profile information was kept confidential.

11.2.2 Inclusion criteria of sample

The unbalanced participants (two male learners) were disqualified from participating in this study (N = 30 – 2). The exclusion criterion was followed to ensure consistency and regularity in engagement with instructions and participation in the planned activities. Thus, the sample had only twenty eight participants in the study ($N = 28$).

11.2.3 Experimental and control groups

Twenty-eight of the chosen participants were equally divided into two groups for the study: experimental group ($N = 14$, $M = 9$) and control group ($N = 14$, $M = 9$). Language proficiency in the experimental group consisted of fourteen participants, comprised of a few participants (3) with prior proficiency in English. Their medium of instruction had been English and English as a subject of the study. For the remaining 11 learners, although they studied English as a subject, their medium of instruction was Hindi. The control group comprising fourteen participants similarly had only a few participants (4) who were reasonably proficient in English with English medium of instruction and English as a subject, while the other ten participants received education in the Hindi language. These learners of English were non-native speakers with only exposure to a second language as a curriculum subject.

11.2.4 Settings, materials and tools

A large room was identified, and it was equipped with teaching aids such as a green chalkboard, a raised platform to provide added height to the instructor to ensure clear visibility to learners seated in the room. The learners were assigned comfortable chairs close to the instructor's dais. The learning environment amenities were identical and accessible to both instructors who were given a group to deliver module content (English speaking skills) at different times. The learning sets up a positive atmosphere that relaxes the learner and reduces negative emotions, stress, and anxiety (Dewaele *et al* 2019). Experimental-group participants were exposed to pre-designed lectures infused with prosocial words and positive emotion words, while the control group participants had the instructor delivering courses with neither prosocial nor positive emotion words.

11.2.5 Instructional engagement for control and experimental groups

The language learning module for an English speaking program designed for both groups was identical. The content engagement was pre-planned and commenced with an introduction to learning English to improve the English-speaking skills of the learners. Only the style of lecture delivery was purposefully varied based on including or excluding pre-designed prosocial and positive emotion language to be employed by the instructor for experimental and control groups, respectively. Furthermore, even the instructions for the activity after delivering module content distinctly differed due to the language used by the two instructors for their assigned group. The pre-planned selection of positive-prosocial vocabulary was adopted from Frimer *et al*'s (2015) list, specifically for the instructor's interaction with the learners from the experimental group. Frimer's list words (Frimer *et al* 2015) were chosen to suit and complement the module content aptly to initiate and sustain emotional associations between the instructor and learners from the experimental group. Conversely, the instructor used regular communicative language devoid of prosocial words to maintain 'no subjective connection' with the learners from the control group. The experimental and control groups were given formal instructions and received module content, considering each group's pre-planned and intended learning environment by their respective instructors. Both instructors followed a 45–60 min duration for each segment of the five-part module. Recordings of each learner's response (relating to behavioural habits) for both groups were similar, and response data was collected through a questionnaire given to every ($N = 28$) learner before and after each interactive engagement and speaking skill related to the activity.

11.2.6 Written consent and evaluation form

11.2.6.1 Socio-economic profiles of the participant-learners

Participants had to provide their socio-economic particulars such as their title, name, gender, date of birth, educational qualification, medium of instruction during education, the mono-bi-multi-lingual competency and proficiency. In addition, a written consent statement form was given to each learner along with a questionnaire for both group learners before the commencement of the first learning engagement with the instructor.

11.2.7 Assessment sheet to quantify responses on self-measured habits

A valuation sheet documenting the learners' self-assessment was adapted and designed with a Likert scale of seven-pointer scores. The scale of scores ranged from 'very unsatisfactory', which was equated to one on the score sheet, to 'outstanding', which was represented by seven on the score sheet. In addition, the pre-designed self-rating valuation form contained the pre-meditated score scale to collect learners' self-rating scores concerned with examining changes in their behavioural habits. The learners filled out these forms twice: first, before instructional engagement as in pre-valuation, and second, after the instructional meeting, that is, post-valuation.

The content for the self-rating form was prepared by extrapolating Covey's (2013) two primary habits (i.e., emotional reserves and productivity potential), as presented in table 11.1. In addition, we also preserved the seven essential habits of successful individuals (modified as simple meaning-based ideas, i.e., take the lead, goal-oriented, prioritising, solution-oriented, empathy, cooperation and honing skill).

11.2.8 Extrapolating critical habits of successful individuals

Nine habits of successful individuals (Covey 2013) were extrapolated to gather self-rated valuation scores from the learner participants for the current study purpose:

a. Emotional reserves refer to the display of thoughtfulness and compassion towards others' sentiments.
b. Productivity potential: balancing personal life and work commitments.
c. Taking the lead: manage oneself and take responsibility.

Table 11.1. Primary habits extrapolated in the context of learners (Covey 2013).

Covey's primary habits	Adapted behavioural habits extrapolated for learners	Meanings ascribed to behaviours/ habits
Emotional reserves	Emotions—inducing positive-prosocial interactive behaviour: prosocial self	Emotional reserves leading to positive outcomes—within oneself or in others (trustworthy, empathetic, thoughtfulness, teamwork, self-esteem)
Productive potential	Effortfulness	Productive effort devoted towards task accomplishment

d. Goal-oriented: identify goals to accomplish in life.
e. Prioritise: design plans to achieve set goals.
f. Solution-oriented: extend cooperation for resolving conflict that benefits all.
g. Empathy: empathise and comprehend others' perspectives.
h. Synergise: innovate and collaborate on improved ideas to resolve problems.
i. Sharpen the skill: discover life-purpose and pursue satisfaction in life.

Furthermore, Covey's nine habits originally written as long-phrases in the text: i.e., *emotional justification* (emotional reserve); *productive equilibrium* (productivity potential); *be proactive* (taking the lead), and so on, were transcribed to simple vocabulary replacements such as prioritise, goal-oriented, solution, empathy, cooperate, take the lead and so on. This process of modifying phrases was intended to facilitate quick self-rating valuations of behaviour habits by the participants prior and post-interaction and instructional engagement. The extrapolated nine habit classification details (Covey 2013), specifically for participants' self-rating scores of their participation and performances, are given in table 11.2.

Keeping in line with the current study objectives, participants filled in self-rating valuation forms of their behaviour habits twice, using their understanding and best judgement for every statement, once prior and second, post instructional engagement with the instructor.

11.2.9 Data collection method

Regardless of the learner group, the participants were thoroughly informed through the preliminary interaction session about the anticipated learning outcome that would minimise their anxiety and fear of speaking English in the English learning class. However, these learners were not provided with any insight or information regarding the pre-designed and pre-meditated lecture content, including prosocial and positive emotion language for their spoken English class-lecture and activity. This practice was adopted to ensure natural data of unbiased self-assessment responses for analysis and comparative study.

Table 11.2. Critical habits of successful individuals (Covey 2013), incorporated and extrapolated for collecting participants self-rating scores.

Seven key habits	Domain attributes: public and social-self or private and personal self	Adapted behavioural habits extrapolated for participants in the current study	Equated meaning of the behaviour/habits
Habit 1: Take the lead (*be proactive*)	Personal-self	Proactive—being responsible or taking initiative.	• Towards personal empowerment, • Taking onus for oneself, • Active self-improvement, and • Being self-sufficient and self-motivated.
Habit 2: Goal-oriented (*begin with the end in mind*)	Personal-self	Goal-oriented: having clarity of vision and values	• Foresighted, contemplative and planning with a goal in mind.
Habit 3: Prioritise (*put first things first*)	Personal-self	Planning (integrity/execution)	• Possess the potential to plan and prioritise before execution.
Habit 4: Solution-oriented (*think win-win*)	Public and social-self: positive interpersonal connections: creating co-dependent partnerships	Resolution of concerns (shared benefits and reciprocal respect)	• A win-win situation. • Finding solutions linked to selflessness in proactive interaction than the competition.
Habit 5: Empathy (*seek to understand, before being understood*)	Public and social-self: positive interpersonal connections—creating cooperative partnerships	Empathy leading towards mutual understanding	• Building interpersonal rapport based on active listening skills to enhance empathy.
Habit 6: Cooperate (*synergize*)	Public-social self: effective interactive, interpersonal relationship—creating synergetic co-dependent relationships	Creative potential leading to inspired cooperation	• Create team synergy; • Bonding; • Inspired cooperation; • Tolerance; • Being approachable; and • Solution-oriented; • Creativity and satisfaction are associated with learning.
Habit 7: Honing skills (*sharpen the saw*)	Positive-prosocial self: private and personal-self and public-social self	Satisfaction and rediscovering or renewal of self	• Happiness is linked with: ○ eagerness; ○ self-empowerment; ○ self-development; ○ overall wellness; ○ self-reliance to conquer hurdles; ○ being hardworking; and ○ achieving goals.

Before the first instructional engagement, participants of both study groups were made to fill the consent form. After that, instructions to read all the statements on habit carefully before circling the apt number that indicated their current emotion and the measure for each habit performance, with the given seven-point Likert Scale (very poor = 1, and outstanding = 7). This exercise was carried out twice: at the beginning of this study; for the first time before the first-time instructional engagement (lecture) and subsequently at the end of the study, and the second time was after the final interactive meeting (fifth segment of the five-part module-based interaction with learners). We instructed each participant to complete the valuation self-rating forms before instructional engagement sincerely and subsequently after each speaking skill performance-based activity. Further, the participants were directed to be attentive and focused while receiving the module content during the instructional and interactive engagements with the instructor. After each interactive speaking skill-based activity, the participants had to fill out the self-rating forms before their interactive arrangements. The primary purpose was to examine the extent of influence that instructor's positive-prosocial communicative language has on learners' emotional wellness and overall behavioural-habit outcome. We fulfilled the goal by using the self-rating valuation form with a seven-point Likert scale to measure the learners' performances and emotional changes. The instructor–learner interaction, instructional engagements of the instructors, speaking skill-based learners' activities, and learners' responses were documented on an audio-visual camera.

11.2.10 Statistical framework for data analysis

The collected raw data of the recordings were saved on the laptop for transcription and analysis of the instructor's pre-designed and pre-planned positive emotion and prosocial language explicitly employed for learners in the experimental group.

Correspondingly, the instructor's natural and neutral language style employed for the control group content was saved post-recording and transcribed for study. Furthermore, both study groups self-rating response scores were individually charted on an excel-sheet to derive the collated data for both groups separately. The numerical data were collected (using the self-rating score on a 7-point Likert scale) from every participant of both groups, then changed to derive average values for each habit.

11.3 Results

Our study incorporated essential habits (taking the lead, goal-oriented, prioritising, resolution, empathy, productivity, and satisfaction) across the two study groups (control and experimental) and two performance evaluations (pre- and post-interaction engagement). It revealed a robust main-effect of habits ($p \leqslant 0.03$). The patterns of satisfaction, empathy, productivity and resolution had higher scores than effort, goal-oriented and prioritising. These response scores of the participant-learners suggest an improvement in their relationship with fellow learners. The higher scores explain the participant's ability to perceive better others' viewpoints by developing solutions and creative ideas for others' benefit. Further, our analysis identified substantial two predominant effects ($p \leqslant 0.05$) of valuations, which signify higher scores for after interaction and instructional engagement than before interaction and instructional engagement. Finally, we identified the interaction between seven essential habits (taking the lead, goal-oriented, prioritising, resolution, empathy, productivity and satisfaction) × two evaluations (pre-and post-interactional engagement). This interaction was significant ($p \leqslant 0.045$) between the goal-oriented and joy conditions, wherein self-rating scores were higher for post-test lecture than pre-test lecture, as illustrated in figure 11.2.

The Tukey analyses procedures in post-hoc analysis revealed the habit of goal-oriented had a significant increase in assessment scores post-lecture ($p \leqslant 0.018$) and satisfaction ($p \leqslant 0.047$). Furthermore, the exposure to instructional engagement was infused with prosocial and positive emotional language. This mindful participation by the learners not only rendered the participants function better with improved planning, organising and preparing towards their desired goal accomplishments but also enabled them to be more cooperative towards others while resolving their conflicts to benefit others.

The interactive results between two habits (taking the lead, empathy) × 2 study groups × 2 valuations (pre- and post-interactive engagements) indicated a strong main effect of habits ($p \leqslant 0.005$), furnishing the more significant score for empathy than taking the lead. Furthermore, ANOVA defined a substantial interaction between habits (taking the lead, empathy) × two identified study groups ($p \leqslant 0.056$), thereby validating assessment scores for behaviour habit of empathy being higher than taking the lead, equally for two study groups, as illustrated in figure 11.3.

This investigation explained that learners' enhanced empathy skills would respond positively besides seeing others' perspectives. The comparisons established a maximum score for empathy over taking the lead for participants of the

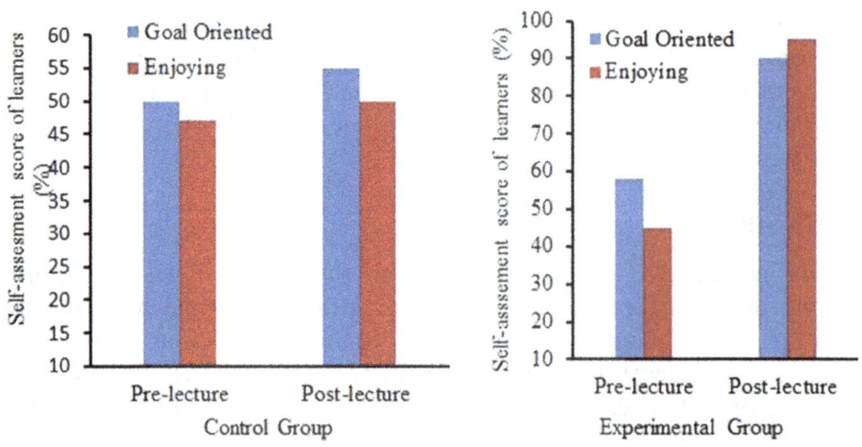

Figure 11.2. The self-assessment scores relating to goal-oriented and enjoyment are higher for the experimental group than the control group after the pre-designed lecture with prosocial and positive language.

experimental group ($p \leqslant 0.000\,01$) and control group ($p \leqslant 0.003$). According to mean variances, more significant scores were evident for the control group only for behavioural—the habit of taking the lead ($p \leqslant 0.003$), but not for empathy ($p > 0.637$) as compared to experimental group scores. Further, neither were any of the differences robust that were observable for the predominant effect in the control and experimental group ($p > 0.537$) and valuations (pre- and post-interactive engagement) ($p > 0.094$) nor any noteworthy outcome indicated due to these two interactive factors ($p > 0.143$). We found only three interactive elements reached significant ($p > 0.867$) scores: (i) behavioural habits: taking the lead and empathy; (ii) between two study groups of participants: control and experimental groups; and (iii) valuations of the two pre- and post-interactive engagements.

Subsequently, we carried out the mean scores of two habits (resolution, empathy) × two study groups × two valuations (pre- and post-interactive engagements), and found no robust effect ($p > 0.621$). Nevertheless, the factors between two habits (solution, empathy) and two valuations (pre- and post-interactive engagements) revealed considerable interaction ($p \leqslant 0.0390$), observable as the maximum mean score for behavioural-habit of empathy post-interactive engagements. Furthermore, post-analysis indicated a substantial variation between pre- and post-instructional engagement for English learning, which correlated with the behavioural habit of 'empathy', $p \leqslant 0.000\,39$, although it failed to demonstrate the behavioural habit of 'resolution' ($p > 1.00$). Comparatively, the post-interactive engagement score of empathy was much more than the post-interactive engagement score for solution ($p \leqslant 0.000\,92$).

As anticipated, the mean score of two essential habits (emotion, effort) × two study groups × two valuations (pre- and post-interactive engagements) identified substantial interaction effect, $p \leqslant 0.005$, revealing the higher score for emotion than effort post-instructional engagement lecture only for the experimental group. Post-hoc analysis employing Tukey procedures further ascertained significant differences between after instructional engagement (post-test) scores of control and experimental groups, $p \leqslant 0.001$, which were found to be greater for emotion than effort. Nonetheless, the average score was considerably higher for 'effort' before the instructional engagement lecture (pre-test) for the experimental group, $p \leqslant 0.000\,01$; and for the control group before instructional engagement lecture, $p \leqslant 0.001$ and after instructional engagement lecture (post-test), $p \leqslant 0.01$. This suggests that learner participants from the control group were sure to assist others but had no interpersonal connection and thus were emotionally detached from others. Hence, both before and after the scores of the control group and experimental groups, where learners were not exposed to positive emotion and prosocial languages, exhibited higher scoring for effort than emotions. Furthermore, the interactions between habits (emotion, effort) and valuations pre- and post-instructional engagement lecture (pre-test, post-test) was significant ($p \leqslant 0.032$) and was found to generate a higher score for emotion than effort for post-instructional engagement lecture only, but not for prior-instructional engagement lecture. Additionally, the mean comparisons affirmed substantial differences between scores for emotion only ($p \leqslant 0.0001$) and not for effort ($p > 0.801$). Nonetheless, the average scores comparisons between effort and emotion revealed a

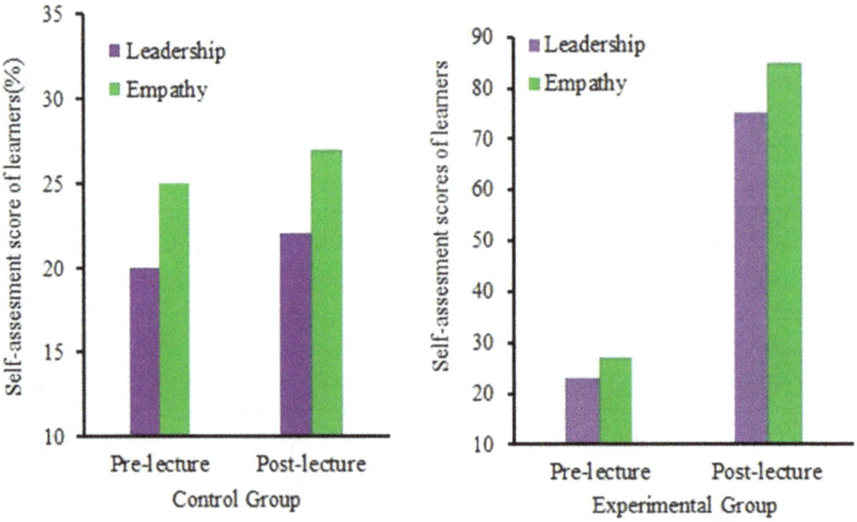

Figure 11.3. The self-assessment scores relating to taking the lead (leadership) and empathy habits are significantly increased for the experimental group compared to the control group learners only after the lecture (post-lecture).

higher score for the calculation than emotion ($p \leqslant 0.0008$) before the instructional engagement of English learning.

11.4 Discussion

This study explored the efficacy of instructors' prosocial and positive language in altering and transforming the behaviour and habits of learners towards learning, such as a language speaking skill proficiency (English) and the effect of this approach. The findings of this study have established the influence prosocial language has in altering and modulating emotions, showing empathy, increasing the spirit of interdependence and learners' well-being during the activities. We found the interactive communication content infused with pre-designed positive emotion and prosocial vocabulary does enhance the learners' habits related to empathy, satisfaction, productivity, resolution, goal-orientation, taking the lead, prioritising and planning. The outcome of our study confirms the effect of positive emotion priming on enhancing emotions (Kühne *et al* 2011) and cognitive appraisal in the learners (Sutton and Wheatley 2003). The experimental group exhibited the association of prosocial words of learners to their perceptiveness, thoughtfulness, and open-mind towards learning with higher scores for empathy and satisfaction than for solutions and productive effort. The generation of positive behavioural habits (consideration, respect, commitment and mindful deliberation), prosocial-self, emotional regulation and increased empathy in learners is induced by emotionalised learning practices. Overall, this study finds an altered and transformative effect is likely to be observed in learners (improvement in knowledge, skill, and a desire towards positive emotional, functional and social outcomes) with the

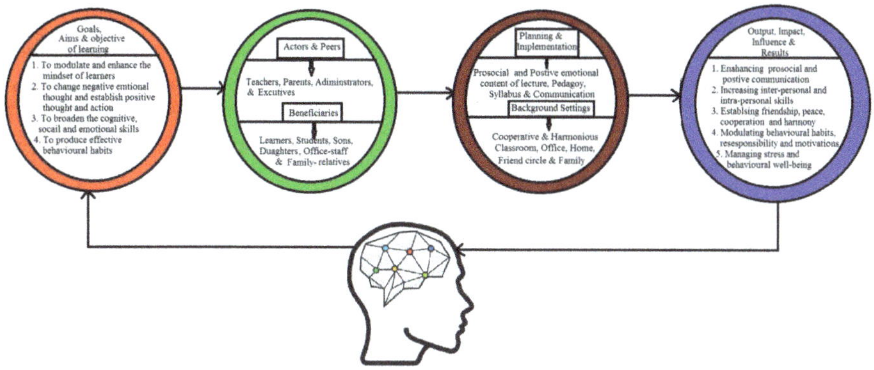

Figure 11.4. The input and output interactive models of behavioural changes are presented with respect to teaching–learning of prosocial and positive languages.

introduction of pre-planned instructors' interaction incorporating prosocial language, as the inputs and outputs are presented in figure 11.4.

With its behavioural habit analysis of the participant learners, the study confirms the effect of positive emotion on altering habits in the learners. Post-instructors' interaction, these learners are inclined to interact with their instructor, be proactive, take the initiative and responsibility. In the context of instructing and learning, the framework of positive psychology validates generating well-being and positive emotion (Seligman 2011, 2018, Klimova and Pikhart 2020). Adherence to positive psychology constructs demonstrates learners' enhanced inclination to participate due to positive emotion, which predisposes them to activities and discussions (Oxford 2015, 2020). The increase in the interpersonal relationship between instructor and learners occurs with positive psychology and emotional science (Bar-On 2010), and it further correlates with EI advocated by Covey (2013). The outcome relates closely to Covey's (2013) habits and an early study of Buckmaster (1994) on primary school children, wherein the study established that the inclusion of positive interactive activity minimised high levels of competitiveness and encouraged a congenial environment. Empathy and EI are interlinked, and the arousal of understanding and empathy towards others begets prosocial changes about social skills such as effective communication, sharing, compassion and cooperation (Brackett *et al* 2019). Our findings equally confirm the inclusion of positive emotion and prosocial words in the pre-designed interaction of instructors, generate positive results in physical, emotional, mental and spiritual attributes in the habits of the learners.

11.4.1 Efficacy of positive emotion and prosocial language changes habits of learners

Positive consequences are generated when positive emotions transform and alter the thoughts, attitudes and behaviours of learners. Similar outcomes were identified and observed in previously established literature in socio-emotional influence (Atkinson 2014, Atkinson *et al* 2018) and positive psychology (Mercer *et al* 2016). The learners experiencing a safe and fostering environment are active, relaxed, demonstrate prosociality and develop competencies specifically in the meaningful relational condition generated by the instructor. The impact of an individual's social relationships and interactions directly influences the brain structurally and functionally and consequently the behaviour (Immordino-Yang *et al* 2019, Jones *et al* 2019). The results in the current study, specifically the response scores after the lecture, mirrored the transformation in learners' behaviours. There was an enhanced response in habits of creativity, solution, understanding and enjoyment in the learners. An increased level of enjoyment was particularly noticeable when activity was performed in front of peers and instructor (Dewaele and Alfawzan 2018, Dewey *et al* 2018, Dewaele *et al* 2018). Such performances amongst peers spark the interactional instinct and generate a proactive attitude towards every positive stimulus encountered by the learner therein (Dewaele 2011, Baudoin and Galand 2017). Consequently, even in English language learning, the learners responded proactively and exhibited willingness and enthusiasm to perform in the planned activities. Thus, our study's findings corroborate the established evidence of previous studies that state emotional learning experiences essentially enhance the efficacy of learning.

Furthermore, this study incorporates the RULER approach or SEL (social and emotional learning) based instructional engagement for better learning. The 'recognising, understanding and labelling' is followed by the instructor in handling the learners, and 'expressing and regulating' emotions mindfully by the instructor, to establish a warm nurturing environment and promote learning for the learners of the experimental group (Brackett *et al* 2019, Elias 2019). The findings of this study validate the relevance of positive emotion in broadening the scope of learning and acquiring skills, besides corroborating the previous research on emotional and cognitive interaction (Oxford 2015). The emotion-oriented learning experience is enhanced with prosocial and positive language (Oxford 2020). The results of this study correlate to Schumann's neurobiological standpoint, established psychological paradigms lead to emotional stimulus appraisal (Schumann 1997, Tarai *et al* 2019); and to Zinsser *et al*'s (2016) study on socialisation process influencing and impacting the efficacy of socio-emotional learning.

11.4.2 Emotional efficacy and proactive effort are shaped by prosocial language

We found that learners' level of empathy was altered and increased response scores when they received prosocial language-based interactions. This evidence validates the prosocial effect language has on transforming behaviour and changing learners' learning mindset. The learning is enhanced due to the emotional appraisal or, in other words, emotional state is innately embedded at the core of cognition. The current findings reveal transformational changes with improved emotional, social skills and prosocial behaviours in the experimental group of learners (Aknin *et al* 2018) that induces an empathetic response as learners begin to comprehend and perceive from others' standpoint (Buckmaster 1994).

However, the learners belonging to the control group exhibited higher scores for proactive effort (self-awareness) than empathy (social skills). This level of response, devoid of social skill development, is accounted for by the absence of prosocial and emotional vocabulary during the instructor–learner interaction. Thus, the control group displays a lesser degree of helpfulness and social skills in the learners. Although instructional style and interactive approach generate co-dependence amongst learners and augment social connections towards being proactively prosocial, cooperative learning is enhanced to understand the benefits of following the synergetic interactive path towards improving behavioural outcomes (Premo *et al* 2018). The instructors' skills implicate the quality of interaction between instructor–learner during interpersonal connection, effective instructional practices and motivation; consequently, the learners' behaviour and learning are qualitatively emotional (Davis 2003). The interpersonal relationship between instructor and learner is explicated by cognitive appraisal theory and the shared neural coupling during instructional engagement and learning (Jin and Dewaele 2018, Nguyen *et al* 2021). However, the understanding depends on the learners' cognitive and linguistic abilities and social knowledge (Li and Jeong 2020). The likelihood of joint attention to stimulus during shared understanding underlies coupled neural responses during social interaction (with embodied real-life activities to integrate sensory-motor information to enable performance action), whereby learning is facilitated through embodied communication (Li and Jeong 2020, Nguyen *et al* 2021). The developmental and educational psychology findings also affirm that learning and social skills competency occur through guidance, practice, and active engagement with the development of the brain, or learning occurs through advice, training, and interaction with others. This reinforces the development of knowledge and understanding of others by observing their emotional states and social interaction (Mercer 2013). The interpretation and processing in the brain (information on emotional state and social interaction) is through the psychological tool of language. Therefore, creative language is instrumental in generating change within the learner as personal-self as well as public-social-self. Positive and prosocial verbal and non-verbal language create emotional priming, leading to improved interpersonal interaction, nurturing positive emotion, and creating a supportive condition (Kühne *et al* 2011).

Here are few examples of the instructor's positive responses, reproduced from transcripts of the lectures:

'***Instructor***—*Yes, that was a good answer.*

Instructor—*Yes, very good.*

Instructor—*First talk about your strength child, then talk about your weakness. L……, speak slowly, take your time, yes, continue talking.*

Instructor—*That was quick. Why don't you elaborate on what is your strength and explain a little, also say why it is your strength?*'

These findings also substantiate previously established evidence on the influence of prosocial language in eliciting a favourable opinion from the public towards the political parties (Frimer *et al* 2015, Decter-Frain and Frimer 2016). Emotional priming and cognitive stimulus appraisal enhance prosocial behavioural attitudes apparent in the learners of the experimental group. The role of positive psychology is significant in reducing anxiety, augmenting self-perception, generating positive social-interpersonal connections, empathy, intimacy, improved social engagement and finding solutions (Jin and Dewaele 2018, Dewaele *et al* 2019). The instructor's prosocial language use creates a supportive environment and activates cognition which generates eagerness towards learning and induces well-being. The transformed social, behavioural attributes of the experimental group of learners found in the study are prosocial language, which creates positive emotional valence (Rintell 1984, Pennebaker 2017, Tarai *et al* 2019).

Furthermore, positive behaviours and instructor and learner interaction are heightened when instructors' communication (verbal and non-verbal) convey vocalic emotions amounting to compassion, appreciation, respect and warmth (Kwitonda 2017, Sauter 2017). The regular practice of authentic communication for the learners looking to enhance speaking skills, such as using subjective experiences and executing role-plays, will facilitate the acquisition of expressing and effectively communicating emotions (Dewaele 2011). The recall of memory associated with language learning proficiency is better when the learner is exposed to naturalistic real-world utterances, observations, and interactional participation with embodied experiences (Jeong *et al* 2010, Ellis 2019, Culbertson *et al* 2020, Liand Jeong 2020). Therefore, our study gives substantial consideration to the instructor's language and the activity. To elicit responses, promote participation, encourage language proficiency and develop communication skills in the learners, the extempore topics for the training specifically focused on learners' subjective experiences: *My Role-model; Experiences of a day at college or work; My life's memorable experience; Favourite food; An expression of gratitude or vote of thanks speech; An apology, and lastly, a conversational interaction among participants—'Getting to know the Stranger'.*

The instructor's positive communicative language that transformed behavioural outcomes and habits observable in the learners from the experimental group are quoted below:

*'**Instructor**—S……, excellent. You have improved compared to the last performance. Have you all (to the other learners) noticed? And the best part is he has started speaking English. He was nervous, yet he performed, did not give up.*

Let us all clap for him.

S…., you have understood the technique, now you have to continue it to improve your speaking skill.'

The instructor's mindful behaviour and actions of cognitive engagement (self-regulation) sustain proactive behaviour in the learners, such as improving the focus, responsibility, and willingness and minimising learners' anxiety and fear (Illés and Akcan 2017, Jagers *et al* 2019). Learners from the experimental group corroborate this construct's post-interactional engagement outcome when they tend to get a positive emotion and embodiment of experiential learning. The enhanced prosocial and positive interactional behaviour of the instructor contributes to the learners' enhanced emotional and cognitive outcome; as the instructor fosters learners' interest, fires enthusiasm and satisfaction of enjoyment with motivation towards learning, a desire to participate due to emotional contagion (Dewaele *et al* 2018, King and Chen 2019). Furthermore, the instructors' efforts to replace emotionally uninteresting learning routines with interesting challenges facilitate enjoyment; thus, while participating in extempore speaking, the learners are keen to speak about their subjective and emotional experiences. Consequently, the instructors' personality attributes and EI (emotional intelligence) promote emotional competence and regulation, vital to learners' holistic growth (Rodrigo-Ruiz 2016, Brackett *et al* 2019). Given the interlinking paradigm of empathy and emotional intelligence, the current outcome confirms pre-designed and conscious delivery of positive and prosocial instructional engagements or content create enhanced understanding between instructor–learners.

Sharing emotional experience and an enhanced interpersonal connection generates greater trust and reinforces empathy towards all (Kuykendall 1993, Brackett *et al* 2019). It is widely acknowledged that language impacts thoughts, emotions and behaviours. The substantial evidence on the power of words harnessed in communicative language exists in the domain of politics (Frimer *et al* 2015, Decter-Frain and Frimer 2016, Pennebaker 2017). Current study outcomes mirror the transformations induced through the instructor's specifically chosen and deliberate use of words during instructional engagement and validate the prevalence of prosocial language as an effective stimulus to modulate change. For instance, fostering interpersonal relationships, prosocial behaviour, and generating empathy and trust, encouraging social appreciation and interactive connection are underpinned by inclusive pronouns form ('we, us, our'). The instructors' prosocial behaviour and personal attitude mirrored substantially through inclusive pronouns (Boyd and Pennebaker 2015), predominantly modulate learners towards empathy, positive emotional arousal and stimulate prosocial behaviour (Aknin *et al* 2018), besides demonstrating the instructors own emotional regulation, endurance, well-being and consequently reducing emotional labour and burnout (Gkonou *et al* 2020).

The examples to substantiate the mindful usage of inclusive pronouns incorporated in the instructor's communicative language style are cited as follows:

'***Instructor***—*Why do we talk to someone?*

Yes, we express our thoughts. Good! What else do we say?

Instructor—*Yes, correct, we discuss matters. Let us list out what we thought and concern, and we share information, we share ideas, we share thoughts and something more …. facts and emotion. What one person shares with another person is communication.*

Where do we use verbal communication?

Instructor—*Yes, excellent. We use verbal communication in writing and speaking. Speaking is oral communication.*'

A warm and emotionally safe atmosphere for learning is reflected when the instructor is actively involved in instructional clarity; displays enthusiasm is encouraging besides exhibiting care and concern towards the learners and their education. The positive motivational valence mirrored through words fosters a positive approach while negative valence stimulates withdrawal response (Moors and Houwer 2001). A Canadian study on emotional strategies employed to promote learning was devoid of any changes in self-efficacy or enhancement in performance on account of learners' pre-existing positive emotional threshold (Rossiter 2003). Therefore, it is appropriate to suggest that the instructor's language enables a warm, supporting, positive, approachable, connecting, interactive and relaxed environment for learning. Furthermore, instructors' positive approach sustains and encourages prosocial behaviour to create proactive interpersonal connection, all of which converge towards an emotion-based and socio-cognitive value-based learning (Schumann 1997). In a nutshell, this study primarily validates that learners are transformed when exposed to prosocial and positive emotion-based language that creates a safe learning environment; secondly, the study also reflects learners improved emotional and understanding levels and altered behaviour with empathy, consideration and dedicated individuals with positive and prosocial attributes.

11.5 Conclusion

This chapter offers valuable insights into the multidisciplinary and multi-level frameworks of positive psychology, neurobiology, language learning and cognitive neurosciences, highlighting the importance of social and emotion-based learning. Literature that accounts for the cognisance of taking the socio-cultural context and emotional and social factors is systematically discussed, referring to cognition and behaviour (Avila 2019, Brackett *et al* 2019, Immordino-Yang *et al* 2019, Jagers *et al* 2019, Jones *et al* 2019, Klimova and Pikhart 2020, Zhang *et al* 2020).

Language, as a socio-cultural and psychological and communicative tool, is significantly associated with the social brain. The relationship between effective use of language to facilitate learning through the use of positive and prosocial language and the implications on the social brain is evident in the study findings. Our study validates the previous research that has demonstrated the impact of socially and emotionally catalysed epigenetic changes in brain structure and functioning in the context of cognition, social-emotional functioning, behavioural changes and learning. The findings of this study have come to establish the quantitative information and provide additional insights regarding the influence of the prosocial and optimistic language of the instructor or trainer in effectively mentoring and directing learners to improve English language proficiency. The framework of positive psychology and social-emotional learning is discussed in great detail; the analysis of study results has identified and established the influence of prosocial and positive emotion in instructors' instructional practices. This chapter has adapted and incorporated seven habits identified by Covey to validate and support the impact of positive psychology and SEL in influencing learning and modulating learners' changes through the deliberate use of prosocial language by instructors and trainers for any skill training or competencies.

Furthermore, we observe that the habits and behaviours of learners changed, and the efficacy of language learning was enhanced with the usage of prosocial language in the interactional engagement between instructor and learner. Therefore, we can conclusively state that the instructor's strategic prosocial practices and positive communicative language augment the learners' self-reliance, socio-emotional development, and learning. Thus, the implication of 'how' (style) and 'what' (content) to communicate, as the style of communication sustains considerable influence on emotions, thinking, habits and behaviour of learners. Therefore, the significance of prosocial language is substantial as it impacts learning in addition to instilling self-efficacy. Thus, the future study can observe, examine and explore strategic and mindful use of language to enhance and improve teamwork, leadership, mental health and mentoring of learners.

References

Aknin L B, Van de Vondervoort J W and Hamlin J K 2018 Positive emotion reward and promote prosocial behavior *Curr. Opin. Psychol.* **20** 55–9

Aragão R 2011 Beliefs and emotions in foreign language learning *System* **39** 302–13

Atkinson D 2014 Language learning in mind body world: a sociocognitive approach to second language acquisition *Lang. Teach.* **47** 467–83

Atkinson D, Churchill E, Nishino T and Okada H 2018 Language learning great and small: environmental support structures and learning opportunities in a sociocognitive approach to second language acquisition/teaching *Modern Lang. J.* **102** 471–93

Avila M O C 2019 Exploring teachers' and learners' overlapped turns in the language *Stud. Second Lang. Learn. Teach.* **9** 581–606

Barcelos A M F and Aragão R C 2018 Emotions in language teaching: a review of studies on teacher emotions in Brazil *Chin. J. Appl. Linguist* **41** 506–31

Barcelos A M F 2015 Unveiling the relationship between language learning beliefs, emotions and identities *Stud. Second Lang. Learn. Teach.* **2** 301–25

Bar-On R 2010 Emotional intelligence: an integral part of positive psychology *S. Afr. J. Psychol.* **40** 54–62

Baudoin N and Galand B 2017 Effects of classroom goal structures on student emotions at school *Int. J. Educat. Res.* **86** 13–22

Blake S, Bird J and Gerlach L 2007 *Promoting Emotional and Social Development in Schools: A Practical Guide* (New York: SAGE Publications)

Boyd R L and Pennebaker J W 2015 A way with words: using language for psychological science in the modern era *Consumer Psychology in a Social Media World* (London: Routledge) pp 250–64

Brackett M A, Bailey C S, Hoffmann J D and Simmons D N 2019 RULER: a theory-driven, systemic approach to social, emotional, and academic learning *Educat. Psychol.* **54** 144–61

Bubbico G, Chiacchiaretta P, Parenti M, Di Marco M, Panara V, Sepede G, Ferretti A and Perrucci M G 2019 Effects of second language learning on the plastic aging brain: functional connectivity, cognitive decline, and reorganisation *Front. Neurosci.* **13** 423

Buckmaster L 1994 Effects of activities that promote cooperation among seventh graders in a future problem solving classroom *Elem. Sch. J.* **95** 49–62

Cain G and Carnellor Y 2008 Roots of empathy: a research study on its impact on teachers in Western Australia *J. Stud. Wellbeing* **2** 52–73

Castillo R, Fernández-Berrocal P and Brackett M A 2013 Enhancing teacher effectiveness in Spain: a pilot study of the RULER approach to social and emotional learning *J. Educat. Train. Stud.* **1** 263–72

Castillo-Gualda R, García V, Pena M, Galán A and Brackett M A 2017 Preliminary findings from RULER approach in Spanish teachers' emotional intelligence and work engagement *Electron. J. Res. Educ. Psych.* **15** 641–64

Chen J 2019 Efficacious and positive teachers achieve more: examining the relationship between teacher efficacy, emotions, and their practicum performance *Asia-Pacific Educat. Res.* **28** 327–37

Constantinou E, Van Den Houte M, Bogaerts K, Van Diest I and Van den Bergh O 2014 Can words heal? Using emotion labeling to reduce the effects of unpleasant cues on symptom reporting *Front. Psychol.* **5** 807

Covey S R 2013 *The Seven Habits of Highly Effective People: Powerful Lessons in Personal Change* (New York: Simon and Schuster)

Culbertson G, Andersen E and Christiansen M H 2020 Using utterance recall to assess second language proficiency *Lang. Learn.* **70** 104–32

Davis H A 2003 Conceptualising the role and influence of student-teacher relationships on children's social and cognitive development *Educ. Psychol.* **38** 207–34

Decter-Frain A and Frimer J A 2016 Impressive words: linguistic predictors of public approval of the US congress *Front. Psychol.* **7** 240

Dewaele J M and Alfawzan M 2018 Does the effect of enjoyment outweigh that of anxiety in foreign language performance? *Stud. Second Lang. Learn. Teach.* **8** 21–45

Dewaele J M 2011 Reflections on the emotional and psychological aspects of foreign language learning and use *Anglistik: Int. J. English Stud.* **22** 23–42

Dewaele J M, Chen X, Padilla A M and Lake J 2019 The flowering of positive psychology in foreign language teaching and acquisition research *Front. Psychol.* **10** 2128

Dewaele J M, Witney J, Saito K and Dewaele L 2018 Foreign language enjoyment and anxiety: the effect of teacher and learner variables *Lang. Teach. Res.* **22** 676–97

Dewey D P, Belnap R K and Steffen P 2018 Anxiety: stress, foreign language classroom anxiety, and enjoyment during study abroad in Amman, Jordan *Annu. Rev. Appl. Linguist.* **38** 140–61

Elias M J 2019 What if the doors of every schoolhouse opened to social-emotional learning tomorrow: reflections on how to feasibly scale up high-quality SEL *Educ. Psychol.* **54** 233–45

Ellis N C 2019 Essentials of a theory of language cognition *Modern Lang. J.* **103** 39–60

Frijda N H 2016 The evolutionary emergence of what we call 'emotions' *Cogn. Emot.* **30** 609–20

Garner P W 2010 Emotional competence and its influences on teaching and learning *Educ. Psychol. Rev.* **22** 297–321

Gholamrezaee S and Ghanizadeh A 2018 EFL teachers' verbal and nonverbal immediacy: a study of its impact on students' emotional states, cognitive learning, and burnout *Psychol. Stud.* **63** 398–409

Gkonou C and Mercer S 2017 Understanding emotional and social intelligence among English language teachers *Discussion Paper* British Council ELT Research Papers

Gkonou C, Dewaele J M and King J 2020 *The Emotional Rollercoaster of Language Teaching* (Bristol: Multilingual Matters)

Gläser-Zikuda M, Stuchlíková I and Janík T 2018 Emotional aspects of learning and teaching: reviewing the field – discussing the issues *Orbis Scholae* **7** 7–22

Goetz T, Lüdtke O, Nett U E, Keller M M and Lipnevich A A 2013 Characteristics of teaching and students' emotions in the classroom: investigating differences across domains *Contemp. Educat. Psychol.* **38** 383–94

Green Z A and Batool S 2017 Emotionalized learning experiences: tapping into the emotional domain *Evaluat. Program Plann.* **62** 35–48

Greitemeyer T 2009 Effects of songs with prosocial lyrics on prosocial behavior: further evidence and a mediating mechanism *Pers. Social Psychol. Bull.* **35** 1500–11

Hagenauer G, Hascher T and Volet S E 2015 Teacher emotions in the classroom: associations with students' engagement, classroom discipline and the interpersonal teacher-student relationship *Eur. J. Psychol. Educ.* **30** 385–403

Henry A and Thorsen C 2018 Teacher–student relationships and L2 motivation *Modern Lang. J.* **102** 218–41

Henry A and Thorsen C 2019 Weaving webs of connection: empathy, perspective taking, and students' motivation *Stud. Second Lang. Learn. Teach.* **9** 31–53

Illés É and Akcan S 2017 Bringing real-life language use into EFL classrooms *ELT J.* **71** 3–12

Immordino-Yang M H, Darling-Hammond L and Krone C R 2019 Nurturing nature: how brain development is inherently social and emotional, and what this means for education *Educ. Psychol.* **54** 185–204

Jagers R J, Rivas-Drake D and Williams B 2019 Transformative social and emotional learning (SEL): toward SEL in service of educational equity and excellence *Educ. Psychol.* **54** 162–84

Jennings P A and Greenberg M T 2009 The prosocial classroom: teacher social and emotional competence in relation to student and classroom outcomes *Rev. Educ. Res.* **79** 491–525

Jeong H, Li P, Suzuki W, Sugiura M and Kawashima R 2021 Neural mechanisms of language learning from social contexts *Brain Lang.* **212** 104874

Jeong H, Sugiura M, Sassa Y, Wakusawa K, Horie K, Sato S and Kawashima R 2010 Learning second language vocabulary: neural dissociation of situation-based learning and text-based learning *Neuroimage* **50** 802–9

Jin Y X and Dewaele J M 2018 The effect of positive orientation and perceived social support on foreign language classroom anxiety *System* **74** 149–57

Jones S M, McGarrah M W and Kahn J 2019 Social and emotional learning: a principled science of human development in context *Educ. Psychol.* **54** 129–43

King J 2016 'It's time, put on the smile, it's time!': the emotional labour of second language teaching within a Japanese university *New Directions in Language Learning Psychology* (Cham: Springer) pp 97–112

King J, Dewaele J M and Gkonou C 2020 Concluding thoughts on the emotional rollercoaster of language teaching *The Emotional Rollercoaster of Language Teaching* (Bristol: Multilingual Matters) ch 16 pp 288–95

King R B and Chen J 2019 Emotions in education: Asian insights on the role of emotions in learning and teaching *Asia-Pacific Educ. Res.* **28** 279–81

Klimova B and Pikhart M 2020 Current research on the impact of foreign language learning among healthy seniors on their cognitive functions from a positive psychology perspective—a systematic review *Front. Psychol.* **11** 765

Kühne R, Schemer C, Matthes J and Wirth W 2011 Emotional priming in political campaigns: how campaign-induced emotions prime political opinions *Int. J. Public Opin. Res.* **23** 485–507

Kuykendall J 1993 "Please," "Thank You," "You're Welcome": teacher language can positively impact prosocial development *Day Care Early Educ.* **21** 30–2

Kweldju S 2019 Educational neuroscience for second language classrooms *J-ELLiT* **3** 37–45

Kwitonda J C 2017 Foundational aspects of classroom relations: associations between teachers' immediacy behaviours, classroom democracy, class identification and learning *Learn. Environ. Res.* **20** 383–401

Li P and Jeong H 2020 The social brain of language: grounding second language learning in social interaction *NPJ Sci. Learn.* **5** 1–9

MacIntyre P D and Mercer S 2014 Introducing positive psychology to SLA *Stud. Second Lang. Learn. Teach.* **4** 153–72

MacIntyre P D and Vincze L 2017 Positive and negative emotions underlie motivation for L2 learning *Stud. Second Lang. Learn. Teach.* **7** 61–88

McKeown S and Taylor L K 2018 Perceived peer and school norm effects on youth antisocial and prosocial behaviours through intergroup contact in Northern Ireland *Br. J. Soc. Psychol.* **57** 652–65

Meirovich G 2012 Creating a favorable emotional climate in the classroom *Int. J. Manag. Educ.* **10** 169–77

Méndez López M G and Peña Aguilar A 2013 Emotions as learning enhancers of foreign language learning motivation *Profile: Issues Teach. Prof. Dev.* **15** 109–24

Mercer N 2013 The social brain, language, and goal-directed collective thinking: a social conception of cognition and its implications for understanding how we think, teach, and learn *Educ. Psychol.* **48** 148–68

Mercer S, Oberdorfer P and Saleem M 2016 Helping language teachers to thrive: using positive psychology to promote teachers' professional well-being *Positive Psychology Perspectives on Foreign Language Learning and Teaching* (Cham: Springer) pp 213–29

Moors A and Houwer J D 2001 Automatic appraisal of motivational valence: motivational emotional priming and Simon effects *Cognit. Emot.* **15** 749–66

Nguyen M, Chang A, Micciche E, Meshulam M, Nastase S A and Hasson U 2021 Teacher-student neural coupling during teaching and learning *Social Cogn. Affec. Neurosci.*

Oxford R 2015 Emotion as the amplifier and the primary motive: some theories of emotion with relevance to language learning *Stud. Second Lang. Learn. Teach.* **3** 371–93

Oxford R L 2020 The well of language teachers' emotional well-being *The Emotional Rollercoaster of Language Teaching* (Bristol: Multilingual Matters) ch 14 pp 247–68

Padilla-Walker L M and Carlo G (ed) 2015 *Prosocial Development: A Multidimensional Approach* (Oxford: Oxford University Press)

Pennebaker J W 2017 Mind mapping: using everyday language to explore social & psychological processes *Procedia Comp. Sci.* **118** 100–7

Premo J, Lamb R and Cavagnetto A 2018 Conditional cooperators: student prosocial dispositions and their perceptions of the classroom social environment *Learn. Environ. Res.* **21** 229–44

Rintell E M 1984 But how did you feel about that?: The learner's perception of emotion in speech *Appl. Linguist.* **5** 255–64

Rodrigo-Ruiz D 2016 Effect of teachers' emotions on their students: some evidence *J. Educ. Soc. Pol.* **3** 73–9

Rossiter M J 2003 The effects of emotional strategy training in the ESL classroom *Tesl-Ej* **7** 1–20

Ruth N 2019 'If you wanna make the world a better place': Factors influencing the effect of songs with prosocial lyrics *Psychol. Music* **47** 568–84

Sauter D A 2017 The nonverbal communication of positive emotions: an emotion family approach *Emot. Rev.* **9** 222–34

Schonert-Reichl K A 2019 Advancements in the landscape of social and emotional learning and emerging topics on the horizon *Educ. Psychol.* **54** 222–32

Schumann J H 1997 *The Neurobiology of Affect in Language* (Boston, MA: Blackwell)

Schumann J H 2001 Learning as foraging *Motivation in Second Language Acquisition* (Honolulu: University of Hawai'i) pp 21–8

Seligman M 2018 PERMA and the building blocks of well-being *J. Posit. Psychol.* **13** 333–5

Seligman M E 2011 Flourish: a visionary new understanding of happiness and well-being *Policy* **27** 60–1

Sieberer-Nagler K 2016 Effective classroom-management and positive teaching *English Lang. Teach.* **9** 163–72

Srinivasan P 2015 Exploring the influences of teacher's intelligence and emotional intelligence on students' academic achievement *Am. J. Educ. Res.* **3** 1159–62

Sutton R E and Wheatley K F 2003 Teachers' emotions and teaching: a review of the literature and directions for future research *Educ. Psychol. Rev.* **15** 327–58

Tarai S, Mukherjee R, Qurratul Q A, Singh B K and Bit A 2019 Use of prosocial word enhances the processing of language: frequency domain analysis of human EEG *J. Psycholinguis. Res.* **48** 145–61

Teimouri Y 2017 L2 selves, emotions, and motivated behaviors *Stud. Second Lang. Acquisit.* **39** 681–709

Thierry G and Rebuschat P 2020 An introduction to the cognitive neuroscience of second and artificial *Lang. Learn.* **70** 5–19

Wentzel K R 2019 Introduction to the special issue on social and emotional learning *Educ. Psychol.* **54** 127–8

Zhang J, Teo T and Wu C 2019 Emotion words modulate early conflict processing in a flanker task: differentiating emotion-label words and emotion-laden words in second language *Lang. Speech* **62** 641–51

Zhang J, Wu C, Yuan Z and Meng Y 2020 Different early and late processing of emotion-label words and emotion-laden words in a second language: an ERP study *Second Lang. Res.* **36** 399–412

Zinsser K M, Denham S A, Curby T W and Chazan-Cohen R 2016 Early childhood directors as socialisers of emotional climate *Learn. Environ. Res.* **19** 267–90

IOP Publishing

Neurocognitive Perspectives of Prosocial and Positive Emotional Behaviours
Theory to application
Shashikanta Tarai and Arindam Bit

Chapter 12

Neurocognitive mechanisms of prosocial and antisocial language incongruency: theorising behavioural results and ERP components

Shashikanta Tarai and Arindam Bit

This chapter is based on the electroencephalographic (EEG), paradigm to examine the neurocognitive mechanisms involved in prosocial positive and antisocial negative congruency and incongruency in English sentences. Participants are judged for prosocial positive and antisocial negative nouns or adjectives, which are either congruent or incongruent with the following prosocial positive and unsocial negative verbs in a sentence. Results of this chapter demonstrate the distinct event-related potential (ERP) markers, such as the early P100 and the late P300 components, which are associated with the processing of unsocial and prosocial sentences, respectively. Furthermore, the incongruent sentences show more significant reduction of N400 amplitudes than their congruent counterparts. Finally, most of these ERP incongruence results are discussed and interpreted in the light of current literature, focusing on the neurocognitive mechanisms of prosocial language that play a significant role in developing human cooperation, communication and joint attention for their survival.

12.1 Introduction

Social interactions define the prosocial nature of who we are and what we do as humans (Melis and Semmann 2010, Hamilton 2015, Silk and House 2016). Humans are prosocial beings from the evolutionary point of view. We prefer prosocial and social behaviours over unsocial ones, following the moral values of compassion and empathy (Singer and Klimecki 2014, Rodríguez-Gómez *et al* 2020). The conceptual theorisation of prosocial behaviours like helping, sharing, cooperating, donating, and volunteering that benefits others has attracted researchers of diverse fields,

doi:10.1088/978-0-7503-3383-2ch12

including sociology, anthropology, and psychology (Malti *et al* 2016, Martí-Vilar *et al* 2019). Sociopsychological and political studies have confirmed that prosocial behaviours enhance public support, social approval, tolerance, and solidarity among people (McDonald and Messinger 2011, Wang and Hamilton 2013). Prosocial behaviours that have been developed through evolutionary processes, are considered as survival strategies of humans based on societal cooperation (Henrich and Henrich 2006, Darwin 2008, Chudek and Henrich 2011, Tomasello 2019). However, the violence, aggression, hostility, lying and stealing that accounts for the antisocial behaviours harm others and thus invite the consequence of destruction, horror and terror (Lambert *et al* 2017). Whether prosocial or antisocial/unsocial, these behaviours are loaded, segmented, processed, and transmitted chiefly through language. Language is designed to signal prosocial and antisocial behaviours of others. For example, the study of Wang and Hamilton (2013, 2014) shows the first-person and third-person perspectives of prosocial sentences ('John gives Laura a warm and affectionate hug'; 'I share sweets with Lola and her friends'). It also shows the first-person and third-person perspectives of anti/unsocial sentences ('I cruelly bullied Stephanie about her weight problem'; 'Eric plays loud music to interrupt Sarah studying') at the behavioural level. Persuasive language fosters prosocial communication contrary to aggression within and outside of the group. Contrastively, antisocial communication has resulted in the group's pessimistic, negative, destructive and unsupportive behaviour (Eisenberg *et al* 1983). However, some research based on behavioural, neuroimaging and EEG investigations has studied the influence of prosocial and antisocial behaviours (Frimer *et al* 2015, Tusche *et al* 2016, Balconi *et al* 2019, Tarai *et al* 2019), but very few studies have tested the incongruity of prosocial and unsocial or antisocial words from neuro-cognitive perspectives in English sentences.

12.1.1 Prosocial communicative behaviours

Studies suggest that a correlation exists between prosocial behaviour and language at the developmental phase (Ensor and Hughes 2005, Rhee *et al* 2013). Language adds to prosociality and societal coordination (Dunfield *et al* 2011, Girard *et al* 2017). Similarly, the language of kindness and love promotes inter- and intra-personal sensitivity among speakers and listeners (Williams *et al* 2018). Prosocial verbal communication receives more significant social approval (Kacewicz *et al* 2014). A recent study has shown that the minimum use of prosocial language captures a low public support rate in the US Congress debate (Frimer *et al* 2015). Governments and individuals can achieve public support and social approval by using prosocial words like help, cooperation and sympathy. However, such a prosocial communication strategy fails to accommodate liars, criminals and terrorists, having antisocial personalities and destructive behaviours and is instrumental to antisocial language. Prosocial behaviours are used to oppose unsocial or pro-self behaviours (Eisenberg *et al* 2014). Prosocial and antisocial languages usually do not go together in social discourse as prosocial actions counter unsocial behaviours and vice-versa (Redondo-Pacheco *et al* 2016). The mismatch between prosocial and antisocial or unsocial words in communication may increase response time and demand more neurocognitive resources in interpreting the meaning of mismatch in the sentences. This chapter aims to study the neurocognitive phenomena involved in solving congruent and incongruent prosocial and unsocial words in English sentences by performing an EEG experiment.

12.1.2 Processing of semantic ambiguities

Several ERP studies have consistently revealed the negative-going N400 component of brain potential over centro-parietal, temporoparietal and parieto-occipital regions, when our brain processes the lexico-semantic incongruent written or spoken sentences (e.g., I drink my tea with milk and socks.) (Kutas and Federmeier 2011, Schindler and Kissler 2016, 2017). N400 was also observed to be more significant when participants were told to read such words in sentences related to the disobedience or violation of social norms, conventional beliefs, racial and gender stereotypes (Hehman *et al* 2014, Schindler *et al* 2015, Molinaro *et al* 2016). Even in the case of false political statements, the effect of N400 is more significant (Bornkessel-Schlesewsky and Schlesewsky 2013). During the processing of incongruent sentences, Kiehl *et al* (2002) and Martín-Loeches *et al* (2012) have reported increased cerebral activity in the inferior medial-temporal, bilateral inferior-frontal and bilateral motor-cortex. By employing the acquisition of intracranial events method during the assessment of incongruent sentences, the early research has found large activation in both the hemispheric sides of the frontal (inferior) and temporal (anterior) cortex for incongruent sentences than for congruent ones (McCarthy and Nobre 1993, McCarthy *et al* 1995). However, some other studies provide evidence of the processing of incongruent sentences in the brain's frontal, parietal, temporal and central regions, but no EEG and fMRI research has investigated the processing of prosocial and unsocial incongruent sentences in English.

12.1.3 Neuroimaging studies on prosocial behaviours

Neuroimaging studies have primarily focused on positive social beliefs, gratitude and empathy that are related to non-linguistic aspects of human. For example, the neuroimaging investigation on gratitude identified the prefrontal, the medial prefrontal cortex (mPFC) and frontal regions (Sui and Han 2007, Immordino-Yang *et al* 2009, Chiao *et al* 2010) and right side of the anterior temporal cortex (Wood *et al* 2008). The prefrontal cortex was found more active when performing cooperative tasks (Funane *et al* 2011, Cui *et al* 2012). The mPF cortex is a crucial region that regulates prosocial behaviours (Masten *et al* 2011, Rameson *et al* 2012, Zaki and Mitchell 2013, Wang and Hamilton 2014). The basic perceptual and complex conflict-related processing of moral judgements are triggered through the anterior cingulate cortex (ACC) (Botvinick *et al* 2004, Braem *et al* 2017). This ACC is associated with affective limbic areas and prefrontal regions (Greene *et al* 2004). Therefore, the prosocial perspective and decision abilities are processed in the medial as well as in dorsomedial prefrontal cortex (mPFC, dmPFC), temporal sulcus (pSTS) and the superior posterior junction (TPJ) in the temporo-parietal regions

(Majdandžić *et al* 2016, Kral *et al* 2017). Additionally, the temporal lobe is responsible for assessing others' emotions, beliefs and empathy (Morelli *et al* 2014). These studies have only focused on brain regions linked with prosocial behaviours without reference to unsocial incongruent stimulus functional in the domain of language. Furthermore, the violence stimuli are processed in the frontal lobe that primarily involves the executive functions (Soderstrom *et al* 2002). A very low volume of grey-matter is found in the prefrontal cortex of individuals with antisocial personality behaviour (APB) as compared to individuals with the non-APB (Ferguson 2010). Additionally, studies on psychopathic offenders have reported an impaired executive function in dorsolateral prefrontal dysfunction (Kandel and Freed 1989, Lapierre *et al* 1995). Most of these neuroimaging researches have emphasised the prefrontal and temporal regions of the brain that are engaged during the prosocial cooperative and antisocial non-linguistics tasks. In the language domain, the current chapter investigates the various ERPs with the help of EEG, measuring the latency and amplitudes, and concerning time (ms) and magnitude (μν), during the processing of prosocial and unsocial sentences having congruent and incongruent structures.

Electro-cortical signatures associated with antisocial threatening, terrorism and killing acts are still inadequate, limited and inconsistent (Miskovic and Keil 2012). The processing of incongruent prosocial and antisocial words helps to study neural signatures assigned to support social cognition and prosocial decision-making (Mills *et al* 2014). Still, it is unclear how our brain processes incongruent prosocial and antisocial sentences. The question rises here whether any hemispheric laterality effect exists while processing prosocial and antisocial sentences. Do the prosocial and unsocial congruent sentences also process in the same region and ERP components that are linked with positive and negative emotional words? These problems have not been yet addressed in the domain of neuroscience of language and psycholinguistics. Therefore, the current chapter examines the neuro-cognitive signatures associated with prosocial and antisocial words by measuring spatio-temporal ERPs in contexts of congruent and incongruent sentences. We predicted that the incongruent sentences that demand semantic information would be processed in the brain's prefrontal and temporal regions. Notably, in line with the earlier findings (Balconi *et al* 2019) on social cooperation and prosocial donation, this study projected greater activation in the frontal and prefrontal cortex for the incongruent prosocial sentences. We also anticipated that the frontal brain regions and early time courses would be linked with neurocognitive processing of anti/unsocial words. Prosocial and anti/unsocial incongruent sentences could decrease response accuracy (%) and increase the behavioural response time (ms).

12.2 EEG and behavioural methods

Undergraduate students ($N = 20$, $F = 10$) who were bilingual (e.g., proficient in Hindi and English) participated in the experiment. We did not allow any subjects who had impairments and cognitive deficits to join in the investigation. The Indian Council of Medical Research (ICMR-2017) guidelines were followed to conduct the experiment. English sentences were considered as stimuli which were composed by using prosocial-positive and antisocial-negative words. The nominal (e.g., nouns and adjectives) and verbal categories (e.g., verbs and adverbs) of target words were selectively chosen from the study of Frimer *et al* (2015). Each essential stimulus contains 11 words comprising nouns, auxiliaries, verbs, pronouns, complementisers and prepositions. In sentences, nouns were either semantically matched (congruent) or mismatched (incongruent) with prosocial and unsocial verbs. For example, the stimulus is like a sentence: she makes **'relationship'** with others because she wants to **kill** them. However, in this sentence, the nominal category of the word 'relationship' is mismatched with the unsocial word 'kill'. Sentential stimuli are presented on a computer screen to perform the task. Participants read and comprehended the meaning of sentences; they judged whether the sentences were congruent or incongruent. They were instructed to press the 'left-key' for congruent and 'right-key' for incongruent sentences. Figure 12.1 illustrates, the trial structure and time line of stimuli.

Most of the extracranial EEG studies define the spatio-temporal nature of the human brain in terms of ERP components to symbolise the categorisation of different perceptual stages (Haxby *et al* 2000, Wong *et al* 2009, Luo *et al* 2010, Young and Bruce 2011). For this study, we obtained the raw electrical signals of EEG by using EEG ADI instruments with a frequency of 2000 Hz. Two personal

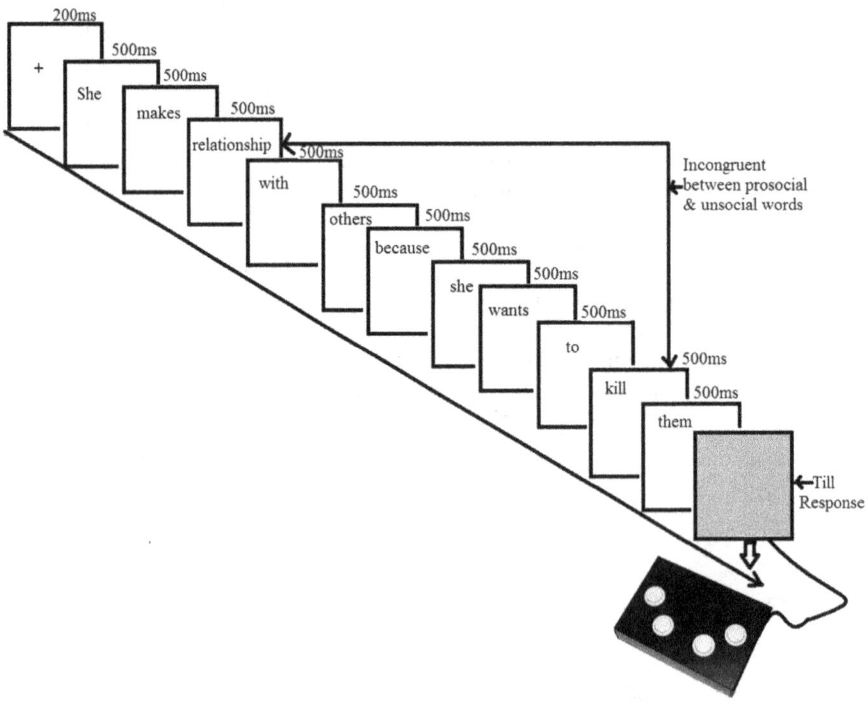

Figure 12.1. The trail structure and time line of stimuli presentation are illustrated with respect to the experimental design.

computers (PC): one for the stimuli presentation and the other for the acquisition of EEG signals were used to complete the task of the experiment; figure 12.2 illustrates the EEG experimental set-up.

The artefacts were removed by filtering the acquired EEG signals with a frequency range from 0.01 to 40 Hz. The total time of ERP was kept at 1000 ms, covering a time window of minus 200 ms before the onset of the stimulus to plus 800 ms after the stimulus. EEG signals were segmented based on four experimental conditions: prosocial congruent and incongruent, and unsocial congruent and incongruent. The average baseline signals were measured to categorise ERPs such as the early ERP (P100, N200) and the late ERP (P300, N400) components. The change of P100 waves stretched from windows 20 to 175 ms, whereas the wave of N200 fell between 176 and 275 ms. However, the late ERP component P300 peaks fall between 276 and 380 ms; the peak of N400 stretches from 400 to 600 ms. The amplitudes ($\nu\mu$) of these components were analysed concerning the four experimental conditions and the hemispheric regions of the brain, such as the left and right sides of the prefrontal, frontal, temporal and parietal lobes. In addition to EEG signals, we also analysed the response accuracy (RA in %) and time (RT in ms). Repeated measures ANOVA were conducted for behavioural and EEG data using the Statistical Package for Social Sciences (SPSS). The experimental procedures and protocols for testing hypothesis are illustrated in figure 12.3.

12.3 Findings and observations

12.3.1 Behavioural findings

The behavioural results that included response time (ms) and response accuracy (%) clearly showed more accuracy and faster response to prosocial ($p \leqslant 0.001$) than

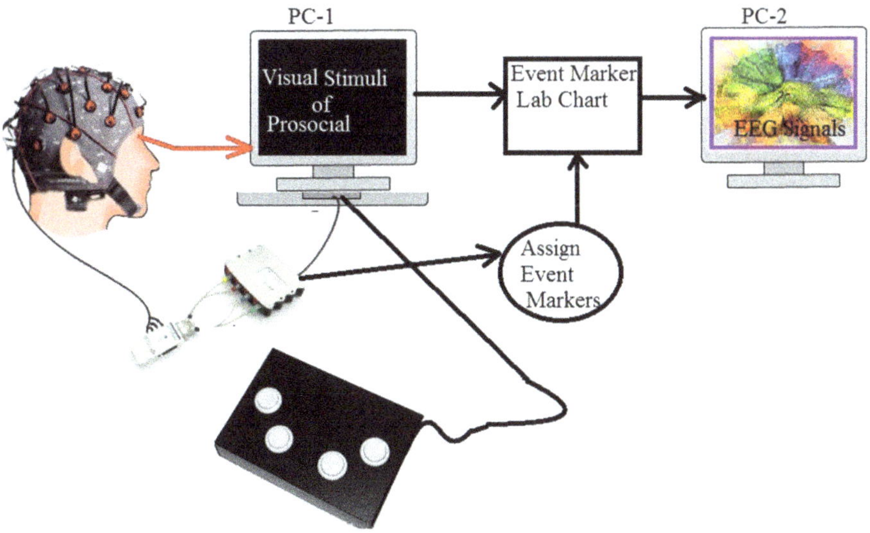

Figure 12.2. The laboratory set-up for conducting EEG is designed to acquire the electrical signals of brain.

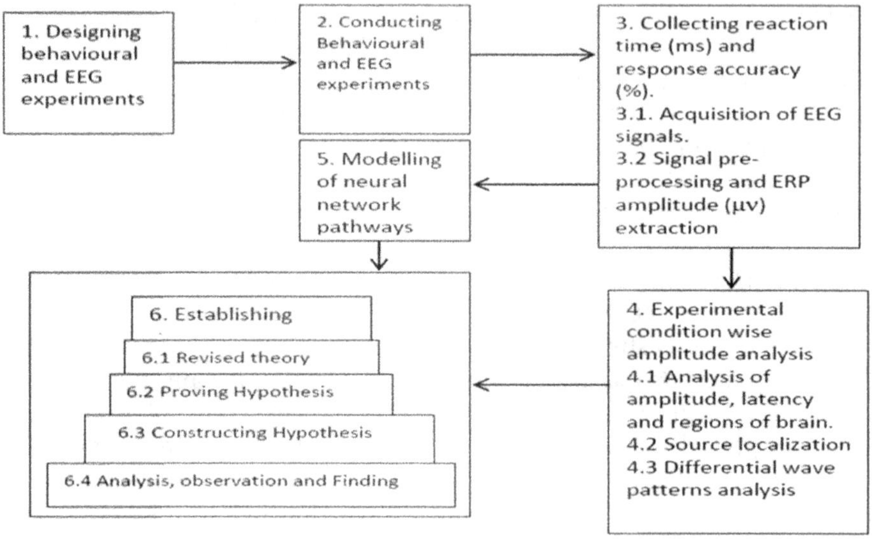

Figure 12.3. The experimental protocols and analysis procedures of EEG and behavioral data are presented in step-by-step sequences.

unsocial sentences irrespective of congruency. The highest accuracy ($p \leqslant 0.04$) and the quickest response time ($p \leqslant 0.02$) were observed in the case of prosocial congruent than prosocial or unsocial incongruent trials. Sentential trials having prosocial words were processed faster with high accuracy than trials having unsocial words.

12.3.2 The early P100 and N200 effects

The unsocial sentences that were processed more slowly with low accuracy showed higher amplitudes ($p \leqslant 0.04$) of early P100 (20–175 ms) in the frontal regions of the brain. Like unsocial sentences, the fearful ($p \leqslant 0.024$) and disgust ($p \leqslant 0.019$) faces elicited larger P100 and N200 amplitude than neutral faces in the occipito-temporal regions of brain (Krusemark and Li 2011, Mendoza-Medialdea and Ruiz-Padial 2021, Ruiz-Padial and Mercado 2021). However, in the left-side of prefrontal regions, the amplitudes of P1 were significantly higher ($p \leqslant 0.04$) for incongruent prosocial than unsocial sentences. Sentences having prosocial words were processed only in the left side of the temporal regions of the brain, as the ERP waves of P100 and topo-map show in figure 12.4. However, the negative deflection of N200 (176–275 ms) showed high negative amplitudes ($p \leqslant 0.05$) for unsocial sentences in the left-side of frontal regions. The incongruent unsocial sentences showed higher amplitudes of N2 than congruent ones in the temporal regions of the brain. The congruency effect yielded significant value only in the case of antisocial sentences but not for prosocial sentences. No significant effect of congruency was observed in P100 and N200 components.

12.3.3 The late P300 and N400 effects

Like the early P100, the amplitudes of late positive deflection of P300 (276–400 ms) were higher for prosocial than unsocial sentences in the prefrontal ($p \leqslant 0.05$) and

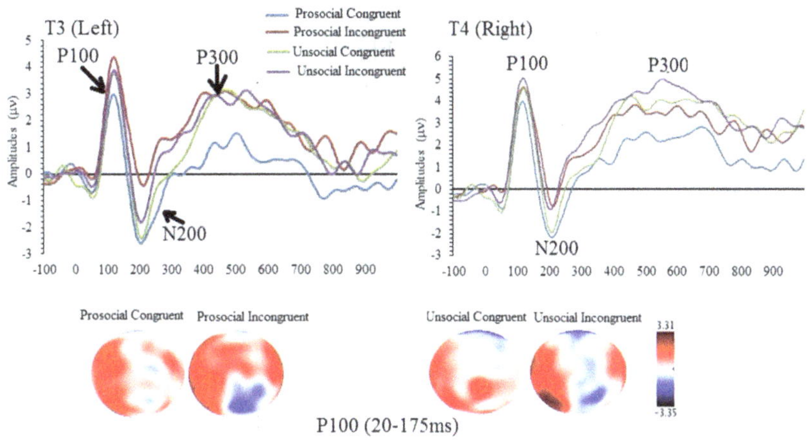

Figure 12.4. Shows the ERP waves of P100 in which the prosocial incongruent is having higher amplitudes than unsocial incongruent in the left-side of temporal regions of brain.

frontal ($p \leqslant 0.02$) regions. The positive P3 peak for prosocial congruent was higher ($p \leqslant 0.03$) in the left-side than right-side of the frontal brain. Even the prosocial incongruent sentences ($p \leqslant 0.01$) showed higher amplitudes of P3 than unsocial incongruent sentences in the mid-central regions of the brain. However, the late negative N400 deflection (400–600 ms), which was higher in the temporal ($p \leqslant 0.03$) and parietal ($p \leqslant 0.04$) regions, showed higher amplitudes for incongruent than congruent sentences. This result is well-matched with the earlier findings that the unsocial-fortunate and prosocial-unfortunate incongruent stimuli ($p \leqslant 0.043$) elicited a higher negative amplitude of N400 (375–500 ms) than the unsocial-unfortunate and prosocial-fortunate stimuli in the left parietal regions (Rodríguez-Gómez *et al* 2020). The incongruence or discordance between music and language stimuli is elicited ($p \leqslant 0.032$) in the N400 in the right-side of temporal regions (Proverbio and Russo 2021). Another study has also found the N400 effect, which is significant ($p \leqslant 0.001$) during the processing of conflicting violations between meaningful and pseudowords integration efficiency (Martin *et al* 2016). The regions of interest showed a significant effect ($p \leqslant 0.001$) of incongruence and semantic anomaly ($p \leqslant 0.006$) in N400 in the fronto-central (FC1, FCz and FC2), central (C1, Cz and C2) and centro-parietal (CP1, CPz and CP2) regions (Dwivedi and Selvanayagam 2021, Hernández-Gutiérrez *et al* 2021). However, we have not found any significant correlation between N400 and pro/unsocial sentences. This means that our study is silent about the earlier hypothesis that the amplitudes of N400 are higher for negative emotion than positive emotion (Chwilla *et al* 2011).

12.4 Discussion and interpretation of findings

Our study examined the neurocognitive mechanisms involved in the interpretation of prosocial and unsocial words in congruent and incongruent sentences. It explored the behavioural response time, accuracy and brain activities in contexts of ERP during semantic anomaly tasks. As anticipated, we observed a more significant behavioural advantage of prosocial sentences over antisocial ones. Prosocial sentences are responded to very fast with high accuracy. Notably, the congruency effect was observed only in prosocial sentences, suggesting quicker response time with higher accuracy for prosocial congruent sentences than incongruent ones. We conceptualised that the presence of prosocial words facilitates much faster than antisocial words. This effect could be observed because prosocial words, like prosocial behaviours, widen the affective bond within society (Balconi *et al* 2019). For antisocial information, the early P100 amplitudes were sensitive, whereas, in processing of prosocial information, the late P300 amplitudes demonstrated larger amplitudes. The congruency effects modulated the amplitudes of N400. In the case of incongruent sentences, we observed higher amplitudes than congruent sentences. This congruency effect is consistent and regular with the N400 in the case of emotional faces and prosody, and the prosody and words congruency stimuli (Paulmann and Pell 2010, Wang *et al* 2011, Tarai and Srinivsan 2019).

12.4.1 Unsocial sentences processed in P100

The higher response time with a low accuracy rate in recognising unsocial sentences was matched with high amplitudes of P100 in the brain's frontal areas. Early P1 amplitudes were sensitive to antisocial English sentences because the brain might suppress antisocial behaviours in the early component. The antisocial apprehensive and fearful information are processed in ERP early component near 50 ms following the onset of the stimuli (Mueller and Pizzagalli 2016). Further, violent behaviours are strongly corroborated with the brain's frontal regions (Critchley *et al* 2000). In antisocial and fearful behaviours, the prefrontal cortex, which is also responsible for cost-benefit analyses and cognitive controls, shows higher activation than other regions of the brain (Tabibnia *et al* 2008, Van Petten and Luka 2012, Lambert *et al* 2017). These brain regions are also concerned with human violence. Damage in the prefrontal region, specifically in the orbitofrontal and ventromedial lobes, increases violent acts, aggression, anger, hostility, and terror (Grafman *et al* 1996, Anderson *et al* 1999). A similar effect is also observed in the context of violent subjects, compared to non-violent controls in the brain's prefrontal areas (Davidson *et al* 2000). The blood flow and glucose metabolism increase dramatically in the prefrontal and frontal regions when antisocial individuals, violent psychiatric inpatients and murderers plead not guilty to others (Wong *et al* 1997). Considering these supportive findings, we suggest that early inhibition and top-down processing of unsocial sentences enhances the amplitudes of the brain's frontal regions.

12.4.2 Prosocial sentences processed in P3

The detailed processing of prosocial meaning occurs in the late P300 in the prefrontal areas of the brain. Prosocial words are usually positive and pleasant in meaning that explicitly prefers processing in the late component. This finding supports earlier studies that happy or friendly terms are linked with a larger LPC or a late positive component (Herbert *et al* 2008). This late ERP is also connected with the explicit and detailed processing of the valence dimensions of emotions in a situation when the job is to recognize independent emotional against non-emotional words, pictures or faces (Citron 2012). In contrast to non-emotional words, the emotional words elicit larger amplitudes (450–700 ms) in the LPC or late positive-complex waves (Dillon *et al* 2006). A physiological study demonstrates the LPC component, which is induced due to the processing of joyful and pleasant emotions and music (Paulmann *et al* 2013). Contrarily, a similar ERP study has elaborated the distinctive electrophysiological markers such as the processing of language induced sadness and fearful stimuli, which occur in P300 and N400 components, respectively (Cuthbert *et al* 2000, Proverbio and Russo 2021). Overall, the latency of P300 is mainly affected by the preferred positive linguistic stimuli (Haupt *et al* 2008). This argument is also justified under the broaden-and-build theory that reveals the advantage of positive emotions (Fredrickson 2001). Like happy emotions, prosocial sentences enlarge the thought and action repertoires of humans. Contrarily, like anger or other negative emotions, the antisocial sentential information narrows down the thoughts and actions to specific action-tendencies like escape, attack and expel (Fredrickson 2004). Studies under this theoretical framework have argued that cognitive processing of positive influence integrates diverse materials (Borod *et al* 2000) that widen the mental scope of attention and action.

Consequently, like happy or pleasant words, the prosocial sentences demonstrate larger P3 amplitudes in comparison to antisocial terms because the attentional scope for prosocial stimuli is much broader than unsocial sentences. A study revealed that P300 amplitudes consistently increase during the processing of global compared to local stimuli (Lithfous *et al* 2016). By considering the advantage of positive emotions and global processing, this chapter claims that prosocial words or lexicons widen the global attentional networks, demanding explicit processing in the P3 component of the brain.

12.4.3 Effect of congruency in N4

As expected, the significant effect of semantic congruency for prosocial and antisocial words enhanced the amplitude of N4 for incongruent sentences over congruent ones in the temporal region of the brain. This N4 result is consistently observed in the earlier research on lexico-semantic integrational violations that occur at the syntactic or discursive level in the central and parietal areas (Chwilla *et al* 2011, Borovsky *et al* 2012). The manipulation of socially situated contexts that provides semantic incongruent or anomaly is processed in the N400 component (Dwivedi and Selvanayagam 2021). Even during sentence comprehensions, the incongruency between the contextual meaning and voice is also induced in N400 (Bornkessel-Schlesewsky and Schlesewsky 2013, Jouralev *et al* 2019). For example, a sentence like ‘Every evening I drink some *wine* before I go to sleep’ is uttered in a male child voice, an N400 effect is observed in centro-parietal regions (Van Berkum *et al* 2008). This late negative component essentially responds to the semantic incongruency stimuli based on the previous word meaning (Kutas and Federmeier 2011, Payne *et al* 2015). The brain topography shows a higher N400 peak in the centro-parietal and parietal regions of the brain (Van Petten 2014, Schöne *et al* 2018). The incoherent and non-emotional words demonstrate high N4 amplitudes (Kutas and Schimitt 2003). Such discourse incoherent, semantic violations and interference effects were regularly observed in prosody and word conflict. Studies suggest the interference of prosody over the synonyms of word (Schirmer *et al* 2005, Ishii *et al* 2010) and the prosody intervention on emotion-showing face in the late negative N400 (Paulmann and Pell 2010). The emotional and linguistic incongruence or discordance occurs in N400 (Wang *et al* 2011, Proverbio and Russo 2021). Furthermore, the N4 is considered a conflict and violation control component associated with a great detail and explicit semantic processing in the domain of language (Elmer *et al* 2010, Brunellière *et al* 2019). For example, the Parkes *et al* (2016) study demonstrates N400 components during the processing of emotional word-meaning violation or incongruent (e.g., My mother was killed and I felt *great.*). In this direction, our results essentially validate the late semantic violation in N4 temporal regions in the case of processing of prosocial and anti- or unsocial incongruent sentences. A recent study corroborated the N4 component with the incongruent statements when respondents agreed or disagreed with pro- (supporting) and anti- (against) European Union statements (Galli *et al* 2017). In the N400, the brain is susceptible when it processes the incongruence between grip and goal information, revealing the integral incongruent meaning between the two (Decroix *et al* 2020).

12.4.4 Effect of prosocial congruency in P1, P3 and N4

Prosocial incongruent stimuli enhance the amplitudes of N4, P1 and P3 in the prefrontal, frontal-parietal and central regions. It seems that antisocial words were intervened with prosocial words, strengthening the amplitudes of early and late ERP components. Like happy emotional stimuli, prosocial incongruent stimuli are recognised quicker and earlier in the brain. However, the question arises here: why were the prosocial incongruent sentences processed and modulated in prefrontal and frontal regions of the brain in N4, P1 and P3. It may be because the semantic interference of antisocial over prosocial words requires early implicit recognition or identification and late explicit processing. The argument is that the logical features of stimuli, task difficulty, attentional load, selection of an object and item categorization need late P3 processing in the left hemispheric frontal region (Orlandi and Proverbio 2019). This finding is supported by the fact that processing of incongruent, probability and violation of expectation stimulus occurs in the P300 component (Fabiani *et al* 2000). P3 amplitudes were found more positive for inconsistent stimulus than consistent stimulus concerned with prosocial helping actions in the left hemispheric region of the brain (Cunningham *et al* 2005, Leng *et al* 2019). Since positive and prosocial words belong to primary language categories, the positive P3, as the current study expects, is modulated by elaborative tasks of incongruent sentences.

Further, we believe that the prosocial incongruent sentences engage highly logical and pragmatic strategies of communication to retain social aspects of cognition in the late ERP components. Primarily, this assertion is linked with increased cortical activation of the frontal and prefrontal cortices, which are observed in the context of social cognition, cooperative and prosocial behaviours (Balconi and Pagani 2014, Balconi *et al* 2018). Secondly, this claim is supported by the argument of many researchers that the dorsolateral prefrontal cortex (DLPFC) and anterior cingulate cortex (ACC) facilitate the societal and prosocial process of interaction, relationship, exchange, reinforcement and communication (Petrican and Schimmack 2008, Balconi *et al* 2018). Thirdly, antisocial intervention with prosocial words that constitute the prosocial incongruent inhibits or suppresses the semantic violation and enforces the prefrontal cortex to observe the conflict (Baeken *et al* 2011). Fourthly, these arguments support the previous hypotheses regarding the role of frontal and prefrontal cortices in prosocial communication, interpersonal relationship and social processes like helping, empathic and altruistic decisions (Balconi *et al* 2019). Finally, this claim is also supported by the Stroop interference effect that requires executive control of the prefrontal region (Botvinick *et al* 2004). Many investigations have affirmed prefrontal areas' engagement in monitoring and controlling the conflicts (Swick and Turken 2002). We believe that the interference of anti- or unsocial words in the prefrontal to parietal regions followed a transient course of processing that progressed from early P1 to late P3/P4 ERP components. This early and late processing indicate that the brain possessed a social nature stretched from prefrontal to parietal areas, suppresses the effects of antisocial words demanding for joint neural network resources in early and late ERP components. These arguments suggest that the human brain often tend to control selfish information when processing prosocial attitudes (Knoch and Fehr 2007) and hostility and automatic antagonism (Haidt 2001) by enhancing the amplitudes of early and late ERP components.

12.4.5 Effect of unsocial incongruency in N2

Our N2 results revealed that prosocial words intervened with the preceding unsocial words in sentences enhancing higher amplitudes of N2 for incongruent antisocial over congruent in the temporal lobe. This result is compatible with the outcome of previous researches on Stroop tasks that demonstrated a significant effect in the face and prosodic congruency trials in N200 (Kanske and Kotz 2010). The N200 component, whose peak occurs around 200 to 300 ms following the onset of the stimuli, is well recognized as a conflict processing neural marker in fronto-central and parietal areas of the brain (van Veen and Carter 2002, Zinchenko *et al* 2015). Furthermore, the early negative N200, whose peak falls between 130 and 270 ms, is affected more by incongruent than congruent sentences in the anterior regions of the brain (Schauenburg *et al* 2019). Furthermore, emotional incongruity's rapid and initial effect is correlated with automatic, effortless dictation in the area of the anterior cingulate cortex (ACC) (Schauenburg *et al* 2019, 2021). Similarly, we observed the N200 component in the frontal and temporal regions of the brain due to the involvement of incongruent antisocial linguistic structure. This result indicates that antisocial incongruent information created social distance in terms of verbal communication among humans.

12.4.6 Prosocial processed in left and unsocial processed in right hemispheres

Interestingly, our laterality effect in P100 demonstrated larger activation for prosocial sentences on the left side and antisocial on the right side of the temporal regions of the brain. This hemispheric asymmetry for prosocial and antisocial corrections supports the early and automatic processing of emotional words, indicating a correlation of right-hemisphere with happy words and the association of left-hemisphere with angry words in temporo-parietal temporal regions (Leitman *et al* 2010, Tarai and Srinivsan 2019). Furthermore, the laterality effect of prosocial and anti/unsocial sentences is consistent with the asymmetric hypothesis of emotional valences (Davidson 1994). The negative emotions are lateralised towards the right, while the positive emotions are lateralised towards the brain's left hemisphere (Aftanas *et al* 2001). Altogether, our result about early laterality on P1 supports the BVH or behavioural valence hypothesis (Davidson 2003), assigning left-side for positive and right-side for negative emotions. Based on this hypothesis, we assert that temporal regions of the left hemispheric side are highly sensitive to prosocial sentences, and for antisocial sentences, the right hemispheric side is marginally sensitive. In this regard, our study confirms the BVH, which suggests early and automatic recognition of prosocial words is concerned with the left hemisphere. The temporal regions are considered as the primary epicentres for processing the social cues of language uniquely facilitating the understanding of social actions and observations and serving the theory of mind (Yang *et al* 2015).

12.4.7 Left-hemispheric laterality effect in P3

Laterality result is observed in the left rather than in the right hemispheric regions of the prefrontal brain. Language stimuli motivate these left-hemispheric laterality effects. These findings are well-established and associated with the concept that the cognitive domains of language are computed and processed in the left hemispheric areas of the brain (Price 2000), but, right-hemispheric laterality effect concerned with emotion is still unclear and debatable among the researchers (Beraha *et al* 2012). A faction of researchers has observed that the right hemisphere of the brain is responsible for emotions, feelings and sentiments, whereas left-hemispheric regions are allied with the cognitive process (Atchley *et al* 2003, Sim and Martinez 2005). However, another faction of scholars believes that emotional stimuli are processed in both the hemispheric sides of the brain in the case of brain damage (Mandal *et al* 1992). Considering the diametrical arguments, although we agree on the hemispheric laterality hypothesis of emotions, the question arises here whether both hemispheres are aligned with the assessment task of emotional, prosocial and anti- or unsocial words that pose both characteristics of incremental processing of language as well as detailed processing of feelings, selfish behaviours and emotions. Social factors embedded with language largely influence the language processing of congruency and incongruence meaning in P1, N2, P300, LPP and N400 components (Leuthold *et al* 2015, Schacht and Vrtička 2018).

Some studies suggest that both the hemispheres process the meaning of emotional words, but their activation time courses vary from one region to another region of the brain (Naumann *et al* 1992). Early processing is modulated by incremental-processing of scripted words in the left while the right hemisphere activates the emotional sense of the words later (Abbassi *et al* 2011). The frontal and temporal regions of the left-hemispheric side are involved in processing the meaningful and not meaningless words (Gabrieli *et al* 1998). Brain activities are significantly enhanced in the left area of the prefrontal cortex during the processing of semantic information and cognitive behaviour of language that include verb generation, abstract and concrete judgments (Demb et al 1995). In this context, this study shows the dominance of the left hemisphere during sentence processing in the prefrontal regions of the late P3 component irrespective of prosocial and antisocial words.

12.5 Conclusions

This chapter provides an inclusive account of behavioural and neurocognitive mechanisms involving the processing of prosocial and antisocial English sentences in congruent and incongruent sentential stimuli. Our results suggest that, like sad emotional words, the anti/unsocial sentences are processed in early P1, and prosocial sentences are processed in P3 as observed in the case of happy emotional words. Though, prosocial sentences that increase the latency of P3 support the 'broaden-and-build theory of positive emotions' (Fredrickson 2001). The happy feeling is more sensitive to global features of stimuli (Hicks and King 2007, Schwarz and Clore 2007). Like the positive sentiments, the prosocial sentences broaden the global attentional mechanisms, while the antisocial sentences narrow down the local attentional mechanisms. In sum, this study reveals that the sentence's congruent prosocial and antisocial sentences influence the neuro-cognitive mechanisms during language processing. Prosocial incongruency enhances the early (P1) and late (P3 and N4) components as the human brain consciously tends to control top-down computation and neural processing of narrowing selfish and egoist information. This fact is supported by earlier ERP studies that observing or recognising others' pain and establishing sympathy elicit an early response in N1 or N200 component, whereas the later components P3 or LPC are associated with detailed evaluation, judgement and reappraisal computation (Fan *et al* 2011, Coll 2018). This indicates that the volume of societal nature of the brain has extended from prefrontal to parietal areas in early and late ERP components.

However, the anti- or unsocial incongruent was processed in N2 due to its social aloofness or detachment in communication. As anticipated, the incongruent sentences that reinforce the amplitudes of N4 contribute to the semantic violation theory and conflict monitoring in neuroscience. Our early laterality effects in P1 support the BVH, indicating the left-hemisphere for prosocial and the right-hemisphere for antisocial information processing. These findings are significant in conceptualising the neuroscience mechanism of prosocial and anti/unsocial incongruency in language. The congruency task modulates the prosocial and antisocial written language. Arguments of this study open a future scope to establish a symmetric correlation between prosocial–global and antisocial–local stimuli. Recognising and prioritising prosocial capabilities play a crucial role in developing adaptive and survival strategies. These adaptations consequently improve interpersonal communications, social wellbeing and relationships. We must intervene and adopt prosocial and positive linguistic stimuli to attenuate criminal or antisocial behaviours and save civilisation from terror and conflicts. This observation would rationalise the cooperative, kindness and altruistic-based school curriculums which may promote prosocial behaviour, self-regulation, executive function and social-emotional developments of learners.

References

Abbassi E, Kahlaoui K, Wilson M A and Joanette Y 2011 Processing the emotions in words: the complementary contributions of the left and right hemispheres *Cogn. Affect. Behav. Neurosci.* **11** 372–85

Aftanas L, Varlamov A, Pavlov S, Makhnev V and Reva N 2001 Event-related synchronisation and desynchronisation during affective processing: emergence of valence-related time-dependent hemispheric asymmetries in theta and upper alpha band *Int. J. Neurosci.* **110** 197–219

Anderson S W, Bechara A, Damasio H, Tranel D and Damasio A R 1999 Impairment of social and moral behavior related to early damage in human prefrontal cortex *Nat. Neurosci.* **2** 1032–7

Atchley R A, Ilardi S S and Enloe A 2003 Hemispheric asymmetry in the processing of emotional content in word meanings: the effect of current and past depression *Brain Lang.* **84** 105–19

Baeken C, Van Schuerbeek P, De Raedt R, De Mey J, Vanderhasselt M A, Bossuyt A and Luypaert R 2011 The effect of one left-sided dorsolateral prefrontal sham-controlled HF-rTMS session on approach and withdrawal related emotional neuronal processes *Clin. Neurophysiol.* **122** 2217–26

Balconi M and Pagani S 2014 Personality correlates (BAS-BIS), self-perception of social ranking, and cortical (alpha frequency band) modulation in peer-group comparison *Physiol. Behav.* **133** 207–15

Balconi M, Fronda G and Vanutelli M E 2019 Donate or receive? Social hyperscanning application with fNIRS *Curr. Psychol.* **38** 991–1002

Balconi M, Vanutelli M E and Gatti L 2018 Functional brain connectivity when cooperation fails *Brain Cogn.* **123** 65–73

Barbaroux M, Norena A, Rasamimanana M, Castet E and Besson M 2021 From psychoacoustics to brain waves: a longitudinal approach to novel word learning *J. Cogn. Neurosci.* **33** 8–27

Beraha E, Eggers J, Hindi Attar C, Gutwinski S, Schlagenhauf F, Stoy M, Sterzer P, Kienast T, Heinz A and Bermpohl F 2012 Hemispheric asymmetry for affective stimulus processing in healthy subjects—a fMRI study *PLoS One* **7** e46931

Bigelow F J, Clark G M, Lum J and Enticott P G 2021 The development of neural responses to emotional faces: a review of evidence from event-related potentials during early and middle childhood Development *Cogn. Neurosci.* **51** 100992

Bornkessel-Schlesewsky I and Schlesewsky M 2013 Reconciling time, space and function: a new dorsal–ventral stream model of sentence comprehension *Brain Lang.* **125** 60–76

Borod J C *et al* 2000 Relationships among facial, prosodic, and lexical channels of emotional perceptual processing *Cogn. Emot.* **14** 193–211

Borovsky A, Elman J L and Kutas M 2012 Once is enough: N400 indexes semantic integration of novel word meanings from a single exposure in context *Lang. Learn. Develop.* **8** 278–302

Botvinick M M, Cohen J D and Carter C S 2004 Conflict monitoring and anterior cingulate cortex: an update *Trends Cogni. Sci.* **8** 539–46

Braem S, King J A, Korb F M, Krebs R M, Notebaert W and Egner T 2017 The role of anterior cingulate cortex in the affective evaluation of conflict *J. Cogn. Neurosci.* **29** 137–49

Brunellière A, Auran C and Delrue L 2019 Does the prosodic emphasis of sentential context cause deeper lexical-semantic processing? *Lang. Cogn. Neurosci.* **34** 29–42

Chudek M and Henrich J 2011 Culture–gene coevolution, norm-psychology and the emergence of human prosociality *Trends Cogni. Sci.* **15** 218–26

Chiao J Y, Hariri A R, Harada T, Mano Y, Sadato N, Parrish T B and Iidaka T 2010 Theory and methods in cultural neuroscience *Soc. Cogn. Affect. Neurosci.* **5** 356–61

Chwilla D J, Virgillito D and Vissers C T W 2011 The relationship of language and emotion: N400 support for an embodied view of language comprehension *J. Cogn. Neurosci.* **23** 2400–14

Citron F M 2012 Neural correlates of written emotion word processing: a review of recent electrophysiological and hemodynamic neuroimaging studies *Brain Lang.* **122** 211–26

Coll M P 2018 Meta-analysis of ERP investigations of pain empathy underlines methodological issues in ERP research *Soc. Cogn. Affect. Neurosci.* **13** 1003–17

Conway P and Gawronski B 2013 Deontological and utilitarian inclinations in moral decision making: a process dissociation approach *J. Person. Soc. Psychol.* **104** 216

Costa D, Dias C, Sousa T, Estiveira J, Castelhano J, Figueiredo V, Pereira A and Castelo-Branco M 2021 Modulation of early level EEG signatures by distributed facial emotion cues bioRxiv

Crago R V, Renoult L, Biggart L, Nobes G, Satmarean T and Bowler J O 2019 Physical aggression and attentional bias to angry faces: an event related potential study *Brain Res.* **1723** 146387

Critchley H D *et al* 2000 The functional neuroanatomy of social behaviour: changes in cerebral blood flow when people with autistic disorder process facial expressions *Brain* **123** 2203–12

Cui X, Bryant D M and Reiss A L 2012 NIRS-based hyperscanning reveals increased interpersonal coherence in superior frontal cortex during cooperation *Neuroimage* **59** 2430–7

Cuthbert B N, Schupp H T, Bradley M M, Birbaumer N and Lang P J 2000 Brain potentials in affective picture processing: covariation with autonomic arousal and affective report *Biol. Psychol.* **52** 95–111

Cunningham W A, Espinet S D, DeYoung C G and Zelazo P D 2005 Attitudes to the right-and left: frontal ERP asymmetries associated with stimulus valence and processing goals *NeuroImage* **28** 827–34

Darwin C 2008 *The Descent of Man, and Selection in Relation to Sex* (Princeton, NJ: Princeton University Press)

Davidson R J 1994 Asymmetric brain function, affective style, and psychopathology: the role of early experience and plasticity *Develop. Psychopathol.* **6** 741–58

Davidson R J 2003 Affective neuroscience and psychophysiology: toward a synthesis *Psychophysiol.* **40** 655–65

Davidson R J, Putnam K M and Larson C L 2000 Dysfunction in the neural circuitry of emotion regulation--a possible prelude to violence *Science* **289** 591–4

Decroix J, Roger C and Kalénine S 2020 Neural dynamics of grip and goal integration during the processing of others' actions with objects: an ERP study *Sci. Rep.* **10** 1–11

Demb J B, Desmond J E, Wagner A D, Vaidya C J, Glover G H and Gabrieli J D 1995 Semantic encoding and retrieval in the left inferior prefrontal cortex: a functional MRI study of task difficulty and process specificity *J. Neurosci.* **15** 5870–8

Dillon D G, Cooper J J, Grent T, Woldorff M G and LaBar K S 2006 Dissociation of event-related potentials indexing arousal and semantic cohesion during emotional word encoding *Brain Cogn.* **62** 43–57

Dunfield K, Kuhlmeier V A, O'Connell L and Kelley E 2011 Examining the diversity of prosocial behavior: helping, sharing, and comforting in infancy *Infancy* **16** 227–47

Dwivedi V D and Selvanayagam J 2021 Effects of dispositional affect on the N400: language processing and socially situated context *Front. Psychol.* **12** 1045

Eisenberg N, Hofer C, Sulik M J and Liew J 2014 The development of prosocial moral reasoning and a prosocial orientation in young adulthood: concurrent and longitudinal correlates *Dev. Psychol.* **50** 58

Eisenberg N, Lennon R and Roth K 1983 Prosocial development: a longitudinal study *Dev. Psychol.* **19** 846

Elmer S, Meyer M and Jancke L 2010 Simultaneous interpreters as a model for neuronal adaptation in the domain of language processing *Brain Res.* **1317** 147–56

Ensor R and Hughes C 2005 More than talk: relations between emotion understanding and positive behaviour in toddlers *Br. J. Dev. Psychol.* **23** 343–63

Evans J R, Budzynski T H, Budzynski H K and Abarbanel A (ed) 2009 *Introduction to Quantitative EEG and Neurofeedback: Advanced Theory and Applications* (New York: Academic)

Fabiani M, Stadler M A and Wessels P M 2000 True but not false memories produce a sensory signature in human lateralised brain potentials *J. Cogn. Neurosci.* **12** 941–9

Fan Y, Shi F, Smith J K, Lin W, Gilmore J H and Shen D 2011 Brain anatomical networks in early human brain development *Neuroimage* **54** 1862–71

Ferguson C J 2010 Blazing angels or resident evil? Can violent video games be a force for good? *Rev. Gen. Psychol.* **14** 68–81

Fredrickson B L 2004 The broaden-and-build theory of positive emotions *Phil. Trans. R. Soc. London* B **359** 1367–77

Fredrickson B L 2001 The role of positive emotions in positive psychology: the broaden-and-build theory of positive emotions *Am. Psychol.* **56** 218

Frimer J A, Aquino K, Gebauer J E, Zhu L L and Oakes H 2015 A decline in prosocial language helps explain public disapproval of the US Congress *Proc. Natl Acad. Sci.* **112** 6591

Funane T, Kiguchi M, Atsumori H, Sato H, Kubota K and Koizumi H 2011 Synchronous activity of two people's prefrontal cortices during a cooperative task measured by simultaneous near-infrared spectroscopy *J. Biomed. Opt.* **16** 077011

Gabrieli J D, Poldrack R A and Desmond J E 1998 The role of left prefrontal cortex in language and memory *Proc. Natl Acad. Sci.* **95** 906–13

Galang C M and Obhi S S 2020 Automatic imitation does not predict levels of prosocial behaviour in a modified dictator game *Actapsychologica* **204** 103022

Galli G, Sirota M, Materassi M, Zaninotto F and Terry P 2017 Brain indices of disagreement with one's social values predict EU referendum voting behavior *Soc. Cogn. Affect. Neurosci.* **12** 1758–65

Girard L C, Pingault J B, Doyle O, Falissard B and Tremblay R E 2017 Expressive language and prosocial behaviour in early childhood: longitudinal associations in the UK Millennium Cohort Study *Eur. J. Dev. Psychol.* **14** 381–98

Grafman J, Schwab K, Warden D, Pridgen A, Brown H R and Salazar A M 1996 Frontal lobe injuries, violence, and aggression: a report of the Vietnam Head Injury Study *Neurology* **46** 1231–1

Greene J D, Nystrom L E, Engell A D, Darley J M and Cohen J D 2004 The neural bases of cognitive conflict and control in moral judgment *Neuron* **44** 389–400

Gross J, Schmitz F, Schnitzler I, Kessler K, Shapiro K, Hommel B and Schnitzler A 2004 Modulation of long-range neural synchrony reflects temporal limitations of visual attention in humans *Proc. Natl Acad. Sci.* **101** 13050–5

Güntekin B and Basar E 2007 Emotional face expressions are differentiated with brain oscillations *Int. J. Psychophysiol.* **64** 91–100

Haidt J 2001 The emotional dog and its rational tail: a social intuitionist approach to moral judgment *Psychol. Rev.* **108** 814

Hamilton A F D C 2015 EPS prize lecture: cognitive underpinnings of social interaction *Q. J. Exp. Psychol.* **68** 417–32

Haupt F S, Schlesewsky M, Roehm D, Friederici A D and Bornkessel-Schlesewsky I 2008 The status of subject–object reanalyses in the language comprehension architecture *J. Mem. Lang.* **59** 54–96

Haxby J V, Hoffman E A and Gobbini M I 2000 The distributed human neural system for face perception *Trends Cogni. Sci.* **4** 223–33

Hehman E, Volpert H I and Simons R F 2014 The N400 as an index of racial stereotype accessibility *Soc. Cogn. Affect. Neurosci.* **9** 544–52

Henrich J and Henrich N 2006 Culture, evolution and the puzzle of human cooperation *Cogn. Syst. Res.* **7** 220–45

Herbert C, Junghofer M and Kissler J 2008 Event related potentials to emotional adjectives during reading *Psychophysiology* **45** 487–98

Hernández-Gutiérrez D, Muñoz F, Sánchez-García J, Sommer W, AbdelRahman R, Casado P, Jiménez-Ortega L, Espuny J, Fondevila S and Martín-Loeches M 2021 Situating language in a minimal social context: how seeing a picture of the speaker's face affects language comprehension *Soc. Cogn. Affect. Neurosci.* **16** 502–11

Hicks J A and King L A 2007 Meaning in life and seeing the big picture: positive affect and global focus *Cogn. Emot.* **21** 1577–84

Hudac C M *et al* 2021 Modeling temporal dynamics of face processing in youth and adults *Soc. Neurosci.* **16** 345–61

Immordino-Yang M H, McColl A, Damasio H and Damasio A 2009 Neural correlates of admiration and compassion *Proc. Natl Acad. Sci.* **106** 8021–6

Ishii K, Kobayashi Y and Kitayama S 2010 Interdependence modulates the brain response to word–voice incongruity *Soc. Cogn. Affect. Neurosci.* **5** 307–17

Jouravlev O, Schwartz R, Ayyash D, Mineroff Z, Gibson E and Fedorenko E 2019 Tracking colisteners' knowledge states during language comprehension *Psychol. Sci.* **30** 3–19

Kacewicz E, Pennebaker J W, Davis M, Jeon M and Graesser A C 2014 Pronoun use reflects standings in social hierarchies *J. Lang. Soc. Psychol.* **33** 125–43

Kamarajan C, Rangaswamy M, Chorlian D B, Manz N, Tang Y, Pandey A K, Roopesh B N, Stimus A T and Porjesz B 2008 Theta oscillations during the processing of monetary loss and gain: a perspective on gender and impulsivity *Brain Res.* **1235** 45–62

Kandel E and Freed D 1989 Frontal-lobe dysfunction and antisocial behavior: a review *J. Clin. Psychol.* **45** 404–13

Kangassalo L, Spapé M, Ravaja N and Ruotsalo T 2020 Information gain modulates brain activity evoked by reading *Sci. Rep.* **10** 1–10

Kanske P and Kotz S A 2010 Modulation of early conflict processing: N200 responses to emotional words in a flanker task *Neuropsychologia* **48** 3661–4

Kiehl K A, Laurens K R and Liddle P F 2002 Reading anomalous sentences: an event-related fMRI study of semantic processing *Neuroimage* **17** 842–50

Kilner J, Bott L and Posada A 2005 Modulations in the degree of synchronisation during ongoing oscillatory activity in the human brain *Eur. J. Neurosci.* **21** 2547–54

Knoch D and Fehr E 2007 Resisting the power of temptations: the right prefrontal cortex and self-control *Ann. NY Acad. Sci.* **1104** 123–34

Kopell N, Ermentrout G B, Whittington M A and Traub R D 2000 Gamma rhythms and beta rhythms have different synchronisation properties *Proc. Natl Acad. Sci.* **97** 1867–72

Kral T R, Solis E, Mumford J A, Schuyler B S, Flook L, Rifken K, Patsenko E G and Davidson R J 2017 Neural correlates of empathic accuracy in adolescence *Soc. Cogn. Affect. Neurosci.* **12** 1701–10

Krusemark E A and Li W 2011 Do all threats work the same way? Divergent effects of fear and disgust on sensory perception and attention *J. Neurosci.* **31** 3429–34

Kutas M and Federmeier K D 2011 Thirty years and counting: finding meaning in the N400 component of the event-related brain potential (ERP) *Annu. Rev. Psychol.* **62** 621–47

Kutas M and Schmitt B M 2003 *Language in Microvolts* (New York: Lawrence Erlbaum Associates)

Lambert B, Declerck C H, Emonds G and Boone C 2017 Trust as commodity: social value orientation affects the neural substrates of learning to cooperate *Soc. Cogn. Affect. Neurosci.* **12** 609–17

Lapierre D, Braun C M and Hodgins S 1995 Ventral frontal deficits in psychopathy: neuropsychological test findings *Neuropsychologia* **33** 139–51

Leitman D I, Wolf D H, Ragland J D, Laukka P, Loughead J, Valdez J N, Javitt D C, Turetsky B and Gur R 2010 'It's not what you say, but how you say it': a reciprocal temporo-frontal network for affective prosody *Front. Human Neurosci.* **4** 19

Leng H, Wang Y, Li Q, Yang L and Sun Y 2019 Sophisticated deception in junior middle school students: an ERP study *Front. Psychol.* **9** 2675

Leuthold H, Kunkel A, Mackenzie I G and Filik R 2015 Online processing of moral transgressions: ERP evidence for spontaneous evaluation *Soc. Cogn. Affect. Neurosci.* **10** 1021–9

Lindberg N, Tani P, Appelberg B, Naukkarinen H, Rimón R, Porkka-Heiskanen T and Virkkunen M 2003 Human impulsive aggression: a sleep research perspective *J. Psychiatr. Res.* **37** 313–24

Lithfous S, Tromp D, Dufour A, Kemp J, Sellal F and Després O 2016 Differential processing of hierarchical visual stimuli in young and older healthy adults: an event-related potentials (ERP) study *Neuropsychology* **30** 600

Luo Y, Zhang Y, Feng X and Zhou X 2010 Electroencephalogram oscillations differentiate semantic and prosodic processes during sentence reading *Neuroscience* **169** 654–64

Majdandžić J, Amashaufer S, Hummer A, Windischberger C and Lamm C 2016 The selfless mind: how prefrontal involvement in mentalising with similar and dissimilar others shapes empathy and prosocial behavior *Cognition* **157** 24–38

Malti T, Ongley S F, Peplak J, Chaparro M P, Buchmann M, Zuffianò A and Cui L 2016 Children's sympathy, guilt, and moral reasoning in helping, cooperation, and sharing: a 6-year longitudinal study *Child Dev.* **87** 1783–95

Mandal M K, Asthana H S, Tandon S C and Asthana S 1992 Role of cerebral hemispheres and regions in processing hemifacial expression of emotion: evidence from brain-damage *Int. J. Neurosci.* **63** 187–95

Martin C D, Molnar M and Carreiras M 2016 The proactive bilingual brain: using interlocutor identity to generate predictions for language processing *Sci. Rep.* **6** 1–8

Martín-Loeches M, Fernández A, Schacht A, Sommer W, Casado P, Jiménez-Ortega L and Fondevila S 2012 The influence of emotional words on sentence processing: electrophysiological and behavioral evidence *Neuropsychologia* **50** 3262–72

Martí-Vilar M, Serrano-Pastor L and Sala F G 2019 Emotional, cultural and cognitive variables of prosocial behaviour *Curr. Psychol.* **38** 912–19

Masten C L, Morelli S A and Eisenberger N I 2011 An fMRI investigation of empathy for 'social pain'and subsequent prosocial behavior *Neuroimage* **55** 381–8

McCarthy G, Nobre A C, Bentin S and Spencer D D 1995 Language-related field potentials in the anterior-medial temporal lobe: I. Intracranial distribution and neural generators *J. Neurosci.* **15** 1080–9

McCarthy G and Nobre A C 1993 Modulation of semantic processing by spatial selective attention *Electroencephalogr. Clin. Neurophysiol.* **88** 210–19

McDonald N M and Messinger D S 2011 The development of empathy: how, when, and why. Moral behavior and free will: a neurobiological and philosophical approach pp 333–59

Mendoza-Medialdea M T and Ruiz-Padial E 2021 Understanding the capture of exogenous attention by disgusting and fearful stimuli: the role of interoceptive accuracy *Int. J. Psychophysiol.* **161** 53–63

Melis A P and Semmann D 2010 How is human cooperation different? *Phil. Trans. R. Soc.* B **365** 2663–74

Mills K L, Lalonde F, Clasen L S, Giedd J N and Blakemore S J 2014 Developmental changes in the structure of the social brain in late childhood and adolescence *Soc. Cogn. Affect. Neurosci.* **9** 123–31

Miskovic V and Keil A 2012 Acquired fears reflected in cortical sensory processing: a review of electrophysiological studies of human classical conditioning *Psychophysiology* **49** 1230–41

Molinaro N, Su J J and Carreiras M 2016 Stereotypes override grammar: social knowledge in sentence comprehension *Brain Lang.* **155** 36–43

Morelli S A, Rameson L T and Lieberman M D 2014 The neural components of empathy: predicting daily prosocial behavior *Soc. Cogn. Affect. Neurosci.* **9** 39–47

Mueller E M and Pizzagalli D A 2016 One-year-old fear memories rapidly activate human fusiform gyrus *Soc. Cogn. Affect. Neurosci.* **11** 308–16

Naumann E, Bartussek D, Diedrich O and Laufer M E 1992 Assessing cognitive and affective information processing functions of the brain by means of the late positive complex of the event-related potential *J. Psychophysiol.* **6** 285

Niedermeyer E and Lopes da Silva F H 2005 *Electroencephalography: Basic Principles, Clinical Applications and Related Fields* (Baltimore, MD: Lippincott Williams & Wilkins)

Orlandi A and Proverbio A M 2019 Left-hemispheric asymmetry for object-based attention: an ERP Study *Brain Sci.* **9** 315

Özgören M, Başar-Eroğlu C and Başar E 2005 Beta oscillations in face recognition *Int. J. Psychophysiol.* **55** 51–9

Panteleeva Y, Courvoisier D S, Glowinski D, Grandjean D M and Ceschi G 2021 Effects of emotionally incongruent musical excerpts on memory retrieval *Psychol. Music* 03057356211034571

Parkes L, Perry C and Goodin P 2016 Examining the N400m in affectively negative sentences: a magnetoencephalography study *Psychophysiology* **53** 689–704

Pasion R, Fernandes C, Pereira M R and Barbosa F 2018 Antisocial behaviour and psychopathy: uncovering the externalising link in the P3 modulation *Neurosci. Biobehav. Rev.* **91** 170–86

Paulmann S, Bleichner M and Kotz S A 2013 Valence, arousal, and task effects in emotional prosody processing *Front. Psychol.* **4** 345

Paulmann S and Pell M D 2010 Contextual influences of emotional speech prosody on face processing: how much is enough? *Cogn. Affect. Behav. Neurosci.* **10** 230–42

Payne P, Levine P A and Crane-Godreau M A 2015 Corrigendum: somatic experiencing: using interoception and proprioception as core elements of trauma therapy *Front. Psychol.* **6** 423

Petrican R and Schimmack U 2008 The role of dorsolateral prefrontal function in relationship commitment *J. Res. Person.* **42** 1130–5

Price C J 2000 The anatomy of language: contributions from functional neuroimaging *J. Anat.* **197** 335–59

Proverbio A M and Russo F 2021 Multimodal recognition of emotions in music and language *Psychol. Music* 0305735620978697

Rameson L T, Morelli S A and Lieberman M D 2012 The neural correlates of empathy: experience, automaticity, and prosocial behavior *J. Cogn. Neurosci.* **24** 235–45

Ray W J and Cole H W 1985 EEG alpha activity reflects attentional demands, and beta activity reflects emotional and cognitive processes *Science* 750–2

Redondo-Pacheco J, Inglés-Saura C J, Parra-Galvis L K, Nieto-Barroso L M and Navarro-Galvis M L 2016 Prosocial behavior: theoretical perspectives *Int. J. Psychol. Res.* **11** 299–320

Rhee S H *et al* 2013 Early concern and disregard for others as predictors of antisocial behavior *J. Child Psychol. Psych.* **54** 157–66

Rivera B and Soylu F 2021 Incongruity in fraction verification elicits N270 and P300 ERP effect *Neuropsychologia* **161** 108015

Roberts J W, Bennett S J and Hayes S J 2018 Impression or expression? The influence of self-monitoring on the social modulation of motor contagion *Q. J. Exp. Psychol.* **71** 850–8

Rodríguez-Gómez P, Martín-Loeches M, Colmenares F, Ferreiro M V R and Moreno E M 2020 He had it comin': ERPs reveal a facilitation for the processing of misfortunes to antisocial characters *Cogn. Affect. Behav. Neurosci.* **20** 356–70

Rothbart M K, Sheese B E and Posner M I 2007 Executive attention and effortful control: linking temperament, brain networks, and genes *Child Dev. Persp.* **1** 2–7

Ruiz-Padial E and Mercado F 2021 In exogenous attention, time is the clue: brain and heart interactions to survive threatening stimuli *PLoS One* **16** e0243117

Schacht A and Vrtička P 2018 Spatiotemporal pattern of appraising social and emotional relevance: evidence from event-related brain potentials *Cogn. Affect. Behav. Neurosci.* **18** 1172–87

Scharinger M, Monahan P J and Idsardi W J 2016 Linguistic category structure influences early auditory processing: converging evidence from mismatch responses and cortical oscillations *NeuroImage* **128** 293–301

Schauenburg G, Aryani A, Hsu C T, Schröder T, Conrad M, von Scheve C and Jacobs A M 2021 Conflict detection in affective language content: affective incongruency in semantically correct sentences describing social interactions activates the anterior cingulate cortex (Preprint)

Schauenburg G, Conrad M, von Scheve C, Barber H A, Ambrasat J, Aryani A and Schröder T 2019 Making sense of social interaction: emotional coherence drives semantic integration as assessed by event-related potentials *Neuropsychologia* **125** 1–13

Scherer K R and Moors A 2019 The emotion process: event appraisal and component differentiation *Annu. Rev. Psychol.* **70** 719–45

Schindler S and Kissler J 2017 Getting social-the impact of social presence on our perception, thoughts and behavior *Psychophysiology* **54** S19

Schindler S and Kissler J 2016 Selective visual attention to emotional words: early parallel frontal and visual activations followed by interactive effects in visual cortex *Hum. Brain Mapp.* **37** 3575–87

Schindler S, Wegrzyn M, Steppacher I and Kissler J 2015 Perceived communicative context and emotional content amplify visual word processing in the fusiform gyrus *J. Neurosci.* **35** 6010–19

Schirmer A, Tang S L, Penney T B, Gunter T C and Chen H C 2005 Brain responses to segmentally and tonally induced semantic violations in Cantonese *J. Cogn. Neurosci.* **17** 1–2

Schnitzler A and Gross J 2005 Normal and pathological oscillatory communication in the brain *Nat. Rev. Neurosci.* **6** 285–96

Schöne B, Köster M and Gruber T 2018 Coherence in general and personal semantic knowledge: functional differences of the posterior and centro-parietal N400 ERP component *Exp. Brain Res.* **236** 2649–60

Schwarz N and Clore G L 2007 Feelings and phenomenal experiences *Social Psychology: Handbook of Basic Principles* ed E E Higgins and A Kruglanski 2nd edn (New York: Guilford)

Silk J B and House B R 2016 The evolution of altruistic social preferences in human groups *Phil. Trans. R. Soc.* B **371** 20150097

Sim T C and Martinez C 2005 Emotion words are remembered better in the left ear. Laterality: asymmetries of body *Brain Cogn.* **10** 149–59

Singer T and Klimecki O M 2014 Empathy and compassion *Curr. Biol.* **24** R875–8

Soderstrom H, Hultin L, Tullberg M, Wikkelso C, Ekholm S and Forsman A 2002 Reduced frontotemporal perfusion in psychopathic personality *Psych. Res.: Neuroimag.* **114** 81–94

Sui J and Han S 2007 Self-construal priming modulates neural substrates of self-awareness *Psychol. Sci.* **18** 861–6

Swick D and Turken U 2002 Dissociation between conflict detection and error monitoring in the human anterior cingulate cortex *Proc. Natl Acad. Sci.* **99** 16354–9

Tabibnia G, Lieberman M D and Craske M G 2008 The lasting effect of words on feelings: words may facilitate exposure effects to threatening images *Emotion* **8** 307

Tarai S and Srinivasan N 2019 Emotional prosody Stroop effect in Hindi: an event related potential study *Prog. Brain Res.* **247** 193–217

Tarai S, Mukherjee R, Qurratul Q A, Singh B K and Bit A 2019 Use of prosocial word enhances the processing of language: frequency domain analysis of human EEG *J. Psycholinguist. Res.* **48** 145–61

Tomasello M 2019 *Becoming Human* (Cambridge, MA: Harvard University Press)

Tomasello M 2009 *Why We Cooperate* (Cambridge, MA: MIT Press)

Turner B M, Van Maanen L and Forstmann B U 2015 Informing cognitive abstractions through neuroimaging: the neural drift diffusion model *Psychol. Rev.* **122** 312

Tusche A, Böckler A, Kanske P, Trautwein F M and Singer T 2016 Decoding the charitable brain: empathy, perspective taking, and attention shifts differentially predict altruistic giving *J. Neurosci.* **36** 4719–32

Van Berkum J J, Van den Brink D, Tesink C M, Kos M and Hagoort P 2008 The neural integration of speaker and message *J. Cogn. Neurosci.* **20** 580–91

Van Petten C 2014 Examining the N400 semantic context effect item-by-item: relationship to corpus-based measures of word co-occurrence *Int. J. Psychophysiol.* **94** 407–19

Van Petten C and Luka B J 2012 Prediction during language comprehension: benefits, costs, and ERP components *Int. J. Psychophysiol.* **83** 176–90

Van Veen V and Carter C S 2002 The anterior cingulate as a conflict monitor: fMRI and ERP studies *Physiol. Behav.* **77** 477–82

Vartanov A V and Suyuncheva A R 2020, November Comparison of brain induced potentials in internal speech in studied and unknown languages *Biologically Inspired Cognitive Architectures Meeting* (Cham: Springer) pp 547–552

Volman I, Toni I, Verhagen L and Roelofs K 2011 Endogenous testosterone modulates prefrontal–amygdala connectivity during social-emotional behavior *Cereb. Cortex* **21** 2282–90

Wang L, Bastiaansen M, Yang Y and Hagoort P 2011 The influence of information structure on the depth of semantic processing: how focus and pitch accent determine the size of the N400 effect *Neuropsychologia* **49** 813–20

Wang Y and Hamilton A F D C 2015 Anterior medial prefrontal cortex implements social priming of mimicry *Soc. Cogn. Affect. Neurosci.* **10** 486–93

Wang Y and Hamilton A F D C 2014 Why does gaze enhance mimicry? Placing gaze-mimicry effects in relation to other gaze phenomena *Q. J. Exp. Psychol.* **67** 747–62

Wang Y and Hamilton A F D C 2013 Understanding the role of the 'self'in the social priming of mimicry *PLoS One* **8** e60249

Williams P B, Poljacik G, Decety J and Nusbaum H C 2018 Loving-kindness language exposure leads to changes in sensitivity to imagined pain *J. Posit. Psychol.* **13** 429–33

Wong C H, Birkett J, Byth K, Dexter M, Somerville E, Gill D, Chaseling R, Fearnside M and Bleasel A 2009 Risk factors for complications during intracranial electrode recording in presurgical evaluation of drug resistant partial epilepsy *Acta Neurochir.* **151** 37–50

Wong M, Fenwick P, Fenton G, Lumsden J, Maisey M and Stevens J 1997 Repetitive and non-repetitive violent offending behaviour in male patients in a maximum security mental hospital–clinical and neuroimaging findings *Med. Sci. Law* **37** 150–60

Wood S J, Berger G E, Wellard R M, Proffitt T, McConchie M, Velakoulis D, McGorry P D and Pantelis C 2008 A 1H-MRS investigation of the medial temporal lobe in antipsychotic-naïve and early-treated first episode psychosis *Schizophr. Res.* **102** 163–70

Yang D Y J, Rosenblau G, Keifer C and Pelphrey K A 2015 An integrative neural model of social perception, action observation, and theory of mind *Neurosci. Biobehav. Rev.* **51** 263–75

Yang Y F, Brunet-Gouet E, Burca M, Kalunga E K and Amorim M A 2020 Brain processes while struggling with evidence accumulation during facial emotion recognition: an ERP Study *Front. Human Neurosci.* **14** 340

Young A W and Bruce V 2011 Understanding person perception *Br. J. Psychol.* **102** 959–74

Zaki J and Mitchell J P 2013 Intuitive prosociality *Curr. Direct. Psychol. Sci.* **22** 466–70

Zinchenko A, Kanske P, Obermeier C, Schröger E and Kotz S A 2015 Emotion and goal-directed behavior: ERP evidence on cognitive and emotional conflict *Soc. Cogn. Affect. Neurosci.* **10** 1577–87

CPSIA information can be obtained
at www.ICGtesting.com
Printed in the USA
BVHW010039080322
630126BV00007B/28

9 780750 333818